The Psychology of Religion and Coping

THE PSYCHOLOGY OF RELIGION AND COPING

Theory, Research, Practice

Kenneth I. Pargament

THE GUILFORD PRESS
New York   London

To Aileen,
who warms her world
with love

© 1997 The Guilford Press
A Division of Guilford Publications
72 Spring Street, New York, NY 10012

Printed in the United States of America

This book is printed on acid-free paper.

Last digit is print number: 9   8   7   6

Library of Congress Cataloging-in-Publication Data

Pargament, Kenneth I. (Kenneth Ira), 1950–
    The psychology of religion and coping / Kenneth I. Pargament.
        p.   cm.
    Includes bibliographical references and index.
    ISBN 1-57230-214-3   (hc.)   ISBN 1-57230-664-5   (pbk.)
    1. Psychology, Religious.   2. Adjustment
(Psychology)—Religious aspects.   I. Title.
BL53.P228   1997
200′.1′9—dc21   97-9599
                                                                            CIP

ACKNOWLEDGMENTS

I don't think I will be writing many books in my lifetime. The process has been exciting, even exhilarating at times, but it has also been very hard. I have wondered with amazement at some of my colleagues whose words seem to flow so effortlessly. Personally, I've felt more in common with columnist Red Barber who once said: "Writing is easy. All you do is sit down in front of a typewriter, open a vein, and bleed."

I thought I knew a lot more about religion and coping when I started this book than I did. Grappling with phenomena so deeply important, yet so hard to comprehend, has been humbling. In the process of writing, I discovered that my brain is made of Swiss cheese; trying to fill in some of the holes is one reason why the book took twice as long to write than initially envisioned. But in the process I also learned a great deal. My hope is that you too will find the material in this book informative and helpful.

Although I spent many hours writing alone, this book has not been a solitary effort. Along the way I developed a strong sense of kinship with many people from many walks of life—theologians, social scientists, religious leaders, health and mental health professionals, and men and women struggling with the greatest challenges of living. In some instances, I was touched by people who spoke to me over thousands of miles and thousands of years. Reading their thoughts and sentiments, I found myself wishing that I had met them personally, maybe had them over for dinner. Instead, I was given the chance to get to know them through their words. I want to acknowledge their contributions to my own work, and express my gratitude for being able to join them in the search for significance.

I would also like to thank the hundreds of participants in my research studies and my psychotherapy clients for teaching me so much about the richness of religion and our capacity to face life's most stressful moments with courage and integrity. Throughout the book I draw on their experiences and insights. Although some of the details of their stories and their identities were changed to protect their anonymity, the essential themes remain unchanged.

If awards were given for the most numbers of coauthors on papers and publications in the psychology of religion, I would probably be a strong contender—it is something I am proud of. Over the past 17 years, I have been very fortunate to work with an exceptionally talented group of graduate students at Bowling Green State University who have shared my interest in the study of religion. Learning with them has been a two-way street. Their energy, stimulation, and support have made the research process not only enlightening, but also a lot of fun. Particular thanks go to a number of students, some of whom assisted me with the innumerable hassles and details in putting this book together, and others who took the risk of giving me critical, but very valuable feedback on my writing: Timothy Belavich, Curtis Brant, Eric Butter, Brenda Cowell, Lisa Friedel, Kathy Hipp, Tracey Jewell, Lisa Perez, Mark Rye, Cheryl Taylor, Allie Scott, Eric Scott, Jill Zerowin, and Brian Zinnbauer.

A number of colleagues were kind enough to devote many hours to a review of an earlier draft of this book. Their comments were very helpful to me, and I tried to take them to heart as best I could. My thanks go to: Donald Capps, William Hathaway, Ralph Hood Jr., Richard Jenkins, Annette Mahoney, Susan McFadden, Edward Shafranske, Bruce Smith, Catherine Stein, and my mentor, Forrest Tyler. Meliha Duncan was also tremendously helpful in the preparation of this manuscript.

And finally, I want to express my deepest gratitude to my family. They have supported and sustained me in countless ways with their love and care. The support has come in many guises: a phone call from my parents wondering how it's going, with a joke or two from my father, Sol, and a vote of confidence from my mother, Florence; the good-natured acceptance by my sons, Jonathan and Ben, of those times when "Dad is working on the book"; and my wife, Aileen's, unselfish willingness to take on the burden of so many of the details of family life while I was upstairs writing or downstairs worrying. Aileen's extraordinary wisdom, her unwavering support in my moments of doubt, and her willingness to confront me when I got carried away helped me keep my work in perspective and my life in balance. More than anyone, she has taught me what it means to be wise, compassionate, and strong. I would like to dedicate this book to her.

CONTENTS

APPENDICES

Chapter One

———◆◆◆———

AN INTRODUCTION TO
THE PSYCHOLOGY OF
RELIGION AND COPING

On July 19, 1989, Flight 232 on route from Denver to Chicago
encountered serious problems. An explosion on the tail of the plane
destroyed one of the engines and crippled the hydraulic systems. For the
next hour the crew struggled to keep the plane in the air. The passengers
also struggled in their own ways with this threat to their lives. Shortly
after the crash landing, many of the survivors were interviewed by *Life*
magazine ("Here I Was . . . ," 1989). For most of these survivors, the
disaster elicited beliefs, feelings, or practices related to religion in one
way or another. Here are a few excerpts:

> After the flight attendant explained emergency landing procedures, we
> were left with our thoughts. That's when I began praying. I closed my
> eyes and thought, "Dear Lord, I pray that you'll guide the pilot's
> hands." I also thought that if God wanted to take my life, that it was
> O.K. with me. I was full of peace. Here I was sitting on the edge of
> eternity. I wasn't facing the end of my life.

> The plane smelled like a house after a fire. I was exhilarated to be
> alive but deeply grieved when I could see and smell death. It was like
> being at the doorstep of hell. I pulled my Bible out of my bag. That's
> all I wanted.

I don't believe there is a kindly Supreme Being who responds to people one on one. People ask me if I am still a nonbeliever after my life was saved. If everybody had had his life saved except the bad people on the plane, maybe I'd believe a little more. But that's not what happened. Mothers of young children died.

I did what I needed to do to prepare to die. My thought at the time was that I wanted to be reborn into a family where I would be able to hear the teachings of Buddha. I'd done a lot of Buddhist meditation in my life, and this trained me to become one pointed in my awareness. I was totally focused on the brace position.

A lady came up to me the other day. She had seen me on television. She asked if I had thanked the Lord that I had survived. I said, "Yes," but I was thinking, "Cool it, lady. I don't need this." (pp. 29–31, 33, 38)

Few of us go through life without encountering critical moments. Only rarely are these events as dramatic as a plane crash. More often our critical periods involve the regular trials and transitions of life. They take the form of family quarrels, personal conflicts, employment problems, financial troubles, births, illnesses, and deaths. At times, larger social problems such as poverty, racism, or the threat of nuclear war also force themselves into our lives. Whether they are expected or unexpected, short-lived or long-lasting, individual or collective, these moments can push us beyond our capabilities. In these periods of crisis, as we hear from many of the survivors of Flight 232, religion can be intimately involved.

To some this may come as a surprise. For many years there has been talk of a decline of religiousness in the industrialized world. While the activities of cults, televangelists, or religious upheavals in distant parts of the globe occasionally make the headlines, they can be dismissed with a shake of the head as aberrations in a world that is turning away from the supernatural. However, there are other indicators, less dramatic and more subtle, to suggest that religion remains a potent force in the lives of many, if not most, people. For example, in 1988, 9 out of 10 Americans said they have never doubted God's existence; 82% believe that God works miracles today; 79% report that they are sometimes very conscious of God's presence in their lives; and 71% believe in life after death (Gallup & Castelli, 1989). While membership in mainline Protestant denominations has declined, this decline has been offset by increases in evangelical, non-Western, and new religious groups. These indicators suggest that religion is far from extinction.

Perhaps the most dramatic signs of religious life come from times of stress. That religion is closely tied to pivotal periods in life should not be particularly startling. Hardship, suffering, and conflict have been centers of concern for the major religions of the world. Each, in its own way, acknowledges the fact that life can be perilous. Within Buddhism, it is believed that existence is first experienced *as* suffering (*Dukkha*), a term that embodies physical pain and mental anguish, negative changes, and a lack of freedom (Gard, 1962). Within Judaism, suffering in the world is explicitly recognized through the commemoration of slavery and oppression and the celebration of freedom. Christianity presents a model of suffering in the world through the Crucifixion of Jesus Christ.

Thus, religions of the world have a deep appreciation for the often painful nature of the human condition. Even more important though, religious traditions articulate their visions of how we should respond to this condition. In the words of the eminent anthropologist Clifford Geertz (1966), any religion must consider "how to suffer, how to make of physical pain, personal loss, worldly defeat, or the helpless contemplation of others' agony something bearable, supportable—something, as we say, sufferable" (p. 19). While different religions envision different solutions to problems, every religion offers a way to come to terms with tragedy, suffering, and the most significant issues in life.

This book is about the roles of religion when people are put to the test. The purpose is not to engage in a comparative analysis of the major religious traditions. Nor will this book try to analyze personal religious beliefs and practices as pure abstractions. The intent here is to focus on something more concrete, the ground where religion meets crisis. The data for this book in "rawest" form come from the experiences of people in these testing times, such as the accounts of the survivors of Flight 232. Their responses are not abstract, detached, or removed from experience. They involve thoughts, feelings, and actions woven into the fabric of critical moments. Neither are these responses simple. Instead, they reveal a rich variety of religious forms and functions.

A "down-to-earth" look at religion in the midst of crisis leads away from simple religious generalizations to a number of questions. When does religion become involved in coping with difficult situations? What purposes does it serve for people? Why does religion appear to be irrelevant to some people in their most stressful moments? What roles does religion play in coping—is it merely a defense, a passive way of coping, a form of denial? How does religion attempt to conserve whatever is significant to people, and, alternatively, how does religion try to transform it? Is religion itself changed through the coping process? In what ways is religion helpful or harmful to people in coping? Finally, how might religion be used more fully to help people in crisis? These are the central questions in this book. They define the domain of religion and coping.

Before going on, let me note that the word "religion" will not be used here in its narrow sense, that is, as institutionally based religious involvement, dogma, and ritual. Instead, religion will be defined in its broad sense, one that includes both institutional religious expressions and personal religious expressions, such as feelings of spirituality, beliefs about the sacred, and religious practices. More will be said about the meaning of religion in the next chapter.

WHY STUDY RELIGION AND COPING?

There are three good reasons to study religion and coping:

1. First, the study of religion and coping has something to teach us about coping. In our most extreme moments, we are unmasked for who we are: "both the swine and the saints" (Frankl, 1984, p. 178). Studying these moments can help correct and complete the picture of human nature drawn from people going about their daily lives. It can reveal the dark side of the human condition: people lost, confused, deluding themselves, willing to sacrifice others to advance their own interests. And it can bring to light humanity's more valiant side: "the persistence, the will to live, the courage, and indeed the heroism that are as much a part of human nature as the retreats, evasions, and petty impulse gratifications that bulk so large our thinking." (White, 1974, p. 64).

Unfortunately, our studies of the human response to crises often neglect the religious dimension. Perhaps because psychologists tend to be less religious than the general population, they underestimate the powerful role religion can play in the coping process (Ragan, Malony, & Beit-Hallahmi, 1980; Shafranske & Gorsuch, 1984). Yet, as we will see throughout this book, religion is often present in the most remarkable times of life, expressing itself in many ways. It has much to say about human strengths and resources, but it also speaks to the most disturbing of our capacities. Any understanding of the human response to extraordinary moments remains incomplete without an appreciation of religion.

2. The study of religion and coping also offers an opportunity to learn more about religion. Religion is often viewed in the abstract, as a system of beliefs, rituals, symbols, feelings, and relationships that has little to do with the particulars of a situation or an individual's life. I recall an interview with a congregation member who was only peripherally involved in his church. He said: "It's not that I dislike coming to

church. It's just that I have a hard time connecting the readings, the sermon, and the songs to anything that's going on in my life. I still see myself as a religious person although I'm not quite sure how." This man was voicing his difficulty making the abstractions of religious ritual personally meaningful.

There may be no better laboratory for studying and learning about religion in its most palpable forms than times of crisis and coping. This is not to say that crisis triggers a "religious on/off switch." As we will see later in the book, it may be more accurate to suggest that people bring a reservoir of religious resources with them when they face stressful times. For many, the depth and nature of this reservoir is unknown. Like the church member just quoted, they may have difficulty fully articulating the way religion manifests itself in their lives. However, when people are stressed, the religious reservoir is often tapped and revealed for whatever it does (or does not) hold. In the shift from abstract to concrete, from potential to actual, the nature of religion comes into sharper focus. Perhaps partly for this reason, many of the central students of religion from Saint Augustine and Maimonides to William James and Paul Tillich have turned their attention to the roles of religion in the most perplexing, difficult times of life. These times provide one of the clearest windows into religious experience.

3. Finally, the study of religion and coping has some practical implications. People and problems are often most malleable during hard times. This notion has been around for a long time. In fact, many religious and therapeutic approaches are built on this concept and intentionally try to "shake people up" as a prelude to change. For example, within the Zen tradition of Buddhism, novices are exposed to a paradoxical, Alice-in-Wonderland world that challenges their usual modes of perception and understanding: "An ancient master, whenever he was asked the meaning of Zen, lifted one of his fingers. That was his entire answer. Another kicked a ball. Still another slapped the inquirer in the face" (Smith, 1958, p. 141). These "stress-inducing" experiences are intended to break through the novice's existing view of the world to a more complete transcendent awareness of all things.

The key point is that crises are pivotal periods. They destabilize "tried and true" methods for dealing with problems and call for new solutions. Painful as they may be, stressful periods represent a crossroads, a point at which the individual may have to choose among paths that lead in very different directions.

Religion does not stand idly by when it comes to this choice of direction. It provides guidance about where to go and how to get there. Of course, not all religious guidance is alike. There are, as we will see, many religious responses to problems, some better than others. In studying religion and coping, we learn about some of the better pathways and destinations of coping and some of the poorer ones. As importantly, we learn more about the *full* range of ways (religious and nonreligious) to help people along in their journey.

WHY A *PSYCHOLOGY* OF RELIGION AND COPING?

This book will approach religion and coping from an integrative psychological perspective. Psychology has no exclusive rights to this topic. Artists, philosophers, theologians, sociologists, anthropologists, clergy, and many people from many other communities have had a deep interest in and a lot to say about these matters. To paraphrase Allport (1968), a "narrowly conceived" psychology, one that ignores these contributions from other areas, can make only a narrow contribution to the study of religion and coping. When possible, then, I hope to enrich this psychological perspective by drawing on insights from other disciplines. However, it is well beyond my abilities to cover this deep and rich body of work thoroughly, so psychology will be my central focus here—a broadly conceived psychology that acknowledges and welcomes other perspectives.

What, if anything, does a psychology of religion and coping have to offer? I will suggest here that a psychological study of religion and coping provides a much needed bridge between isolated communities. At the end of the book the reader will be in a better position to evaluate this claim for him- or herself.

Scientists, mental health professionals, clergy, and members of religious communities often live in different worlds, speak different languages, and follow different customs. In spite of their differences, I believe these groups have some things to learn about, learn from, and contribute to each other. This kind of exchange is difficult, though, without connecting points or meeting grounds. These have been in short supply. This is where the psychology of religion and coping comes in. It offers a way to bridge psychological and religious worlds of thought, practice, and study.

Bridging Worldviews And Practices

Mention psychology to many people and what comes to mind are couches, inkblots, and talk shows. Psychology is best known as a form of practice, a way of helping people with problems. But psychologists are new to the neighborhood. As just noted, the religions of the world have been concerned about suffering and its amelioration for thousands of years. Yet, the relationships between professional psychological and religious communities have often been tense. Psychology has accused religion of everything from dogmatism and intolerance to social repression and mental illness (e.g., Ellis, 1986). Psychology has, in turn, been accused of arrogance, elitism, amorality, and selfishness (e.g., Vitz, 1977). Regardless of their accuracy, these accusations point to the rift between psychological and religious disciplines.

Why should there be so much tension between the two when they share a concern about the human condition? Perhaps the most compelling explanation is that psychology and religion have become, for many, competitors. Peter Berger (1967) notes that at one time religion was the source of meanings so plausible and compelling that they bound people into a common view of the universe. Within Western culture, however, the scope of the sacred in reality has shrunk over the last several hundred years. Phenomena once commonly understood as religious in nature (e.g., eclipses, disasters, illness) have been redefined as naturalistic. In this process, religion has lost some of its authority as a source of absolute indisputable meaning. Reality has become more of a subjective personal concern, more of a concern for psychology.

In this sense psychology has become a rival to religion within Western societies. It offers another way of looking at the world with its own views of the "good life" and its own mechanisms for solving problems. In place of confession we have psychotherapy. In place of conversion we have personal growth. In place of sins and virtues we have ethics. We could push the point even further by noting how psychology parallels religion in its rituals, rites of passage, traditions, use of symbols, and charismatic leaders. I do not want to call psychology a religion, for that would only cloud the meaning of religion, but it would not be inaccurate to say that, in its theories and practices, psychology functions *like* a religion.

Although there are, in fact, important differences in worldviews and practices between psychology and religion, they are not necessarily irreconcilable. Psychology might be generally characterized as a profession that attempts to help people gain more control over what they have not controlled. Making the unconscious conscious is the hallmark of psychodynamic approaches. Behaviorally oriented psychology has developed treatments to help people overcome a variety of conditions they feel unable to handle, from fearful situations and undesirable physiological reactions to difficult people and addictive behaviors. Cognitive approaches emphasize control of thoughts and feelings as the path to greater self-efficacy and competence in life. Community-oriented psychology tries to empower those with fewer resources (Rappaport, 1981). While there are important exceptions, it may not be too much of an exaggeration to say American psychology is a psychology of personal control.

In contrast, religion generally helps people appreciate what they themselves cannot control. It highlights the limitations of material goods, personal desires, and individual lives. Not only that, it offers a way to come to grips with these limitations through frameworks of belief that go beyond oneself. Religion speaks a language unfamiliar to psychology. Terms such as forbearance, faith, finitude, surrender, suffering, hope, and transformation, so central to religion, convey this appreciation for the incomprehensible, the unfathomable, and the uncontrollable. William James (1902) put it this way: "There is a state of mind, known to religious men, but to no others, in which the will to assert ourselves and hold our own has been displaced by a willingness to close our mouths and be as nothing in the floods and waterspouts of God" (p. 47). This willingness to surrender, he asserted, is the essence of religion. But religion does not end with the act of surrendering. Paradoxically, the giving up of total control is said to pave the way to greater mastery in living. Religion offers its own practices to help people along this road. Spiritual support, religious reframing, purification rituals, rites of passage, and conversion are just a few of these practical religious approaches. Thus, it may not be too much of an exaggeration to say that an appreciation for the limits of human agency lies at the heart of religion.

In short, while psychology and religion are both concerned with the problem of personal control, their assessment of the problem and their solutions are quite different. The psychological world says that we are not as powerless as we imagine ourselves to be; we have resources within ourselves that can be tapped more fully. The religious world says that in fact we are powerless in important ways and that we must look past ourselves alone for answers to important questions. I am suggesting, in a very general way, that the psychological world helps people extend their personal control, while the religious world helps people face their personal limitations and go beyond themselves for solutions.

Different as these perspectives are, they are not necessarily contradictory. *Problems are likely to come up only when we focus on our capacities or our limitations to the exclusion of the other.* For example, ecological crises have resulted from the assumption that air, forests, oil, the sea, and other physical resources represent inexhaustible supplies of energy. Similarly, a greater risk of heart disease has been tied to attempts to take control of uncontrollable situations (e.g., Glass, 1977). On the other hand, if there has been one common criticism of religion, it has been of the failure of religion to encourage change in the world when change is possible. Religions have been accused of ignoring, avoiding, or submitting to reality when personal action is possible to bring about change.

There is much to be gained from bridging the worldviews and practices embedded in psychological and religious perspectives. Human capacities and human limitations *complement* rather than *contradict* each other. In times of crisis and coping both the possible and the impossible become visible. Breznitz (1980) has put it nicely: "It is in the gray area between the possible and the futile that the battle of coping with stress has to be fought" (p. 265). The psychology of religion and coping can weave a respect for the possible together with an appreciation for the futile. It bridges a deep psychological tradition of helping people take control of what they can in times of stress with a rich religious tradition of helping people accept their limitations and look beyond themselves for assistance in troubling times.

Bridging Methods of Knowing the World

Even though psychology is best known as a profession, it is the attempt to ground the practice of psychology within a scientific foundation that makes this discipline truly distinctive. Of course, psychologists are not the only ones struggling to make some sense out of life. Theologians, poets, novelists, and many other groups try as well, and some are every bit as insightful and articulate as psychologists, if not more so. But psychologists should be able to do a better job of describing how they came to their understanding; through the methods of science, psychologists try to create public blueprints of their work for others to follow. Psychologists should also be acutely aware of the biases and limitations in the ways people process information and form conclusions about the world; through the methods of science, psychologists try to offer some measure of insight beyond the limits of our ordinary understanding of reality.

Religion has its own methods of knowing the world. Revelation is sought through prayer, meditation, sacred literature, rituals, communal worship, tradition, reason, art, intimate human relationships, social compassion, and any number of other practices that have developed over the millennia (Streng, 1976). These methods and the inspiration they induce have a validity of their own. As Bertocci (1972) notes: "Biblical writers do not argue for the existence of God any more than most men argue for the existence of the world. Their problem is to understand their relation to the God they feel in their bones" (p. 5).

Much has been made of the differences between scientific and religious methods. Science is said to be objective, religion subjective. Science is said to be limited to matters of fact and religion restricted to matters of value. These distinctions, however, have been overdrawn (see Barbour, 1974). Values, subjectivity, and judgment are bound up in science—from the choice of subject matter and the criterion for statistical significance to the ways data are interpreted and theories revised. Religion, on the hand, does not divorce itself from critical reflection or evaluation of the observable world. Its focus goes beyond empirical reality, but it remains vitally interested in the connection between metaphysical matters and the immediacies of existence (e.g., Oden, 1983). The differences between science and religion are real, but they are not so great as to preclude dialogue and exchange. In fact, this dialogue could enrich both disciplines.

Enriching Religion through Psychological Study

Religion has much to gain by opening itself up to scientific psychological inquiry. Not that psychology can demonstrate the absolute truth of religious claims. We have no tools to "measure God." We cannot prove the presence of an afterlife, the authenticity of Biblical miracles, or whether the essential character of people is good or evil. On the other hand, we cannot invalidate theological claims, either. Fears that science will remove the mystery from religion seriously overestimate the power of science. "Science is," Bronowski (1973) once pointed out, "a very human form of knowledge" (p. 374). It can illuminate the workings of the world, but it falls short of absolute answers to puzzling questions. Some mysteries will remain.

What psychology can offer are important insights into the footprints left by religion. These insights do not speak to religion's truth, but they do help us understand its manifestations and consequences. A scientific look into religion and coping will poke some holes in common religious stereotypes: that religion is only a crutch, that there are no atheists in foxholes, that religion is simply a form of denial. The closer we get to religious life, the more intricate it will become, and the more we will encounter unexpected twists and turns. We will see that religion adds a unique dimension to the coping process, one that cannot be described simply as good or bad. Instead, we will find that religion has the potential to help people through their hardest times and it also has the potential to make bad matters worse.

The knowledge gained from this scientific approach could be a powerful resource for religious individuals and communities. Because the scientific study of religion and coping is so rooted in concrete experience and critical problems of living, it is easier to make the jump from research to practice. It is not too much of a leap from evaluations of the efficacy of religious coping methods to applications of these findings by educators, clinicians, and pastors. The knowledge gleaned from this research will not translate into easy answers to difficult problems. In fact, cookbook solutions are likely to create problems of their own. What the scientific approach can suggest is some answers to difficult questions that are more closely attuned to the richness of religion and coping.

Concerns have been raised from religious quarters that research cannot do justice to the uniqueness of religious experience and the sacredness of each individual. These concerns are not ungrounded. We will see that many social scientists have reduced religious experience to what is assumed to be more basic social and psychological motivations. Belief in God is said to be, at root, a source of comfort and a defense against anxiety. Public worship is basically a way of bringing a community of people together. This type of reductionism, however, says more about the implicit assumptions and worldviews of these researchers than about research per se. Different assumptions are equally plausible, including those that treat spirituality as a legitimate motivation in its own right. There is no reason why researchers cannot approach religion with an eye to what makes it potentially unique. In fact, I believe, an openness to the distinctive character of religious life will only strengthen psychology as a science.

Enriching Psychology through Religious Study

The study of religion can enrich a psychologist's way of knowing the world. The traditional hallmarks of science—a focus on observable behavior, control of unwanted variables, and simplicity in theory and measurement—may be too restrictive to understand religious life. A richness of scientific method is needed to match the richness of religious experience.

Typically, psychologists find their way by focusing on what they can see or, in scientific terms, on directly observable behavior. In the religious world, however, the visible phenomena of most interest are in short supply. The observer can listen to people praying, watch people reading the Bible, witness people experiencing a range of emotions, and notice their interactions with each other. But much of religious experience remains private, subjective, and highly symbolic. It is important then to consider religion not only from the perspective of people who stand outside looking in, but from the phenomenological perspective of those who stand inside the religious world. Both insiders and outsiders have unique but limited perspectives. The outsider may be less able to appreciate the subjective character of religion, the feeling that it is the religious experience which is *really real*, even if it does not square with empirical reality. The insider may be less able to consider a religious approach as one among many possible paths in life with its own advantages and disadvantages. Until they focus on the religious world together, the respective vision of insider and outsider lacks depth (Havens, 1977).

Traditionally, psychologists have also selected their subjects carefully, removed them from their natural settings, and studied them in the laboratory to control for potentially complicating social, situational, and personal factors. When it comes to religion and coping, however, these complicating factors are often the variables of greatest interest. The study of religion in stressful times calls for careful attention to people in the context of their families, organizations, and communities, not removed from them. Admittedly, the study of religion "in context" can be complex and "messy," and yet it may hold a key to religious understanding. Capps (1977) put it this way: "The religious is not elusive because it lurks behind ordinary phenomena but because it is woven into the phenomena" (p. 48).

Mainstream science has not paid much attention to religion. What attention it has received has tended to be cursory and overly simplistic. For instance, one review of major psychiatric journals revealed few systematic studies of religious issues (Larson, Pattison, Blazer, Omran, & Kaplan, 1986). Religion, when it was measured, was usually assessed macroanalytically by one or two global items that ask denomination or degree of religiousness. As we will see, there is quite a bit of evidence to indicate that religion is a multidimensional phenomena. Thoughts, feelings, actions, and relationships are all a part of religious experience. Although psychologists and sociologists of religion have developed a variety of measures that are more sensitive to these varied dimensions of religious life, even these measures have little to say about the ways religion works in specific life situations. Toward this end, religion must be probed more deeply among those struggling with crises. What is called for is a microanalysis. If a widow says that her religion helped her cope with the death of her husband, the psychologist should go on to ask: What does she mean by religion? What aspects of her religion were helpful to her? How was her religion helpful? Were other aspects of her religion difficult to reconcile with her loss?

In other portions of this book, I will present the results of my efforts to look deeply into the roles of religion in coping with negative life events. Some of these results grow out of the Project on Religion and Coping: an intensive analysis of several hundred members of Protestant churches and Roman Catholic parishes who had experienced a major stressful life event within the past year. Through participation–observation in these congregations and interviews with clergy, members, and nonmembers, my graduate students and I developed a comprehensive battery of religious coping measures that reflect a variety of ways religion can express itself in crisis. We administered this battery to the congregation members and then examined the part religious coping plays in times of stress. The findings, which have since been extended to many other groups faced with many other major life crises, offer some important insights into the concrete operations of religion in life's most difficult moments.

The study of religion challenges psychology to stretch itself as a science. Once enriched by its subject matter, psychology will be better equipped to illuminate perhaps the most inscrutable, deeply enigmatic aspects of life. The religious world is too large, too diverse, and too complex to be approached by any single scientific method. It requires a view from the inside and the outside, a willingness to study religion in its social and situational context, and an appreciation for the variety of ways religion can express itself. In short, it requires many tools for study. Bertocci (1972) described it well: "Especially in the area of the psychology of religion, psychologists may be likened to fishermen throwing their lines into an unexplored lake. What fish they catch depends upon the nature of the hook and of the bait used. It seems clear that a wise psychologist will bring with him a variety of hooks and bait, and try to be aware of his own limitations as a fisherman" (p. 38).

In sum, it would be a mistake to assume that science and religion have little to say to each other. As one Presbyterian minister wrote: "To ignore the findings of science is theologically irresponsible and to ignore the deeper impulses of the human spirit is scientifically suicidal" (Henderson, 1988, p. 77). Both science and religion are built upon a desire to expand our understanding of the vast but largely unrecognized order to the universe. Bakan (1966) spoke of this common driving force as the impulse to reach beyond what is manifest in reality to the unmanifest. It is this driving force that has led many scientists from Descartes to Einstein to define themselves as deeply religious. Clearly, science and religion approach the world differently, but their methods may augment rather than detract from each other. The psychology of religion and coping offers one bridge between these ways of knowing the world.

This discussion has considered how a psychology of religion and coping may unify perspectives, practices, and methods of study that deserve integration. But the psychology of religion and coping cannot do everything. From the outset it is important to note some limitations of this approach.

WHAT THE PSYCHOLOGY OF RELIGION AND COPING CANNOT OFFER

A Complete Accounting of Religious Life

The child with a new hammer discovers that the world is in need of a great deal of pounding. This is the Law of the Instrument and it applies to adult psychologists as well as young carpenters (Kaplan, 1964). Armed with a theory, the psychologist may see the world only in terms of that theory. Events that do not fit very well into that theory may be overlooked or twisted and distorted until they do fit. The psychological hammer is swung not just at nails, but at any and all projecting objects.

This is a danger of the psychology of religion and coping. It may be tempting to view religion as merely a way of coping with stress, but that would not do religion full justice. For many people, the sacred is not reserved for times of crisis: it has as much to do with joyful experiences as it does painful ones, the ordinary as much as the extraordinary. Even when we focus on stressful periods, it would be arrogant to suggest that theories of coping can adequately plumb the depths of anguish and suffering described in the classical religious literature. As Beck (1986) put it: "If we were to recommend Job to the nearest seminar for stress reduction we would join the distinguished company of Zophar and Eliphaz in being of absolutely no help" (p. 23).

Important as stress and coping are, they do not make an all-embracing philosophy of life. We do more than cope. Nor will an understanding of stress and coping guarantee good outcomes for people under stress. There are situations in life we cannot cope with successfully. Within the concentration camps of World War II, only 1 out of 600 survived (Benner, Roskies, & Lazarus, 1980). Life and death depended most importantly on factors outside of the person's control. Regardless of how the individual coped, the odds were against making it through the camps alive. An analysis of the coping activities of the inmates could clarify how people sustained themselves psychologically, socially, and spiritually in these desperate conditions, but to focus on coping as a factor leading to individual survival here would be misleading (and possibly also victim blaming).

I will try to avoid the error of the Law of the Instrument in this book and admit from the start that the psychology of religion and coping cannot provide a full accounting of religious life. There is more to religion and life than coping with stress.

An Unbiased Portrayal

Values, imagination, judgment, and creativity enter into every phase of science and practice, including the psychology of religion and coping.

Because it is impossible to detach theories, methods, and practices from personal values and beliefs, it is only fair that the reader know something about my background.

Thoroughly a product of Western culture, I was born and raised in a close, middle-class, Jewish family in a friendly neighborhood in Washington DC. Comfortable as we were, the possibility that things might suddenly and dramatically fall apart never seemed too distant. Stories about the Holocaust, illness, and sudden death were common in our neighborhood. Social unrest added to the sense that danger was always lurking just ahead. Racial tension, the Vietnam war, and poverty were the headlines of my time. Even though I had more than my fair share of very happy experiences, some of these negative events occasionally intruded more directly into my life. Probably the most painful were the experiences my wife and I shared of infertility, miscarriages, Tay–Sachs disease, and premature births.

These and other losses left me with a strong sense of my own limitations. Like many people, I went into psychology in the search for answers and solutions to questions about life (and my own problems). While psychology provided me with some powerful insights, I found some of its answers to be less satisfying, particularly those offered to people faced with the truly uncontrollable.

Somewhat to my own surprise, I found religion to be more helpful in this regard. Although I came from a conservative Jewish family and had attended religious school, I had not thought of myself as personally religious. Nevertheless, I was reassured by the idea that I was a part of something larger than myself. This was more than a belief; it was a feeling that I experienced most strongly in stressful times, outdoors, and, oddly enough it seemed, when my family came together to celebrate religious holidays in synagogue or at home. It took me some time to realize that I was resonating strongly to a central religious theme—that human experience is part of a larger current in the universe. Intrigued by the surprising power of this simple idea, I began studying religion more seriously. Over the past 20 years I have observed, studied, participated, and been welcomed in the religious worlds of many different individuals, groups, and congregations. These experiences have challenged many of my preconceptions and stereotypes and opened my eyes to the richness of religious life. I do not agree with many of the religious answers to life's mysteries, but I feel strongly that religion is struggling with the right questions.

My work has not made me a religious universalist. I remain Jewish, most familiar and identified with my own tradition. The reader will pick up the strains and themes of Jewish "melodies" throughout the book, only a few of which have been deliberately included. However, though my Jewishness represents a "bias," there is nothing inconsistent with it and my efforts to learn about and work together with the members of other religious traditions.

My interest in coping is as much a bias as my interest in religion. I believe it was Robert White who said, "Ennobling visions elevate humanity, degrading visions reduce it." Unfortunately, for people in the business of therapeutic "elevation," psychologists' own visions of the world are not always particularly ennobling. In fact, they may be downright dark and dismal. In psychological writings we can find portraits of people struggling against demonic forces outside or invisible monsters within. As one writer put it cuttingly, the "three horsemen" that loom so large in psychology—Marx, Darwin, and Freud—would have "our circumstances, present and past, conscious and unconscious, genetic and learned, make monkeys of us all" (Bennis, 1989, p. 47). How, I wonder, with our own feet mired in the muddy soil of this assumptive world, can we help our clients who are stuck in theirs? Coping theory, I feel, rests on a broader set of assumptions, one that recognizes the potency of internal and external forces, but one that also recognizes the potential to transcend our personal and social circumstances. I like this kind of thinking. It is also a way of thinking quite compatible with the religious world.

Coping theory also rests on a "common sense" view of life. It assumes that people develop their own perceptions of the world. But it also assumes there is a real world to be perceived. To understand and help people then, it is not enough to work exclusively within their phenomenological worlds. It is also important to consider the degree to which their constructions of the world equip them to deal with reality, even if that reality can never be fully known.

Somehow or another the mixed ingredients of my life have led me to a somewhat paradoxical perspective: to believe that there is a real world "out there," but to see multiple truths in this world; to value the diverse ways we look at and approach life, but to believe that some ways are better than others; to feel we generally do the best we can, but to see that we can be incredibly destructive to ourselves and others; and to treasure our uniqueness as human beings, but to believe that we have to find ways to integrate our competing values, views, and approaches to the world. These are some of the biases that shape this book.

CONCLUSIONS AND PLAN OF THE BOOK

This book represents an integration of theory, research, and practice on religion and coping. There is no attempt here to reduce religion to a matter of coping. Nor does this book attempt to reduce coping to a matter of religion. Instead, I have tried to respect the distinctiveness of each process and the boundaries of each. Yet, in considering the interplay between religion and coping, I believe we will arrive at something more than the sum of its parts. Learning more about religion will teach us more about how people come to terms with their most difficult moments. By learning more about coping we will develop a clearer picture of how religion functions in people's lives. The psychology of religion and coping will, in short, break new ground, deepening and enriching our understanding of both religion and coping. And with that understanding, we will be in a better position to draw on and integrate the worldviews, practices, and methods of many communities concerned about advancing human welfare.

Incomplete and value-laden though it is, I think this book has something worthwhile to say to a variety of groups: health and mental health professionals, human service providers, social scientists, clergy, leaders of religious communities, and educated lay persons. Trying to reach such a diverse group in one book underscores the importance I am attaching to integrating different perspectives and approaches. Of course, a "bridging" book also runs the risk of collapse or of alienating people on all shores. Because the religious, the researcher, and the mental health professional often live in different worlds and speak with different voices, the accent of this book will have to shift at times from the language of one group to that of another. I am hopeful that these variations in tone will blend harmoniously and resonate strongly enough to stimulate further thought, research, interaction, and, ultimately, efforts to help people.

The first section of this book will explore the meanings of religion and coping. New definitions of these constructs will be offered that help organize and integrate much of the material to follow. Specifically, Chapters 2 and 3 will develop and elaborate on a working definition of religion. In Chapters 4 and 5, I will introduce the construct of coping and try to capture the flow of the coping process. Having defined each construct, the second section of the book will examine the ways they come together. Chapter 6 will focus on the questions of when and why religion becomes a part of the coping process. Chapter 7 will challenge some basic stereotypes about religion and illustrate some of the many ways religion expresses itself in the coping process. In Chapters 8 and 9 I will discuss how religion can serve as a force for the conservation and transformation of important human values in coping. The final section of the book will address some more practical issues. Chapter 10 will take an empirical, pragmatic look at the difficult evaluative question: How helpful or harmful is religion in coping? Chapter 11 will focus more specifically on how and why religion goes wrong in the coping process. The book will conclude in Chapter 12 with a discussion of the practical implications of the psychology of religion and coping for our efforts to help people in their times of greatest trouble.

Part One

A PERSPECTIVE
ON RELIGION

Chapter Two

~•~

THE SACRED AND
THE SEARCH
FOR SIGNIFICANCE

ENTERING THE RELIGIOUS LABYRINTH

One Saturday evening a young man, feeling restless, takes a walk. He hears music from a nearby church. Naive about religion but curious, he decides to enter. Seated in the church are several hundred people of all ages listening quietly to a white-robed priest speaking melodically from an altar. When the priest concludes by saying "The peace of the Lord be with you always," the young man is surprised to hear the entire church answer in unison "And also with you." He is even more startled when those seated around him, strangers one and all, shake his hand saying, "Peace be with you."

Attention in the church turns again to the priest who, though it is difficult to tell from a distance, appears to be breaking a piece of wafer and placing it into a cup. As the priest is engaged in his task, the people in the church begin to sing a song. The young man cannot decipher all of the words of the song, but again and again he hears the refrain, "Lamb of God, who takes away the sins of the world."

As the song ends, the church becomes quiet and many people seem to be withdrawn and introspective. A few are quietly mouthing words to themselves. A deeper quiet falls over the church as the priest says:

"Lord Jesus Christ, with faith in your love and mercy I eat your body and drink your blood. Let it not bring me condemnation, but health in mind and body." At this point, the young man is feeling confused; he senses that something very important is happening in the church, but the words, music, and actions are foreign to him.

He sees some people in the church standing up and, assuming that the service is over, he begins to put his coat on. He stops when he sees that the people are walking single-file up to the altar, pausing to stand briefly in front of the priest. Summoning his courage, the young man asks his neighbor what they are doing. The neighbor gives him a long, but not unfriendly, look and replies that they are receiving communion. The young man is struck by the differences in the expressions on the faces of the people as they walk back to their seats: Some appear serene, some seem to be concentrating intensely, some are gazing above, some have no expression at all, some appear happy, and a few have tears in their eyes. As he leaves the church, the young man wonders about the expression on his own face.

In crossing the threshold of religion we enter a different world, a place set apart from our usual experience. Hammann (1987) put it this way: "Things are no longer what they seem. Everything is something else. This world becomes a parable. It is a meanwhile place. Everything in it points to some other reality or some other process that is hidden to ordinary perception" (p. viii). Like the naive young man in the example, those unacquainted with religious life are likely to find the entry into this alien terrain particularly disturbing.

Psychologists may find the passage to the religious world exceptionally challenging. Why? There are several reasons. First, just as "one must have musical ears to know the value of a symphony," one must have some degree of religious familiarity to appreciate religious experience (James, 1902, p. 371). Psychologists, however, are among those least acquainted with religion. Second, religion elicits powerful emotions, positive or negative, not only for the general population, but for psychologists themselves. These deep passions can make it difficult to enter the religious world and gain an accurate picture of it once there. Finally, and perhaps most importantly, psychologists are challenged by the complexities of religion, a phenomenon that takes so many shapes and forms.

To venture into the religious labyrinth, psychologists need a map that describes where religion is located and what is likely to be found once inside. In this chapter, we move toward a definition of religion, one that will locate the religious labyrinth and serve as a guidepost for further exploration.

THE MANY MEANINGS OF RELIGION

Religion means different things to different people. My colleagues and I conducted a systematic study that underscored this point. Using an idiographic approach known as the Lens Model, developed by the psychologist Egon Brunswik, we developed a booklet of profiles of hypothetical people (Pargament, Sullivan, Balzer, Van Haitsma, & Raymark, 1995). The people described in these profiles varied along several dimensions, such as how frequently they attend church services, whether they hold traditional Christian beliefs, their feelings of closeness to God, and their knowledgeability about religious matters. For example, a profile of one woman read as follows:

> June is a 45-year-old upper-class woman. She is Protestant and divorced. June attends church services about twice a month. Given her income, she contributes an average amount of money to the church.
>
> When June prays, she feels God is listening to her. She prays alone a few times a week. Though she does not feel her religious beliefs give her much support in everyday life, in times of trouble or crisis she finds them reassuring.
>
> June's religious beliefs developed as a result of intensive thought and, at times, even painful soul-searching. She believes that Jesus is the Son of God and was resurrected from the grave. But she is not generally knowledgeable about the teachings of her faith. She never talks about her religion with others. In the community, June teaches first aid classes without compensation.

The participants in the study rated many profiles such as this one in terms of how religious the person described was. Through statistical analyses, we were able to develop a model of the meaning of religion for each participant: that is, those dimensions the participant used more heavily and less heavily in his or her ratings of religiousness. We then compared the models of the participants to each other.

Initially, Protestant and Catholic undergraduates participated in this study. The majority of the students had reliable, predictable models of religion. The models themselves, however, were different. Only one dimension, church attendance, was weighted strongly by a majority of the participants. Neither did we find much consensus in the religious models of Protestant students or Catholic students. What was striking were the *differences* in religious meaning. For example, one student used only one dimension, altruism, in his model of religiousness. Another student defined religion largely in terms of doctrinal orthodoxy. Yet another gave weight to more experiential elements in her model of religiousness, such as feelings of closeness with God and degree of involvement in personal religious practices.

Now the idiosyncrasies in definitions of religion among these participants could have reflected their level of religious maturity. Perhaps a more mature religious group would hold more similar views. To test this possibility we duplicated our study with a group of Protestant and Catholic clergy. The results of the first study were generally replicated. Once again, the differences in definitions were striking.

On the face of it, a simple word, "religion," has come to mean very different things to different people. These findings may explain, in part, why it can be so hard to *talk* about religion. When two people are having a discussion about the value or nature of religion they may be talking about very different things; one may be speaking of being a good person and having a feeling of closeness to the sacred, the other may be talking about going to church and believing in the truth of religious claims.

Like the more general population, social scientists have defined religion in diverse ways. In 1958, Clark asked 68 social scientists interested in religious study for their definitions of religion. The definitions were far from uniform. Some focused on concepts of the supernatural, others focused on religion as a response to major problems of life. Some of the definitions emphasized religion as a group process and others stressed the creedal and theological elements of religion. None of these definitions was outlandish. Each captured something of the essence of religion, but each described this essence somewhat differently.

TOWARD A DEFINITION OF RELIGION

The myriad definitions of religion reflect the intricacies of religious life. They also mirror the diverse interests and perspectives of those who study and work with it. More than abstractions, definitions of religion direct and guide the focus of study to particular interests and concerns. They suggest what religion is and what religion is not—in short, how to know it when you see it. But because religion is so complex and personal, no single definition is likely to be completely adequate. Different definitions, however, may add important "slants," challenging or complementing other points of view.

It is unnecessary then to argue for an "ultimate" definition of religion. What a relief! The more modest (but still important) task is to construct a definition of religion that is relevant to the phenomena of interest, in this case not only religion itself but the study of coping. This definition should be compared and contrasted with other views of religion. It should be explicit, clear, and understandable enough so we know what we mean when we talk about religion. And it should provide a framework to organize further thought and study.

One overarching question may be helpful in moving toward a definition of religion: What makes religion special?

To study religion systematically, we must know where it begins and ends. Students of religion have tried hard to sift through the unessentials to get to the heart of religion, that which sets it apart from other human experiences. Two types of response have been offered. According to one perspective, the sacred is what makes religion distinctive. Religion is uniquely concerned with God, deities, supernatural beings, transcendent forces, and whatever comes to be associated with these higher powers. According to a second perspective, religion is distinguished by its special function in life rather than by a divine entity. Most typically, religion is said to be especially concerned with how people come to terms with ultimate issues in life. Each of these perspectives, the former known as the substantive and the latter known as the functional, carries with it a set of advantages and disadvantages in efforts to appreciate the special character of religion.

The Substantive Tradition: The Sacred as the Mark of Religion

Religion has been defined as

> the feelings, acts and experiences of individual men in their solitude, so far as they apprehend themselves to stand in relation to whatever they may consider the divine. (James, 1902, p. 32)

> a system of beliefs in a divine or superhuman power, and practices of worship or other rituals directed towards such a power. (Argyle & Beit-Hallahmi, 1975, p. 1)

> an institution consisting of culturally patterned interaction with culturally postulated superhuman beings. (Spiro, 1966, p. 96)

These are some illustrations of substantive definitions of religion. As a group they generally focus on beliefs, practices, feelings, or interactions in relation to a greater Being. Each definition emphasizes different religious elements: James focuses on emotions and experiences; Argyle and Beit-Hallahmi emphasize religious beliefs, practices, and rituals; Spiro stresses religious institutions and interactions. Nevertheless, they share the same point of reference, the sacred.

A key advantage of substantive definitions is their precision. Religion refers to a specific entity, idea, belief, or practice. These views of religion fit fairly well with the everyday ways we talk about religion. Furthermore, the specificity of these definitions makes the task of studying different aspects of religious life appear to be more manageable.

Some of the precision in these definitions, however, is a bit illusory. They do not, for example, specify what is meant by a deity. After all, who could pinpoint a meaning of God applicable to everyone? Similarly, the range of experiences, beliefs, or practices that may have God as their reference point is staggering. As Müller described in 1889 (cited in Spilka, Hood, & Gorsuch, 1985, p. 30):

> Religion is said to be knowledge, and it is said to be ignorance. Religion is said to be freedom, and it is said to be dependence. Religion is said to be desire, and it's said to be freedom from all desires. Religion is said to be silent contemplation, and it is said to be splendid and stately worship of God.

In spite of their apparent precision, substantive views of religion can be quite encompassing, including many experiences beneath the religious umbrella. One solution to this problem would be to define religion even more precisely, specifying particular *kinds* of religious elements and deities. For example, God might be defined theistically, as the creator of the world, both immanent and transcendent. In doing so, however, we run the risk of religious ethnocentrism, focusing on Western forms of expression that emphasize faith, a church, and theism, excluding other approaches, such as Confucianism with its focus on ethical and moral concerns or Buddhism with its emphasis on the experiential search for enlightenment.

A more basic criticism of substantive definitions is that they miss something of the essence of religion. In describing the deities, beliefs, and practices that make it up, substantive definitions of religion take on a static character. They speak to what religion is, not how it works. For some, however, the essence of religion lies in its operation in life. The problems in trying to specify a substance of religion with boundaries broad enough to encompass diverse religious approaches, yet narrow enough to capture the heart of religion have led some to turn in an entirely different direction to answer the question of what makes religion special.

The Functional Tradition: The Struggle with Ultimate Issues as the Mark of Religion

Illustrated below are some functional definitions of religion:

whatever we as individuals do to come to grips personally with the questions that confront us because we are aware that we and others like us are alive and that we will die. (Batson, Schoenrade, & Ventis, 1993, p. 8)

a set of symbolic forms and acts that relate man to the ultimate conditions of his existence. (Bellah, 1970, p. 21)

a system of beliefs and practices by means of which a group of people struggles with these ultimate problems of human life. (Yinger, 1970, p. 7)

Like substantive ones, functional definitions of religion involve beliefs, practices, symbols, and experiences. However, their point of reference shifts from a supernatural force to a process of dealing with fundamental problems of existence. While functional thinkers define these basic problems somewhat differently, they generally focus on the most negative, weighty, seemingly insurmountable facts of life. What makes religion special is its concern with death, suffering, tragedy, evil, pain, and injustice. J. Milton Yinger (1970), a sociologist and articulate proponent of the functional perspective, describes these fundamental concerns in the form of some key questions:

How shall we respond to the fact of death? Does life have some central meaning despite the suffering and the succession of frustrations and tragedies it brings with it? How can we deal with the forces that press in upon us, endangering our livelihood, our health, and the survival and smooth operation of the groups in which we live—forces that our empirical knowledge cannot handle adequately? How can we bring our capacity for hostility and our egocentricity sufficiently under control to allow the groups within which we live—without which our life would be impossible—to be kept together. (p. 6)

Religion not only faces these issues squarely, it prescribes ways of making sense of and responding to these concerns. From a functional point of view, *how* beliefs, symbols, and actions are put into practice in the midst of critical life issues is more important than the character of these religious elements themselves: "it is not the nature of the *belief*, but the nature of the *believing* that requires our study" (Yinger, 1970, p. 11).

This approach to religion has quite a bit of appeal. It captures the sense that religion is something more than a set of concepts and practices; rather, it has to do with life's most profound issues. It also opens up the study of religion to diverse traditions and innovative approaches, for no individual, group, or culture is spared the confrontation with ultimacy.

But the functional approach has some important drawbacks as well. Viewed functionally, religion becomes an exceptionally vast phenomena. Everything from sports, sex, and art to medicine, materialism, and nihilism could represent a response to the fundamental problems of living. Even psychopathology can be seen as a way of struggling with ultimate concerns. Psychiatrist Irvin Yalom (1980) presents striking portraits of people responding to the most basic questions of existence— death, freedom, isolation, and meaninglessness—with a wide range of painful and disruptive problems, including depression, narcissism, over-aggressiveness, promiscuity, workaholism, compulsive heroism, and vegetativeness.

In their overinclusiveness, functional definitions may dilute religious meaning. Sociologist Peter Berger (1974) voices his concern that in these definitions the special transcendent nature of religion is "flattened out . . . absorbed into a night in which all cats are grey" (p. 129). He suggests that this type of definition may, in a subtle way, support a secular worldview, providing a *"quasiscientific legitimation of the avoidance of transcendence"* (p. 128, emphasis in original).[1] Similarly, Stark and Bainbridge (1985) argue that, while many systems are concerned with ultimate issues, the differences among them are very important. Citing Swanson (1960), they suggest "if members of the American Association of Atheists, the Lutheran Church in America, and the Revolutionary Communist Youth Brigade are all defined as members of religious organizations, we lose the conceptual tools we need to explore the constant and profound conflicts among them" (p. 5). Functional definitions still leave us with the question, then, of how religion, as it is commonly understood, differs from other approaches to critical concerns.

Functional definitions can also exclude religious involvement in nonultimate but nonetheless important affairs of living. Batson et al. (1993) write: "Should I ask Sally to marry or shall I wait? Should I go into law or medicine? Such questions may be extremely important and the answers one gives may have lasting effects on one's life. But coming to grips with such questions is not religious, for they do not concern matters of existence" (p. 10). Some have transferred the religious connection with these more immediate kinds of concerns to other realms, such as magic or superstition. The eminent anthropologist Bronislaw Malinowski (1944) said, "Religion refers to the fundamental issues of human existence, while magic always turns round specific, concrete, and detailed problems" (p. 200) such as a dangerous venture, failing crops, or concerns about health.

However, the distinction between the ultimate and the ordinary, the religious and the magical can be overdone. It breaks down when we consider that the response of many religions to ultimate concerns in life translates into ordinary activities. Within Judaism, over 600 commandments are spelled out in the Bible and in even further detail in the Talmud, a summary of the oral law passed down over centuries. They are not exclusively devoted to ultimate concerns; neither are they removed from the mundane. The Talmud deals with the full range of human activities: agricultural laws, holidays and festivals, the relations between husband and wife, civil and criminal law, the preparation of food, and cleanliness and impurity (Steinsaltz, 1976). Yet it would be a mistake to view these laws as simply ordinary. Because they are so intimately linked to God's covenant with the Jewish people, they take on a sacred character. In this sense the daily life of the Jew can be religious in nature. Neither is this process unique to Judaism. Within other religions, it is not at all unusual to find ordinary day-to-day experiences infused with a sense of the sacred. Leuba (1912), one of the early pioneers in the psychology of religion, once wrote, religion "is not concerned only with the objects of the highest, of ultimate, value to the individual or to society, but with the preservation and advancement of life in matters small and great" (p. 51).

To summarize, functional definitions are dynamic. They depict a religion in motion, rather than a religion frozen in time. Furthermore, they tie religion to what touches us most deeply, those issues and concerns of greatest power in our lives. However, functional definitions can be unduly broad, violating common conceptions of where religion starts and stops by incorporating any effort to deal with ultimacy beneath the religious rubric. They can also be unduly narrow in their focus on ultimacy, excluding other kinds of critical issues and important yet nonultimate issues from the religious arena.

Both substantive and functional traditions have their limitations. But the question of what makes religion special won't go away. How can it be resolved?

Bridging the Substantive and Functional Traditions: The Sacred and the Search for Significance as the Mark of Religion

Let me suggest that what makes religion special is both its substance and its function. Both substantive and functional traditions offer important points of religious reference, with neither defining religion in itself. From the substantive tradition we take the sacred and from the functional tradition we generate the notion of a search for significance. Religion lies at the intersection of the two.

The starting point of many of the world's major religious traditions is the report of an encounter between the individual and some form of divine force: the spiritual temptation and fall of Adam and Eve, the testing of Siddhartha Gautama by the Evil One and his subsequent transformation into the Buddha, the visitation by the Angel Moroni directing Joseph Smith to ancient plates later translated into the Book of Mormon, and the experience of the life, death, and resurrection of Jesus Christ. In these encounters the divine force is experienced in very different ways. Similarly diverse are the practices, beliefs, emotions, and institutions that have grown around these primal experiences. But they share a common point of reference, the divine. It is the divine who gives thoughts, actions, feelings, and groups their sacred character and distinguishes them from other pursuits (e.g., sports, the arts, psychology, political groups) that rest on different foundations. The psychologist Paul Pruyser (1968) described it well: "There is no psychology of the artist apart from the artistic work and beauty that is given form; neither can there be a psychology of religion apart from the idea of God and the forms in which holiness becomes transparent" (p. 17).

Inevitably then the question surfaces, how do we define the divine? Most social scientists take a deep breath at this point. (Others do as well. For thousands of years, poets, sculptors, and painters have struggled to find ways to express the quintessence of the holy in more tangible form.) The deep breath comes from the difficulties of trying to say something about a force so powerful to so many people, yet so "empirically unavailable" (Berger, 1974). At the risk of "taking the coward's way out," I will not try to offer a precise definition. But it is important to draw some boundaries, loose as they may be, around the *concept* of God. I stress the *concept* of God to underscore the fact that I am not referring to God's actual nature but rather to a very humanly constructed understanding of God. As Berger (1974) noted, this peculiarly social-scientific God "will always appear in quotation marks" (p. 126).

Lying within the boundary of the divine are notions of a force that created and maintains the universe, a power transcending natural forces, or a personal Being intimately involved in the world. Perfection, omniscience, omnipresence, all-loving, almighty, and eternal are some of the attributes that, singly or in various combinations, capture a sense of God. Certainly, we hold many things precious in our lives—a commitment to social justice, patriotism, a feeling of euphoria, the sense of meaning, the love for a child, addiction to a drug. None of these, however, should be confused with the divine unless *it takes on divine attributes.*[2]

The latter qualification is very important, for attributes of divinity can be attributed to many entities.

> It may be a quality (e.g., wisdom, love), a relation (e.g., harmony, unity), a particular natural entity (e.g., sun, earth, sky, river, animal), a particular individual or group (e.g., king, the dead), nature as a whole, a pure form or realm of pure forms (e.g., Good, Truth, all Ideas), pure being (e.g., One, Being Itself, Ground of Being), a transcendent active Being (e.g., Allah, Yahweh, God). (Little & Twiss, 1973, pp. 64–65)

Any of the very human experiences of the world, from romantic relationships and hero worship to political affiliations and identification with a sports team can also be "sacralized,"—that is, invested with a spiritual, even supernatural, aura (Greeley, 1972). Consider the emotional reactions to burnings of the American flag; flag burning was decried as a "desecration," a violation of something holy. Later, the United States Congress considered a constitutional amendment to protect this "sacred" symbol. Endowed with an aura of the godly, entities, whatever their form, become sacred. Further, they become legitimate foci for study by those interested in religion. Religion is oriented around the sacred, a concept that includes the divine and the beliefs, practices, feelings, and relationships associated with the divine.

Yet there is more to religion than the sacred. Religion is also oriented to *significance.* By significance, I am referring to what is important to the individual, institution, or culture—those things we care about. I will have quite a bit to say about significance in later chapters. Here it is important to note that significance includes life's ultimate concerns—death, tragedy, inequity. However, it does not stop there. It encompasses other possibilities, possibilities that are far from universal, possibilities that may be good or bad. For some, significance takes the form of tangible possessions— money, houses, good looks, drugs. For others, significance is defined in terms of personal well-being, be it peace of mind, meaning in life, personal growth, physical health, or the avoidance of pain. Significance may be self-centered, but it does not have to be. It may focus on intimacy with others or the desire to make the world a better place. Significance may also be defined in terms of the sacred.

Religion does not stand on the sidelines when it comes to matters of significance. How we find or build significance, how we hold on to it, and how we transform it when necessary are issues of great religious importance. In short, the *search for significance* is another essential point of religious reference. Throughout the book, we will see religion shaping the search for significance in many ways.

It is important to stress, however, that significance is a necessary element of religion, not a sufficient element. To put it another way, significance is not, in and of itself, religious. It becomes religious only after it has been invested with sacred character. There are, for example, numerous ways of coming to terms with the pain of unemployment. Emotional support can be sought from family and friends. An aggressive search can be launched for a new job. The lost job may be devalued or reconstrued as a chance to make a new start. None of these responses is necessarily "religious," unless we stretch the meaning of the term beyond recognition. The experience becomes religious only when the sacred is woven into the person's aspirations and responses: when the situation is viewed as an opportunity to get closer to God, when the congregation becomes a source of emotional support and information about job possibilities, when God is blamed for the loss, or when the Bible is read as a way to soothe the pain of joblessness.

A DEFINITION OF RELIGION

So where is religion located? What makes religion special? Religion is found at the junction of two large spheres: the sacred and significance. In more social-scientific language, religion involves a particular substance with a particular function. I define religion as a process, *a search for significance in ways related to the sacred.* Admittedly, this perspective is tailored to the psychological venture. It excludes concerns about the nature of the sacred that have little to do with significant human issues. These issues fall in other provinces, such as theology, rather than the psychology of religion. It also excludes from the religious arena significant experiences disconnected from beliefs, practices, feelings, and relationships associated with the sacred. These latter concerns are the focus of other approaches to life. But by locating religion at the intersection between the sacred and significance, the *special* nature of religious life comes into sharper focus. Religion has to do with building, changing, and holding on to the things people care about in ways that are tied to the sacred.

Because both the sacred and significance can be defined so differently, this definition is not overly restrictive or religiously ethnocentric. In fact, it seems open to the new and the old: evolving expressions of spirituality as well as traditional expressions of faith, involvement in new religious movements as well as participation in established religious traditions, and religiously based social and political action as well as personal acts of mercy and compassion.

In this chapter, we have developed a definition of religion, one that helps us locate the religious labyrinth and begin to make our way through. In the process of bringing religion into sharper focus, we have had to back up a bit and take a look at it from a distance. From this vantage point, it is easier to see what makes religion special, where it begins and ends. But from a distance, religion may look deceivingly uniform. Even the term "religion" may be deceptive, for it suggests that religion is simply one thing. The closer we come to religion though, the more difficult it is to talk about it in the singular. Few have studied religious experience at closer range than William James (1902). As a prelude to his rich and intimate descriptions of mystical and conversion experiences, he said: "Let us not fall immediately into a one-sided view of our subject, but let us rather freely admit at the outset that we may very likely find no one essence, but many characters which may alternately be equally important to religion" (p. 27). In the following chapter we move further into the religious labyrinth, exploring some of the ingredients that make it so rich in character.

Chapter Three

———❖———

RELIGIOUS PATHWAYS
AND RELIGIOUS
DESTINATIONS

We find religion at the crossroads of the sacred and significance. This is the starting point for our exploration of the religious labyrinth. It is, however, only a beginning. In the previous chapter we considered the meaning of the sacred and significance, the two key elements of religion. But the definition of religion says something more as well. Religion is also a process, a *search* for significance in ways related to the sacred. Although it can take many forms, every search involves two things: a destination and a path to reach it. As we venture further into the religious labyrinth, we will see that religion is vitally concerned with both the destinations pursued in life and the pathways taken to reach them. In this chapter, we examine some of these religious pathways and destinations and consider some of the ways they come together to form comprehensive religious orientations to the search for significance.

RELIGIOUS MEANS: PATHWAYS
TO SIGNIFICANCE

All of the world's religions offer their members a pathway to follow in the search for significance. Far from smooth and undemanding, these routes are often portrayed as arduous. The Hindu hears that the path

34

is: "Like the sharp edge of a razor. . . . Narrow it is, and difficult to tread" (*Upanishads*, 1975, p. 20). The Christian is told: "Narrow is the gate and constricted the road that leads to life" (Matthew 7:14). The Buddhist hears the path to salvation likened to the difficulty of fording a roiling stream (Burtt, 1982). But the ultimate rewards awaiting the dedicated traveler, the religions say, are well worth the trek.

The faiths of the world may agree that the way is demanding, but they do not agree on the way itself. Perhaps no one put it more strikingly than Johnson (1959):

> For the sake of religion men have earnestly affirmed and contradicted almost every idea and form of conduct. In the long history of religion appear chastity and sacred prostitution, feasting and fasting, intoxication and prohibition, dancing and sobriety, human sacrifice and the saving of life in orphanages and hospitals, superstition and education, poverty and wealthy endowments, prayer wheels and silent worship, gods and demons, one God and many gods, attempts to escape and to reform the world. (pp. 47–48)

The diversity of religious pathways makes it impossible to focus on any single religious approach without ignoring or oversimplifying the nature of others (Streng, 1976). Neither, however, can we review religious pathways in all of their variety. Here we will simply illustrate some of the paths people take, following the lead of Pruyser (1968), who argued that religion is to be found in every psychological dimension. Emotions, thoughts, actions, and relationships are all parts of the paths people take in their search for significance. It must be stressed that these paths are not devoid of their own sacred value. "Let us beware," Jewish philosopher and scholar Abraham Joshua Heschel (1986) said, "lest we reduce the Bible to literature, Jewish observance to good manners, the Talmud to Emily Post" (p. 231). As means to valued destinations, religious pathways can develop a spiritual significance of their own.

Ways of Feeling, Thinking, Acting, and Relating

Feeling

For many people, the cornerstone of religion is feeling. Theologian Rudolf Otto (1928), in a highly influential book, *The Idea of the Holy*, described the power of religious feeling in dramatic fashion. The essence of religious experience, he said, is a "creature-feeling," an "emotion of a creature, abased and overwhelmed by its own nothingness in contrast to that which is supreme above all creatures" (p. 10). This emotion, *the mysterium tremendum*, also has the qualities of a magnet: "something that captivates and transports [the person] with a strange ravishment, rising often enough to the pitch of dizzy intoxication" (p. 31). For Otto, this feeling cannot be reduced to any other. It flows directly out of an absolutely convincing experience with the "Wholly Other."

The kind of personal encounter with God described by Otto may not be all that unusual. McReady and Greeley (1976) surveyed a representative sample of American adults and found that 37–50% of different religious groups had had an experience in which they felt as though they were very close to a powerful spiritual force. Many people, however, experience the sacred in less emotionally powerful ways. The transcendent may be approached through a more subtle, contemplative process, or as a personal friend or confidante the individual can rely on. The love for God growing out of human reason, knowledge, and comprehension described by Maimonides (Minkin, 1987) and Spinoza (1957) has a flavor to it different from Otto's passionate intoxicating feelings for God. Religion is certainly a way of the heart, but the heart is simply one of the ways of religion.

Thinking

Religion, to many people, is first and foremost a way of thinking. Few cultures have not incorporated religious perspectives, of one sort or another, into their schemas (cf. McIntosh, 1995) for viewing the world. These perspectives connect a conception of the sacred to the nature of people, the way that life should be lived, and the character of this world and whatever may lie beyond it. These are not simply matters for theologians and intellectuals, as even the briefest review of world history will reveal. Whether salvation is earned or predetermined, whether God's nature is singular or tripartite, or whether one has followed or strayed from the true religious path are questions that have had profound implications for individuals, communities, and cultures within the Western world. Yet we cannot stop here either, for religion is more than a way of thinking.

Acting

Joseph Campbell (1988) reported overhearing an American philosopher talking to a Shinto priest in Japan: "We've been now to a good many ceremonies and have seen quite a few of your shrines. But I don't get your ideology. I don't get your theology." The priest responded: "We don't have theology. We dance" (p. xix). Now the priest may have overstated his point. Clearly, he does have a way of thinking about life, the world, and the nature of transcendence. But his "theology" stresses being and action more than thought. Among some groups, religion is less a way of thinking than it is a way of acting.

Actions are a part of all religions, even those that are more doctrinally oriented. Pruyser (1968) put it this way: "Millions of people stand, bend, stretch, fold their hands, move rosary beads, finger books, suppress coughs and sneezes, look their best, and act most solemnly for at least one hour per week, with the feeling that these are appropriate, necessary, or prescribed activities of religious value and relevance" (p. 175). But as Pruyser goes on to note, it is a mistake to view religious practices as simply "behaviors." Religious acts have power by virtue of their connection to the sacred. Careful attention to form and detail is required in religious practice because mistakes or irregularities can reduce their sacred value. In this sense, religious practices have to do with more than simple action, but with *how* one acts. They can become, as Pruyser describes them, a "craft," another way of religious life.

Relating

The focus on feelings, thoughts, and actions could lead to the conclusion that religion is simply a *personal* way of life. Indeed, in our pluralistic culture that values individual freedom and choice, religion is often seen as more a personal matter than a social experience. Bellah and his colleagues (Bellah, Madsen, Sullivan, Swidler, & Tipton, 1985) underscore the powerful current of individualism that has run historically through the stream of religious life in the United States from its founders, such as Thomas Paine who wrote "My mind is my church," to the majority of the population today who agree that religious beliefs should be independent of any religious institution. In their interviews with white, middle class Americans, they find that, for many, the heart of religion lies in the individual's personal relationship with God, a relationship that is ultimately self-centered. To illustrate their point, they cite a nurse who named her faith after herself: "I believe in God. I'm not a religious fanatic. I can't remember the last time I went to church. My faith has carried me a long way. It's Sheilaism. Just my own little voice" (p. 221). Recalling a stressful period in caring for a dying woman, Sheila felt that "if she looked in the mirror [she] would see Jesus Christ" (p. 235).

The religious individualism reflected in Western culture is also reflected in western psychology. Psychologists have generally defined religion as an individual phenomenon. The primary religious force for William James (1902) was personal emotional experience. Social and institutional religious experiences were relegated to secondary status and excluded from his text. With some important exceptions, other psychologists have also tended to see social expressions as poorly developed forms of religion or roadblocks to individual growth. Allport (1954), for example, initially labeled mature and immature forms of religion as interiorized and institutionalized orientations, respectively. Similarly, in developmental models of religiousness, social forms of religion have been defined as "psychologically primitive" and personal forms of religion, autonomous from religious institutions, have been defined as most advanced (Meadow & Kahoe, 1984).

Individualism in religious study has taken a different form in recent years. The term "religion" is being used by scholars in an increasingly narrow sense; its meaning is restricted to institutionally based dogma, rituals, and traditions. In contrast, the term "spiritual" is reserved for an inner, more personal process. Although it is a "fuzzy" concept (cf. Spilka, 1993), spirituality is generally described as a highly individualized search for the sense of connectedness with a transcendent force (e.g., Emblen, 1992; Legere, 1984). Comparisons of religion and spirituality are not made dispassionately. The preference of many writers for a personal spirituality over an organized religion is clear. For example, one author asserts "we must free the soul from organized religion and give it back in all its passion and fullness to the men and women of our time" (Elkins, 1995, p. 83).

This anti-institutional bias is unfortunate for two reasons. First of all, the distinction between spirituality-as-good and religion-as-bad does not stand up well to empirical scrutiny. There are many counterexamples. We will see in a later chapter that not all personal–spiritual expressions are helpful and not all institutional–religious expressions are harmful.

Second, the tension between the individual and the institutional can be overdrawn. Wulff (1997) notes that virtually every element of the "new spirituality" is familiar to traditional organized religions. He goes on to observe that much of the language commonly associated with the "spiritual" (e.g., journey, yearning, doubt, authority, rebirth, maturity) is just as applicable to the "religious." Lay people themselves do not generally appear to have trouble integrating the individual and institutional aspects of religious and spiritual life. In a recent study of diverse groups (e.g., mental health professionals, New Age church members, hospice nurses, nursing home residents, conservative and mainline Christians), Zinnbauer and colleagues asked the participants to select one of four options that best describes them: spiritual and religious, spiritual and not religious, religious and not spiritual, or neither spiritual nor religious (Zinnbauer, Pargament, Cowell, Rye, & Scott, 1996). Seventy-four percent of the participants labeled themselves spiritual *and* religious. Signs of tension between the individual and the institutional were not apparent for the clear majority of this sample. (Interestingly, the sub-sample of mental health professionals were more likely to label themselves "spiritual and not religious" than almost all of the other groups; another indication perhaps of an institutional religious alienation among mental health professionals, an attitude that sets them apart from those they serve).

A smaller proportion of our sample (19%) did label themselves "spiritual and not religious." However, even though this group was less involved than others in congregation-based beliefs and practices, they were more likely than others to participate in nontraditional group activities, such as meditation, healing, or yoga groups. In a similar vein, over 400 new spiritual associations have developed in just the late 1980s (see Hood, Spilka, Hunsberger, & Gorsuch, 1996).

Clearly, a number of people are searching for significance outside of traditional institutions. Far from searching alone, however, they are coming together to form new groups, groups that are supportive of individualized, subjective, and nontraditional experiences related to the sacred. Although it is easy to overlook, the individualization of religious experience is occurring within a social context that encourages a privatization of faith (Berger, 1967). Religion continues to be experienced and expressed not only intrapersonally, but interpersonally as well, by dyads, families, groups, congregations, communities, and cultures.

In this book, I have chosen to rely on the term "religion" in its broadest sense to encompass personal and social, traditional and nontraditional, and helpful and harmful forms of the religious search. When speaking about religion in its institutional sense, I will refer to religious organizations, denominations, and traditions. The term "spirituality" will be used to describe the central function of religion— the search for the sacred. Spirituality and religion are not polar opposites or competitors from this perspective. They are, instead, intimately connected.

Many Shapes, Many Sizes

The ways of emotion, cognition, behavior, and relationship are not independent of each other. They come together to form different kinds of religious pathways. It is somewhat misleading then to speak of religion as *a* way of feeling, thinking, acting, and relating. There are a variety of religious pathways, too many to consider here. But we can examine some of the features that make them so distinctive.

First, religious paths vary in their *connectedness to the sacred*. Through the practice of prayer, the individual attempts to experience the divine directly. Protestant historian Friedrich Heiler (1932) defined prayer in its essence as a "living communion of man with God, bringing man into direct touch with God into a personal relation with Him" (p. 362). Other religious practices, however, center around symbols and rituals that link the individual to God. In similar fashion, religious feelings may be attached directly to the deity, as in Otto's *mysterium tremendum,* or to the beliefs, rituals, practices, symbols, and communities built *around* God. Reading a passage from the Bible, seeking spiritual counseling, genuflecting before an altar, caring for the homeless, visiting a shrine, chanting a mantra—each of these experiences may be one step removed from God, but each can take on a sacred connotation by virtue of its divine associations. And each has the potential to elicit a wide range of feelings, from sorrow, hatred, and fear to surprise, joy, and compassion.

Second, religious paths vary in their *importance and embeddedness in peoples' lives.* Religion can become an overarching way of life, one that connects the sacred to the daily episodes of living, the past to the present, the present to the future, and the person asleep to the person awake (Wuthnow, 1976). Religion can also be restricted to particular points of transition, times of the year, or situations. It may focus on "only the things that seem orderly or pleasant: lovely woods, vales with sheep grazing, but not storms at sea or a forest fire" or "birth, marriage, childbearing, and death, but not the events in between" (Pruyser, 1968, pp. 77–78).

Third, religious paths vary in *the way they are formed.* Brown (1987) concludes his book on the psychology of religious belief by noting that in one sense people seem "to create their own religion and in another they react to what is made available to them" (p. 218). For some, religion grows out of active searching and questioning. Practices are designed and redesigned, old congregations are left behind and new congregations joined, and beliefs are tested and reformed in the laboratory of life experience. For others, religious beliefs, rituals, and affiliations are passively accepted, handed down from generation to generation like other values, traditions, and assumptions about the world.

Fourth, religious paths vary in *the way they are held.* For some, religious rituals and conceptions, once formed, become more a way of *knowing* the world than *thinking about* the world. This is the point Geertz (1966) makes when he describes religious beliefs as "really real," so completely convincing that they become an unquestioned frame of reference that precedes and structures experience rather than follows it. For others, however, religion is not as compelling. It is held more loosely and uncertainly. Consider the ambivalence voiced by an articulate adolescent from Nicaragua:

[I] sometimes doubt whether God really exists or cares. I don't understand why he lets little children in Third World countries die of starvation, of diseases that could have been cured if they would have had the right medicines or doctors. I believe in God and I love him, but sometimes I just don't see the connection between loving God and a suffering hurting world. Why doesn't he help us—if he truly loves us. It seems like he just doesn't care. Does he? (Kooistra, 1990, pp. 86, 88)

Although we may be capturing this adolescent in the midst of religious change, questions and uncertainty can become enduring hallmarks of religion (Batson et al., 1993).

Finally, religious paths vary in their *content*. We could illustrate this point through the strikingly different religious conceptions and practices of the world. But in a culture as religiously diverse as ours, most of us have some appreciation for the fact that the sacred is viewed and worshipped in many ways. On the other hand, few of us are aware of the rich and varied forms of social life to be found in religious systems. Because we rarely step outside of our own religious communities (apart from the brief excursion into another congregation for a wedding, confirmation, or funeral), we may fail to appreciate that religious congregations adopt as many different personalities as individuals do. Some congregations develop complex hierarchical bureaucratic structures that would rival those of the government. Others are simple and communal. Some congregations set themselves apart from the larger community. Others are more a part of the larger society, supporting secular institutions and tolerating different religious perspectives. Some congregations encourage members to share their deepest problems with their fellow members. In other congregations, personal problems are kept to oneself or shared in a private meeting with the pastor. What congregation a person belongs to does make a difference for the mental health, personality, and religiousness of the members (Maton & Rappaport, 1984; Pargament, Tyler, & Steele, 1979a; Pargament, Echemendia, et al., 1987; Pargament, Silverman, Johnson, Echemendia, & Snyder, 1983).

Religious paths come in many shapes and sizes. Having stressed their differences, though, it may be easy to lose sight of what these diverse religious pathways have in common.

Pathways as Functional Mechanisms

All religious pathways are methods of seeking significance. The thoughts, actions, relationships and feelings that make up these pathways are purposeful mechanisms for achieving valued ends. Let us consider a few examples.

The seven sacraments of the Roman Catholic Church offer a way to connect the person to the spiritual realm throughout the lifespan. Each sacrament serves a specific end tailored to the evolving needs of the individual.

> Through baptism we are spiritually reborn; through confirmation we grow in grace and are strengthened in faith. Having been regenerated and strengthened, we are sustained by the divine food of the eucharist. But if we become sick in soul through sin, we are healed spiritually through penance, and healed spiritually as well as physically, in proportion as it benefits with soul, through extreme unction. Through orders the Church is governed and grows spiritually, while through marriage it grows physically. (Denzinger, 1957, cited by Oden, 1983, p. 112)

Relationships are another set of mechanisms in the search for significance. Take the example of pastoral counseling. Although the process may lead in many directions, it is the relationship between the individual and the pastor and between the individual and God that is often central to change. Christian counselor David Carlson (1988) illustrates this point. Building on a biblical story, he asks his clients to imagine that Jesus has come to their house for lunch and that they have the following experience: "You are amazed at how gentle the voice sounds and his face looks. . . . You take this opportunity to tell Jesus how lonely and guilty you feel. He listens and offers encouragement to face who you are and what you have done that makes you feel that way. . . . Jesus, God's son, offers you his love and forgiveness" (p. 208). The purpose in Carlson's story is clear. He is encouraging his clients to experience Jesus Christ as a nurturant, forgiving parent.

Religious feelings, too, can serve as means toward significant ends. Eighteenth-century theologian and preacher Jonathan Edwards does his best to induce fear in his famous sermon "Sinners in the Hands of An Angry God": "The God that holds you over the pit of hell, much as one holds a spider, or some loathsome insect over the fire, abhors you, and is dreadfully provoked" (Faust & Johnson, 1935, p. 164). Once again, there is purpose in the use of religious feeling here. By bringing God's presence frighteningly close to the members, Jonathan Edwards tries to move them to Christian life. Even the *mysterium tremendum* of Otto, this *sine qua non* of religious experience, can serve important purposes. Heschel (1986) writes: "Awe enables us to perceive in the world intimations of the divine, to sense in small things the beginning of infinite significance, to sense the ultimate in the common and the simple; to feel in the rush of the passing the stillness of the eternal" (p. 135).

These are only a few of the many ways in which religion reaches out to the significant in life. Other ways religion conserves and transforms significance in times of stress will be detailed later in the book.

Some Final Thoughts about Religious Pathways

The metaphor of a pathway is almost universal in the world's religions. There are many different kinds of paths and ways to approach them. While some people will never take a religious road, others will cross one at different points in time. Still others will never leave it. Some people will follow a religious course that rarely intersects with other paths, while the religious journey of others will converge with other paths in life. The paths themselves are far from uniform. Neither are they necessarily straightforward. Made up of feelings, thoughts, actions, and relations that combine in many different ways, religious paths are multidimensional and diverse. Many of them are well established, providing identifiable markers for people to follow. Nevertheless, some people prefer to branch off the more heavily traveled trails and go their own way individually or collectively. This process is not easy. It takes time to build religious paths. They grow out of a dynamic meeting of individual, situational, and larger social forces. Diverse as they are, all religious pathways are functional, designed to reach significance, to hold on to it once it is found, and to discover new forms of significance when old ones are lost. But as we will see later, some paths are better designed than others; thus, it is necessary not only to describe and understand religious paths, but to evaluate them as well.

Important as the religious pathways are, they are not the full story. The search for significance in ways related to the sacred involves not only pathways but destinations. In fact, destinations are built into religious pathways. After all, every path must lead somewhere. As yet, however, we have only alluded to some of these destinations. An exploration of the religious labyrinth would not be complete without a discussion of the ends people seek through religion.

RELIGIOUS ENDS: DESTINATIONS OF SIGNIFICANCE

When we talk about significance, we speak the language of value, worth, and motivation. Religious communities throughout the world are well versed in this vocabulary. Every organized religious system provides its members with its own words to describe the ultimate ends of life. In spite of their differences, however, all of the world's great religions describe the sacred as their common end point. Call it a spiritual presence, Nirvana, everlasting paradise, the Kingdom of God, or eternal life, the spiritual realm lies at the heart of the search for significance in the world's religions. Those who hold to these teachings look to the sacred for significance in life. As Johnson (1959) wrote: "It is the ultimate Thou whom the religious person seeks most of all" (p. 70). Developing, maintaining, and fostering the relationship of the individual to the sacred is the essence of religious life.

The Place of the Human, The Place of the Spiritual

If that were all there were to it, then we could stop here. But religions have as much to do with people as they do gods. Where do human aspirations fit in this schema? Psychologists give one answer to this question, and the religions of the world give another. From the traditional psychological point of view, spiritual pursuits are not what they appear to be; the search for the sacred is, in reality, a reflection of more basic psychological and social motives. "Communion with God," Leuba (1912) wrote in one of the first texts in the psychology of religion, "is a way of dismissing the worrying complications of this world, of escaping a dreaded sense of isolation, of entering into a circle of solacing and elevating thoughts and feelings, of forgetting and of surmounting evil" (p. 8). There are, from this psychological perspective, no unique religious motives, only religious means for gratifying *human* needs. At its very heart then, religion is a matter of psychology.

To the religious mind, this kind of analysis is wrong, plain and simple. In the effort to decipher religion, the social scientist has neglected or distorted what is the essence of the religious world. By shaping religious phenomena to fit beneath a secular umbrella, the most important element of religion—the spiritual—has been left out in the rain. Bloom (1987) makes the same point more cuttingly: "These sociologists who talk so facilely about the sacred are like a man who keeps a toothless old circus lion around the house in order to experience the thrills of the jungle" (p. 216).

The religions of the world give a different answer to the question of the place of the sacred and the profane. Building on the firm belief that the sacred is real and that spiritual desire is a motive that can be reduced to no other, the world's faiths insist the search for the sacred takes priority over temporal concerns. The word "Islam" means submission to the will of God, and "Muslim" means one who submits. Hindus and Buddhists are encouraged to look beyond physical desires, psychological want, and worldly goods and to find the transcendent. The covenant of the Jewish people with God is founded on His primacy, a point firmly established in the first prohibition of the Ten Commandments: "Thou shalt have no other gods before Me" (Exodus 20:3). The ultimate priorities in living are made just as clear in the Gospels. Salvation is won not through oneself, others, or matters of this world but through Jesus Christ.

We have two very different answers to the same question. Traditional psychology says the religious quest is illusory; spirituality is actually an expression of more fundamental psychosocial motives and desires. The religious tradition argues back that psychology has replaced the transcendent with the self and, in this sense, elevated the human to the level of the gods. Not only is the sacred real, the religious tradition counters, it must also precede the profane as the directing force in life. Small wonder that psychological and religious worlds can find themselves at such loggerheads.

Fortunately, there are grounds for reconciliation within each tradition. On the psychological side, a few empirical studies have begun to provide a rationale for treating spirituality as a motivation in its own right. Factor analytic studies have identified spirituality as a distinctive motivation. For example, Gorlow and Schroeder (1968) identified eight types of religiously motivated people: Humble Servants, Self-Improvers, Family-Guidance Seekers, Moralists, God Seekers, Socially Oriented Servants, and Intellectuals. Welch and Barrish (1982) found that these different types of motivation were also associated with a distinctive set of religious and nonreligious behaviors. Other studies suggest that spiritual motivation is not inconsistent with other psychological and social purposes. In the Project on Religion and Coping, we presented our participants with a number of possible significant ends they might seek through religion, such as spirituality, meaning, self-esteem, comfort, and intimacy (Pargament, Ensing, et al. 1990). Scores on the spiritual purpose scale were correlated with scores for each of the other purposes. Our sample did not appear to have difficulty integrating the spirit with the flesh. The search for God seemed quite compatible with the search for other personal and social ends.

On the religious side, most faiths offer a way to reconcile the spiritual with the human. According to many traditions, humankind contains a spark of the divine. God resides in the hearts of all beings as the innermost Self, it is said in Hinduism. People are precious, it is said in the Western tradition, because they have been made in God's image, and since human needs and aspirations are an inherent part of the divine creation, they too are worthwhile. From this vantage point there is nothing contradictory about the sacred and the profane. Caring for oneself, justice, love, altruism, meaning, and self-actualization—each of these very human goals can become "spiritualized" through its association with the sacred.

Thus, within many religious traditions, there is nothing inherently wrong with human desires or contradictory about human and spiritual ends. In fact, the two can be difficult to disentangle. Muhammad says: "He who honours the learned, honours me" (Gaer, 1958, p. 238). In Christ's Sermon on the Mount, we hear: "Blessed are the peacemakers; they shall be called God's children" (Matthew 5:9). In the Book of Psalms, the search for God is interwoven with the attempt to satisfy the most basic of human longings. Deep-felt expressions of love and thanksgiving for the Lord are accompanied by pleas for wisdom, for forgiveness, and for comfort and safety.

The sacred, the ultimate end of the world's major religions, is not disconnected from the workings of the world. Most religious traditions are fundamentally concerned about earthly matters, especially humankind, for there is something of the divine in humanity. And just as the advance of the spiritual kingdom advances humankind, the advance of humanity can advance the spiritual kingdom. Human desires, needs, and values of many sorts then can become spiritually significant. Once they do, they take on a different meaning: "The religious man," Viktor Frankl (1986) writes, experiences life "not simply as a task, but as a mission" (p. xv).

We conclude then that there is room for both spiritual and human destinations in the religious search for significance. It is true that the sacred can be sought to the exclusion of the profane. It is just as true that the profane can be sought to the exclusion of the sacred. But the two can be pursued together as well. As we consider some of the psychological and social ends people seek through religion, we will see that the search for personal and social enrichment is not necessarily inconsistent with the search for God.

The Variety of Personal and Social Ends of Religion

William James (1902) was a strong believer in the multiplicity of religious motives. He asked:

> Ought all men to have the same religion? Ought they to approve the same fruits and follow the same leadings? Are they so like in their inner needs that, for hard and soft, for proud and humble, for strenuous and lazy, for healthy-minded and despairing, exactly the same religious incentives are required? Or are different functions in the organism of humanity allotted to different types of man, so that

some may really be the better for a religion of consolation and reassurance, whilst others are better for one of terror and reproof? It might conceivably be so. . . . (pp. 326–327)

Although James had a tremendous impact on the scientific study of religion, the notion that different people seek different things from religion remains surprisingly radical. Typically, theorists in this area have identified a few monolithic functions of religion that they assume to be true for all people (Paden, 1988). In fact, how the ends of religion are conceived is oftentimes one of the most definitive characteristics of the theory.

There is a problem, however, in positing singular, universal religious ends: Religious phenomena of all sorts must be twisted to fit within one particular mold. We run less risk of distorting religious experience if we make a different assumption—that religion serves different purposes for different people. Consider, for example, the responses of our participants in the Project on Religion and Coping to the questions we asked them about the ends they sought from religion. The average scores on the religious purpose scales are shown in Figure 3.1. As can be seen, people looked to religion for more than one thing in life. They did not focus solely on the spiritual purpose. Neither did they look exclusively to any particular personal or social end. Of course, we can raise serious questions about how accurately people are able to identify and report on their own religious motivations. But if there is any merit to these self-reports, then they suggest that there is no single universal religious end.

A comprehensive review of the many possible ends of religion would go well beyond the scope of this book. Having already defined the centrality of the spiritual end of religion, I will now briefly describe some of the significant personal and social destinations commonly, but not universally, associated with religion.

Religion and the Search for Meaning

From the earliest of times, people have tried to find orderliness, beauty, and reason in the world (Boorstin, 1983). The ancient Egyptians visualized the earth as an egg, protected at night by the moon. The ancient Peruvians described the world as a square with a ridge-like roof inhabited by God. The early inhabitants of India believed the earth rested on four elephants standing atop the shell of a great tortoise. Today we see the world in very different ways, but most of us continue to assume that the universe is in fact ordered and intelligible.

The religions of the world share this assumption. Though their visions differ, every tradition depicts a meaningful world and encourages its members to find and live by this meaning. Much of classic religious literature takes the form of a dialogue between the divine and a seeker of meaning, the perplexed individual who wonders why there is evil, pain, and inequity in the world and how one should live amidst so much confusion.

Many people look to religion for meaning. In one study, more than 2,000 people were asked why they were religious. The most common answer was that "religion gives meaning to life" (Braden, cited in Clark, 1958, p. 79). Other researchers have also found that religious involvement is associated with a greater sense of purpose in life (see Paloutzian, 1981) and a belief that the world is just (Rubin & Peplau, 1975; Sorrentino & Hardy, 1974).[1] The number and popularity of books written in the past decade with titles such as "Where Is God When It Hurts," "When Bad

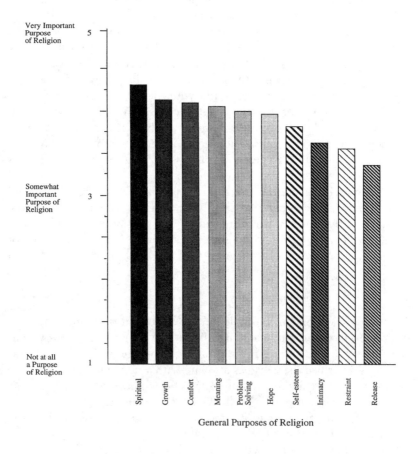

FIGURE 3.1. What people say they look for from religion.

Things Happen to Good People," and "Why Me, Why Anyone" also suggest that many people turn to religion for meaning.

Geertz (1966) believes meaning giving is the most essential function of religion. In his classic paper, entitled "Religion as a Cultural System," he said a minimal definition of religion would not be a belief in God, but a belief that God is not mad. People of different cultures may be able to deal with many conditions in living, but they cannot deal with the uninterpretable—the woman who suffers the deaths of her mother, father, and children or the withdrawal of God from humanity as the result of a small offense. Religions of all kinds ensure that these problems of bafflement, suffering, and injustice are not ultimately incomprehensible. "The effort is not to deny the undeniable—that there are unexplained events, that life hurts, or that rain falls upon the just—but to deny that there are inexplicable events, that life is unendurable, and that justice is a mirage" (pp. 23–24). In essence, religion offers meaning in life.

Religion and the Search for Comfort

Freedom from worry, protection from pain, relief from guilt and self-doubt, reassurance that life will not push the individual beyond the point of endurance—to many minds, these are the primary purposes of religion. This was Sigmund Freud's view. He believed religion offered two kinds of comfort: a protection from the dangers of the world and a protection from the dangers of human impulse itself.

A Shelter from the World

Freud (1927/1961) maintained that people turn to religion, albeit unconsciously, out of a sense of helplessness. Cataclysm, storm, disease, and death mock human efforts at control. Without the gods, people are left to fend for themselves against these superior powers. But with the gods, they can take comfort.

Freud (1927/1961) asserted that religious beliefs and practices provide some respite from tension and anxiety. The outpouring of emotion at a religious gathering, the repetition of behavior in the religious ritual, and the explanation of the workings of the universe within religious dogma all serve to cushion the individual from life's pain and uncertainty. In this sense, he accords a limited value to religion. But, as is well known, Freud felt religion is ultimately a childish, wrong-headed solution to the problems of living; he preferred that people face their state of helplessness head on through an "education to reality" (Freud, 1927/1961, p. 63).

Obviously, organized religions do not share this view. Indeed, they encourage their members to seek and find protection and comfort from the world through their faith. In one early content analysis of about 3,000 Protestant hymns, Young (1926) found that the majority of hymns dealt with one of two motifs. Thirty-three percent focused on the return to a loving, protective God, as we hear in the following hymn:

> Leaning on the everlasting arms,
> Leaning, leaning,
> Safe and secure from all alarms;
> Leaning, leaning,
> Leaning on the everlasting arms.

Twenty-five percent of the hymns reflected the comforts and rewards the individual would experience in the world to come.

A Shelter from Human Impulse

Freud (1927/1961) went one step further, asserting that people look to religion for protection not only from the terrors and cruelty of nature, but from human impulse itself. There are, he held, destructive instincts in everyone. Uncontrolled, these drives pose a threat to the survival of civilization. Unrestrained, these drives also threaten to overwhelm the individual with guilt and worry. The religions, Freud believed, curb the human appetite and, in the process, defend against the social dangers and anxiety rooted in the unmitigated expression of instinct.

That religion encourages people to moderate their impulses seems beyond dispute. As noted earlier in this chapter, the major faiths of the world will not abide self-indulgence. It is, for instance, the theme common to each of the Seven Deadly Sins—pride, envy, wrath, sloth, covetousness, gluttony, and lechery. However, religions generally find fault with human needs not for the psychological and social reasons proposed by Freud, but because, when overindulged, they separate the individual from God. Listen to this admonition about anger in its extreme, taken from the *Zohar*, the Jewish Book of Splendor: "One, who in his ire cares nothing for the welfare of his soul, uprooting it and letting it be replaced by the impure domination, such a man is a rebel against his Lord . . . he tears and uproots his soul in his heedless rage, and allows a 'strange god' to usurp its place within him" (Schimmel, 1980, p. 262). The religions will not tolerate idolatry. There can be no barrier between the individual and God, not even human need. By keeping instinct in its place, God remains in His.

Empirical studies have also tied religious involvement to indicators of impulse control, such as lower rates of premarital and extramarital sexual activity, drug and alcohol abuse, and suicide (see Payne, Bergin,

Bielema, & Jenkins, 1992, for review). Of course, we can only infer from these studies that people seek restraint and relief from their own impulses through religion. Religious involvement could be motivated by the desire for closeness with people rather than the desire for self-control; the improvements in mental health that follow could simply be an unintended but desirable consequence. Or perhaps people seek *both* closeness and comfort. Motivations do not have to be simple or clean. Here we are only suggesting that the search for comfort is one end of religion.

Whether this is the whole story, however, is another question. Religions are far from happily-ever-after storybooks. Fearsome images of hell, vengeance, and slaughter seem to be as plentiful in the religious literatures of the East and West as soothing ones (see Camporessi, 1991). Geertz (1966) puts it this way: "Over its career religion has probably disturbed men as much as it has cheered them; forced them into a head-on, unblinking confrontation of the fact that they are born to trouble as often as it has enabled them to avoid such a confrontation" (p. 18). And empirical studies have found, in some instances, religiousness to be associated with heightened guilt, anxiety, and distress (see Pressman, Lyons, Larson, & Gartner, 1992; Spilka, Hood, & Gorsuch, 1985). In short, while religious involvement can be consoling, it can also raise disquieting questions and demands of its own. The person who looks to religion solely for comfort may go away disappointed.

Religion and the Search for Self

Although religions spurn the arrogance that comes with exclusive self-preoccupation and exaggerated self-opinion, they still see something of the divine within the self. Some important implications follow for the individual:

> He owes himself self-respect, a dignity of thought and action befitting one in whom burns a spark of God.
>
> And he is under the duty to express his individuality. For bearing the divine image, he bears it uniquely.... Therefore he is obliged to discover and develop his uniqueness. Otherwise, to all eternity some aspect of the divine nature shall have been left latent and unfulfilled. (Steinberg, 1975, p. 70)

To find oneself, to respect oneself, and to strengthen and actualize oneself, from this perspective, become religious ends.

These ends are apparent in Erich Fromm's (1950) description of humanistic religion, a religious form he contrasts favorably to authoritarian religion. The latter, Fromm said, represents an indulgence in dependency, a projection of the best of ourselves onto God at the expense of the strengths we do have. To appreciate one's limitations is one thing, but to demean ourselves and worship the powers we rely on is another. Humanistic religion makes no such demand: "Man's aim in humanistic religion is to achieve the greatest strength, not the greatest powerlessness; virtue is self-realization, not obedience" (p. 37). Fromm finds elements of humanistic religion (and authoritarian religion as well) within many of the world's faiths: the Buddhist precept that knowledge and under-standing must grow out of personal experience; the teaching of Jesus that "the kingdom of God is within you"; and the Jewish biblical tradition of human autonomy and divine accountability.

Some writers feel that Fromm has made a religion out of the self. I do not read him that way. Fromm is not dismissing God here; he simply assigns the divine a different role. God represents an ideal, a vision of what people should strive for in living. In this sense, the self to be realized in humanistic religion is a self intimate with God.

If people involve religion in their search for self, then (to the extent they are successful), we should also find signs of a tie between the two. This is a tricky area of study, however, for the major religions encourage a particular kind of self-development, a self connected to the divine, not a self devoted solely to its own glorification. Watson and his colleagues (Watson, Hood, Morris, & Hall, 1985) have suggested that the equivo-cal and, at times, negative relationships between religiousness and indices of self-esteem and self-actualization may be due to an antireligious bias embedded in the measures of self-functioning. For example, several of the items in the Personal Orientation Inventory, a widely used measure of self-actualization, are antireligious in nature (e.g., "People need not always repent their wrongdoings"; "I am not orthodoxly religious"). Others depict an impulsive, happy-go-lucky person, unfettered by social standards. Not surprisingly, when measured in this fashion, self-actuali-zation is incompatible with religious commitment. However, Watson et al. (1985) find that a different picture emerges when less religiously biased measures of self-functioning are used or when the antireligious dimension is statistically controlled. Then the relationship between self-functioning and religious commitment becomes more positive.

Similarly, when we asked people in the Project on Religion and Coping what they seek from religion, many were not hesitant to say they look to religion for their own development. In fact, the search for personal growth through religion was endorsed by church members to a greater degree than any other end, with the exception of the spiritual purpose. I think it is safe to conclude that self-development is another religious end for many people, but remember that this is often a particular kind of self, a self oriented to the sacred.

It is important to add that the search for self does not take place in isolation. Identity, Erik Erikson (1980) noted, is both a psychological and a social phenomenon: "It connotes both a persistent sameness with oneself . . . and a persistent sharing of some kind of essential character with others" (p. 109). People look to religious groups in part to help "constitute themselves" (cf. Bellah et al., 1985). From the earliest moments in life when the newborn receives a name through religious ceremony to life's latter phases when old roles have been relinquished, religious groups offer opportunities for self-definition and development.

Merely the act of affiliating with a religious group says something important about how people are likely to see themselves and how others are likely to see them. Consider the diverse images and associations members of different religious groups can bring to mind: the conservative Christian, the New Age devotee, the Mormon, the orthodox Jew, the mainline Protestant, the devout Muslim. Identity is defined in part by the groups we belong to. The large majority of people in the United States and Canada affiliate with a religious group (Bibby, 1987; Gallup & Castelli, 1989). Of course, for many people this identification is less than total. Picking and choosing selectively from the teachings and practices of a faith is increasingly commonplace. But religion can be relevant even to those who remain unaffiliated, for what people stand *against* says as much about identity as what they stand for. The social religious context is, in this "anti-sense," critical to the development and maintenance of the identities of the atheist, the spiritual person who rejects organized religious involvement, and the religious woman who is, in most respects, conservative, but takes issue with the church's stand on abortion.

Religious groups provide more than labels for self-definition. Every religious tradition represents a "community of memory" (cf. Bellah et al., 1985) that helps its members find themselves in time and place. Through the stories of the tradition, people learn about who and where they come from. They hear the accounts of exemplary individual and fallen figures who model the way life should and should not be lived. Embedded in the stories and rituals of every religious faith are general templates for living, maps that allow people to locate who they are, who they are not, and how they can best express their distinct identities.

Thus, the search for self through religion should not be seen as a solitary pursuit. Bellah et al. (1985) make the point eloquently: "We find ourselves not independently of other people and institutions but through them. We never get to the bottom of our selves on our own. We discover who we are face to face and side by side with others" (p. 84).

Religion and the Search for Physical Health

People look to religion for physical health as well as psychological and emotional well-being. Prayers for a rapid recovery from illness are nothing out of the ordinary in the religious services of most faiths. In one survey of Protestants and Roman Catholics, 79% indicated that they had asked God to restore someone to health; this was the second most common of all prayers (Stark & Glock, 1970). In other parts of the world, thousands of people have taken religious pilgrimages in the search for healing at sites where miraculous cures are believed to have taken place, such as Lourdes, France, and Tiruchendut, India. Traditionally, people have looked as much to religion in their search for health as they have to medicine.

Religions, new and old, have designed their own roles and structures to facilitate this search. Long before the development of medicine as we know it, shamans were calling on spiritual powers to treat the sick and dying and to protect their communities from illness. Alternative forms of religious healing such as shamanism are not a thing of the past. They remain popular in many parts of the world, including the United States, where interest in faith healing, New Age therapies, and transcendental meditation is high (see McGuire, 1988). Religious roles and structures are also well integrated into the traditional system of health care, as illustrated by the presence of religiously based hospitals, hospital chaplains, and religious orders dedicated to serving the sick within many communities. The role of the physician itself can be vested with spiritual significance. "Value the services of a doctor for he has his place assigned him by the Lord" is a verse from the deuterocanonical Book of Ecclesiasticus (38:1) that many physicians might enjoy posting in their waiting rooms. Finally, as we will see later in the book, organized religions are able to draw on a variety of coping methods to help the sick and frail understand and come to terms with their conditions.

Religious traditions are interested in more than the alleviation of pain and suffering. They promote healthy lifestyles among their members: Mormons are told to stay away from alcohol and caffeine; Jews are instructed to avoid nonkosher foods; Seventh-Day Adventists are taught to be vegetarian; Parsis are directed toward late marriage and strict monogamy (see Levin & Vanderpool, 1989). And there is some evidence that religious groups are successful in their health-promoting efforts. Commitment to religious beliefs and practices has been positively associated with a variety of subjective and objective measures of health status for people affiliated with a broad spectrum of religious groups (see Levin, 1994; Matthews, Larson, & Barry, 1993).

Of course, these positive effects are not necessarily the result of an active search for health through religion. Better physical health could be simply a by-product of other religious goals and processes. Perhaps it is an outgrowth of the individual's attempt to gain social support or behavioral control through a religious group. Perhaps the search for spiritual connectedness, emotional comfort, meaning, or a sense of control has some healthy fringe benefits, such as physiological relaxation (cf. Benson, 1984) or potentially immunosuppression-countering effects (Achterberg, 1985; McIntosh & Spilka, 1990). Or perhaps better health is the result of some combination of factors (Hill & Butter, 1995; McFadden & Levin, 1996).

In any case, there is nothing illegitimate about the search for physical health from the perspective of most religious traditions. It is important to add, however, that this understanding of physical health cannot be separated from broader spiritual concerns. Physical health, as religions view it, is one part of a greater spiritual well-being: Christians are told that their bodies are vessels that contain the spirit of God and, as such, deserve glorification; many eastern religions speak of the unity of body and mind; and healing is defined by alternative religious groups as a process of becoming closer to God. In these ways, the search for physical health becomes more than the pursuit of bodily comfort. Like many seemingly worldly objects of significance, physical health can take on sacred value.

Religion and the Search for Community

For sociologist Emile Durkheim (1915) religions are, at heart, a social rather than a psychological, emotional, or physical matter. They provide a representation of society and of the members' relationships to it. Most importantly, Durkheim maintained, religious beliefs and rituals of all kinds unite the adherents into a common faith. "If religion has given birth to all that is essential in society," he said, "it is because the idea of society is the soul of religion" (pp. 432–433).

It is not difficult to find evidence of Durkheim's unifying function among the faiths of today. Where we find religions, we find temples, mosques, synagogues, meeting houses, pagodas, and churches. In 1991, there were over 350,000 religious congregations in the United States (Jacquet & Jones, 1991). These are the homes of people drawn together by something they hold in common—a heritage, a set of beliefs, a dream for the future, or a distinctive way of life. Within their spiritual communities, people can seek out a sense of intimacy and belongingness. They can also express their desire to make the world a better place.

Intimacy

It seems that many people look to religion in their yearning for closeness. Over the past 15 years, my students and I have provided a program of assessment and consultation to a variety of congregations—Protestant,

Catholic, and Jewish (Pargament et al., 1991). While our findings vary from system to system, one of the recurrent themes has been that members are seeking greater intimacy with other members. Many have established their own families away from the communities and families they grew up in. Caught up in activities that keep them apart from each other, they look to the synagogue or church to reestablish that larger sense of connectedness. Without this sense of closeness, many members feel that something vital in religious life is missing. As the member of one such congregation put it: "Ours is a friendly place," he said. "But I joined here for something more than friendliness. It was familiness I missed and wanted."

There is evidence that religious involvement can, at least in some instances, allay feelings of loneliness and disconnectedness (e.g., Ellison & George, 1994; Johnson & Mullins, 1989; Kennell, 1988). For example, psychologist Joseph Kennell (1988) conducted a 3-year case study of a small church in one of the most depressed, socially fragmented parts of the inner city. Members of the church, he found, had larger social support networks than people not affiliated with an area church. Moreover, the support within the church appeared to be less contingent on the skills and resources of the individual. Among nonmembers, social support was associated with greater interpersonal skill. In contrast, social support was unrelated to interpersonal skill among church members. Even marginal people within the church received the social benefits of church involvement. Over his years of observation, Kennell also noted improvements in the relationships among members, particularly among members of the same family. The church, he concluded, had been quite successful in fostering an oasis of belonging in the midst of an impoverished setting. Of course, the church provided more than simply intimacy to its members; it was also a source of concrete help, comfort, growth, and spirituality. But the feeling of belonging was one of the significant ends many of the members sought and attained. Appropriately enough, the congregation was called the Community Church.

The ties forged between people of like faith are a central part of spiritual life. However, some would take issue with Durkheim's view that the gods exist only to unify their members into a coherent group. From the religious vantage point, the gods are not a way to intimacy; intimacy is both a way to God and a way of God. Philosopher Martin Buber (1970) spoke most eloquently of this process. In his classic book *I and Thou,* Buber located God in relationships. Here Buber referred to a particular kind of interaction, not one between an isolated individual and a discrete object, an I and an It, but rather one involving a vital encounter between two subjects, an I and a Thou who meet and complete each other. Buber wrote: "Man lives in the spirit when he is able to respond to his Thou. He is able to do that when he enters this relation with his whole being. It is solely by virtue of his power to relate that man is able to live in the spirit" (p. 89). In any relationship, Buber asserted—be it with nature, people, or spiritual beings—one can encounter God, the "eternal Thou." However, Buber accorded special significance to relationships with people: "The relation to a human being is the proper metaphor for the relation to God—as genuine address here is accorded a genuine answer" (p. 151).

A Better World

The search for community does not end with a feeling of connectedness to other people. When extended beyond the immediate family, the sense of spiritual kinship may be accompanied by a desire to give to others, to make the world a better place (Batson, 1990). It is this love for others, this concern for a better world, that is a culminating value of most religious traditions. Humanity, they say, is called to share divine blessings with others. Almost every tradition espouses some form of the Golden Rule that, in one way or another, people must care for the well-being of others just as we care for ourselves because God cares for us all. From these religious perspectives, the search for a better world is less of a social value than it is a religious imperative.

When we turn to the exact vision of this better world, we find more differences in points of view. Some see the better world in a radically changed social order liberated from the social ills of our day, such as poverty, discrimination, violence, and the destruction of the environment (Maton & Pargament, 1987). Others see evangelism as the key to the better order. "Win men to Christ," they say, "and injustice and suffering will automatically disappear" (Glock, Ringer, & Babbie, 1967, p. 206). Perhaps most often, the better world is defined in terms of greater compassion and caring among people. Here the focus shifts from radical social change and proselyting activities to social service. It should be added that some people choose to embrace larger worlds than others. The injunction to love thy neighbor has been interpreted to read "love thy like-minded neighbor." It is a sad commentary that the kindness and caring so characteristic of relationships within many religious communities can be paralleled by darker expressions of derision and hostility to those who live outside the boundaries of these narrowly defined religious worlds.

To what extent are people religiously motivated by the desire for a better world? At the institutional level, the evidence of religious giving is indisputable. Churches and synagogues provide more than twice the social philanthropy of foundations and corporations (Jacquet, 1986). Of all the predictors to charitable causes, attendance at weekly religious services is the strongest (*Giving and Volunteering in the United States,* 1988). At the individual level, it is also clear that people who are religiously committed see themselves as contributors to a better world; they describe themselves as more empathic (Watson, Hood, Morris, & Hall, 1984), espouse more prosocial values (Tate & Miller, 1971), and report greater helpfulness to others (see Batson et al., 1993 for review). Whether religious people actually *behave* more compassionately, though, is an unsettled question (Spilka et al., 1985). This is quite an involved literature, too involved to review here; but the general picture that appears to be emerging is that different forms of religion are associated in varying ways with different kinds of helping behavior (see Batson et al., 1989; Bernt, 1989).

Of course, helping activities, religious or otherwise, may be motivated by forces other than altruistic ones. Hundreds of years ago, Maimonides pointed out in his Golden Ladder of Charity that not all acts of charity are equally praiseworthy. The charity of the lower rungs grows out of the desire for personal and social reward; the charity of the higher rungs finds its value in the act of giving itself. Experimental research by Daniel Batson and his colleagues (Batson et al., 1989; Batson & Flory, 1990) also suggests that religious giving is not necessarily based on altruistic motives. Some seemingly selfless religious devotees, they find, are guided not by the desire to help others, but by the desire to see themselves or be seen by others as caring, loving, and compassionate. Other religiously minded individuals may express a more genuine commitment to a better world.

What can we safely say, then, about religion and the search for a better world? History, case study, and empirical investigations seem to suggest that the better world is a destination of religious value for some, but not for all.

Some Final Thoughts about Religious Destinations

When theorists and researchers turn their eyes to religion, they often see very different things. This point holds particularly true when it comes to the underlying purposes of religion. One theorist speaks the language of meaning, another of comfort. Still others talk about religion as rooted in the search for intimacy, self, or a better world. It is not that they ignore other concepts; rather, each attaches a different primacy to them. Theorist X's overarching religious destination is secondary to Theorist Y. What is the central religious theme to Theorist

Y is simply a means to a greater end to Theorist Z. I have not felt compelled to pick among X, Y, or Z here. Instead I have assumed that theorists find diverse purposes in religious life because there are, in fact, diverse purposes in religious life. And different people look to religion for different ends. The extraordinary staying power of the world's religions may have much to do with the fact people of different temperament, need, and situation can find one of many niches for themselves in these living systems.

In this section, some of the ends common to many of these religions have been reviewed. The selection of religious destinations—spiritual, meaning, comfort, self, physical health, intimacy, and a better world—was somewhat arbitrary; virtually any end, good or bad, could become sanctified through its association with the sacred. But, no matter how they are defined and organized, it is a mistake to reduce one significant end to another. The search for meaning, intimacy, self, and a better world are not simply disguises for what all people really seek—personal comfort. The search for closeness with God is something other than the desire for personal and social satisfaction in masquerade. Only by twisting and distorting the character of religious significance can we reduce it to a single expression.

RELIGIOUS ORIENTATIONS TO THE MEANS AND ENDS OF SIGNIFICANCE

We have explored some of the diverse pathways and destinations within the religious labyrinth. Although we have considered them separately, religious means and ends are not isolated from each other. They come together to form comprehensive orientations to life.

There are many possible routes to many possible end points, so many, in fact, that the systematic study of religion may appear to be an impossible task. Fortunately, this is not the case. Religious pathways and destinations are limited in number and kind by the realities of the world and the human condition. There are situations in life few of us can avoid—birth, coming of age, illness, accident, and death. Neither can most of us avoid the basic existential questions these crises and transitions raise. All of these constraining forces make it possible to identify a smaller number of well-trodden paths and aspirations in the religious labyrinth.

The notion of religious orientations helps simplify a potentially overwhelming task. They capture, in efficient form, some of the common pathways people take and destinations they seek through religion. I would define religious orientations as *general dispositions to use particular means to attain particular ends in living*. The religious nature of the orientation comes from the involvement of the sacred in the configuration of means and ends. The term "general" is used to underscore the point that religious orientations do not speak to the particulars of any situation. They are cross-situational phenomena; that is, they describe general tendencies or inclinations to use certain religious means and seek certain religious ends over many situations.

This definition is quite different from other views of religious orientation. Although an exceptionally large portion of current research in the field has been devoted to studies of the relationship between various religious orientations and phenomena such as prejudice, helping behavior, personality, and mental health (see Gorsuch, 1984), the meaning of this concept itself has been cloudy. Religious orientation has been viewed variously as a personality variable, a motivational construct, an attitudinal dimension, or a cognitive style (see Hunt & King, 1971; Kirkpatrick & Hood, 1990, for reviews).

I believe the picture becomes clearer if we assume that religious orientations are, in fact, multidimensional. They are, in part, motivational constructs. They have to do with the ends people generally hope to reach. But they are also cognitive, behavioral, attitudinal, emotional, and relational constructs. They describe the religious pathways people generally follow toward their goals.

Thinking about religious orientations as means and ends is also a departure from the religious and psychological literature that has polarized these two constructs.

The Polarization of the Means and Ends of Religion

The terms "means" and "ends" are often used interchangeably with the "bad" and "good" of religion. The idea that religion can serve as a means to an end brings to mind some unsavory images: the sanctimonious church member who jealously protects his position in the congregation to maintain his self-esteem and status in the community; the political leader who invokes the name of God to support a war that extends his power at the expense of his followers' lives.

These "users" of religion have been contrasted unfavorably with those who look to religion as an end in itself. Compare these two writings from a Talmudic treatise, *The Wisdom of the Fathers* (Goldin, 1957), and its commentaries:

> He who makes use of the crown of Torah, is forever puffing himself up and lording it over people, and demands to be honored by virtue of the crown of Torah, which he can show he has acquired, will perish and be driven out of the world. (p. 68)

He who studies the Torah for its own sake merits many things; not only that, but he is worth the whole world, all of it. He is called beloved friend; he loves God, he loves mankind, he is a joy to God and a joy to man. (p. 226)

Psychologists have portrayed utilitarian approaches to religion in similarly unflattering terms. This point is illustrated most sharply in the seminal work of Gordon Allport (1954), who was interested in the seemingly paradoxical relationship between religion and bigotry toward blacks and Jews. Why, he asked, do the creeds of the world's great religions emphasize the brotherhood of all people while their practices all-too-often produce just the opposite effect? How is it, for instance, that one minister in war-torn Europe martyrs himself to protect the Jews in his village while another wraps his anti-Semitism in the cloak of religion? Throughout his career, Allport devoted a significant amount of thought to this question. Not all religions are alike, he concluded. The religion of brotherhood and compassion must be distinguished from the religion of prejudice and bigotry. Early in this line of work, Allport (1950) developed a richly detailed conception of religion at its best, the religion of maturity, and religion at its most pathological, the religion of immaturity. Later, however, Allport moved to a simpler, more narrow conception of these kinds of religion. He offered two "ideal types" of religious orientation lying on the ends of a continuum spanning the good and the bad of religion (Allport & Ross, 1967).

On the negative end is the extrinsic religious orientation:

A person with an extrinsic religious orientation is using his religious views to provide security, comfort, status, or social support for himself—religion is not a value in its own right, it serves other needs, and it is a purely utilitarian formation. Now prejudice too is a "useful" formation: it too provides security, comfort, status, and social support. A life that is dependent on the support of extrinsic religion is likely to be dependent on the supports of prejudice. . . . (p. 441)

On the positive end is the intrinsic religious orientation:

Contrariwise, the intrinsic religious orientation is not an instrumental device. It is not a mere mode of conformity, nor a crutch, nor a tranquilizer, nor a bid for status. All needs are subordinated to an overarching religious commitment. In internalizing the total creed of his religion the individual necessarily internalizes its values of humility, compassion, and love of neighbor. In such a life (where religion is an intrinsic and dominant value) there is no place for rejection, contempt, or condescension toward one's fellow man. (p. 441)

Allport contrasted a religion of means—a device, an instrument, a tool—with a religion of ends—lived, internalized, totally directive. This polarization of means and ends lies at the heart of the concepts of intrinsic and extrinsic religion: "Perhaps the briefest way to characterize the two poles of subjective religion," Allport said, is "that the extrinsically motivated person *uses* his religion, whereas the intrinsically motivated *lives* his religion" (Allport & Ross, 1967, p. 434). Allport's is not an idiosyncratic position among psychologists. For example, in a reformulation and elaboration on his work, Batson et al. (1993) relabeled the extrinsic dimension "Religion as Means" and the intrinsic dimension "Religion as End." Allport's conceptualization of the intrinsic and extrinsic religious orientations and Batson's reformulation remain the most heavily used framework for psychological studies of religion (Gorsuch, 1984).

It is unfortunate that the means and ends of religion have been cast as archenemies, for every search, religious or otherwise, must necessarily involve both means and ends. Even when religion is sought for its own sake, a way must be found to reach this goal. Indeed, as we have seen, the religions of the world prescribe not only the ultimate ends of life, but pathways to these ends. Through prayer the individual seeks God. Through education, children learn about their religious tradition. Through good deeds, a person lives consistently with God's laws. All of the world's great religions recognize that some method, some instrument, or some way toward these ends is a necessary part of religious life. They find nothing reprehensible about the fact that religion is used, when it is used to reach spiritual goals. In fact, they prescribe instrumental means to attain intrinsic ends (Johnson, 1959). There is, in this sense, nothing inconsistent about both "living" and "using" religion.

If we take a close look at the instrumental kind of religious experience that has been so heavily disparaged, we find that the criticisms have more to do with the *misuse* of religion rather than the use of religion per se. To condemn all religious uses because of some religious misuses, however, is a matter of guilt by association. The critical question is not whether religion is lived or used—most people who define themselves as religious, in some way or another, use religion; instead we have to ask, *how* is religion used in living and to what ends?

The following sections explore the distinctive means and ends associated with the three most commonly studied religious orientations: the intrinsic and extrinsic orientations of Allport and the quest orientation of Batson.

A Means-and-Ends Analysis of Intrinsic, Extrinsic, and Quest Orientations

Intrinsic and Extrinsic Orientations

Although Allport characterized the intrinsic and extrinsic orientations as religions of ends and means respectively, ends and means are a part of both orientations. They are, however, ends and means of a very different kind (see Table 3.1). With respect to ends, Allport said, the intrinsically oriented find their most basic motive in religion (Allport & Ross, 1967). What is this master motive? It centers around God rather than the self. As an illustration, he drew on the words of a clergyman who described the intrinsically oriented as those who "come to church to thank God, to acknowledge His glory, and to ask His guidance" (p. 434). Personal needs may be strong, Allport said, but they are ultimately less important. This is not to say that Allport's spiritual ends are devoid of personal and social significance. While faith is of the highest value to the intrinsic, it is a faith "oriented towards a unification of being" and one which "takes seriously the commandment of brotherhood" (Allport, 1966, p. 455). In this way, Allport appeared to sanctify two of the personal destinations we described earlier: the search for self and the search for a better world. The search for meaning may have been spiritualized as well; one item on the intrinsic religiousness scale developed by Allport and Ross (1967) reads: "Religion is especially important to me because it answers many questions about the meaning of life" (p. 441).

A different set of personal ends was singled out for criticism in Allport's extrinsic religious orientation. Over the years, he tied the

TABLE 3.1. Religious Orientations as Means and Ends of Significance

| | Religious Orientation | | |
	Intrinsic	Extrinsic	Quest
Means	Highly embedded in life Guide for living Convincing	Peripheral Lightly held Passively accepted Compartmentalized Sporadic	Active struggle Open to question Flexible Complex Differentiated
Ends	Spiritual Unification Compassion Unselfish	Safety Comfort Status Sociability Self-justification Self-gain at others' expense	Meaning Truth Self-development Compassion

extrinsic orientation to a variety of personal and social needs, including solace, safety, status and sociability. Implicit in much of his writing was a belief in the antisocial nature of these ends. In 1960 Allport wrote: "Extrinsic religion is a self-serving utilitarian, self-protective form of religious outlook, which provides the believer with comfort and salvation at the expense of outgroups" (p. 257).

In short, Allport set up a clear contrast of ends. The intrinsically oriented individual seeks God, faith, a better world, and unification in living. "Self-serving" needs are transcended. The extrinsically oriented individual seeks personal gain in the forms of comfort, esteem, and sociability, even at the expense of others. Spiritual ends of religion are not a part of this equation.

The two orientations differ in means as well as ends. The religion of the intrinsically oriented, Allport said, is fully embedded in life, informing and guiding the person's thoughts, actions, and feelings. In contrast, the religion of the extrinsically oriented is only "lightly held," a peripheral part of life, passively accepted and used as a crutch only when personal need arises.

The polarization of extrinsic and intrinsic orientations into means and ends has led theorists and researchers to ignore important differences in *kinds* of religious pathways and destinations. A closer analysis of Allport's two orientations, however, makes clear that he was not contrasting a religion of means with a religion of ends. He was contrasting a religion of one set of means and ends with a religion of another.

Quest Orientation

Daniel Batson and his colleagues (Batson et al., 1993) presented a third orientation to religion. This orientation grew out of some dissatisfaction with Allport's work. While they found no fault with Allport's conception and measurement of extrinsic religiousness, they argued that intrinsic religiousness has too much the flavor of a rigid dogmatic approach to faith. As an orientation "embraced" and "followed fully," they said, it leaves little room for several other factors crucial to religious experience: complexity, doubt, and tentativeness. These characteristics form the center of Batson's third orientation: religion as quest, an "open-ended, questioning" approach more interested in the ongoing search for truth than "clear-cut, pat answers" (p. 166). Batson cites Siddhartha Gautama, Mahatma Gandhi, and Malcolm X as exemplars of those who have lived a life of quest.[2]

What are the means associated with this religious orientation? Batson is clear on this point. The quest path is largely a cognitive one; it has to do with the way beliefs are formed and held. "Questions are far more central to my religious experience than are answers" reads one item from the quest scale (p. 170). "It might be said that I value my religious doubts and uncertainties" reads another (p. 170). Quest, Batson maintains, is a way of thinking that involves a willingness to actively confront and struggle with tough issues; an open, flexible stance to learning; a skeptical and doubting attitude toward simple solutions to difficult problems; and a complex, highly differentiated framework for viewing the world.

Where does the quest orientation lead? The religious quest represents a search for truth, a search for meaning in life: "An individual who approaches religion in this way recognizes that he or she does not know, and probably never will know, the final truth about such matters. Still the questions are deemed important, and however tentative and subject to change, answers are sought" (p. 166).

The search for personal growth and development also receive mention as ends of quest, although Batson et al. (1993) are less explicit on this point. As noted earlier, Batson et al. (1989) have suggested that quest may also be associated with a genuine desire to help others and better the world. However, it is not clear whether altruism is viewed as simply a by-product of a quest orientation or as an end in itself.

Implications of a Means-and-Ends Approach

Explaining Some Puzzling Findings

Thinking about religious orientations in terms of means and ends helps sharpen these concepts. The distinctive nature of each orientation stands out with more clarity. Elsewhere, I have suggested that a "means-and-ends" analysis may improve the measurement of religious orientations and offer one way to make sense of some puzzling empirical findings in the literature (Pargament, 1992). One such puzzle is the lack of correlation between the three religious orientations, orientations that have been viewed as if they were irreconcilable approaches to religion (Batson & Schoenrade, 1991b; Donahue, 1985). Recall that Allport, for one, conceived of intrinsic and extrinsic religiousness as polar opposites in an effort to explain how religion could be associated with the bigotry of anti-Semitism and racism on the one hand and the love and compassion of Jesus on the other. To find that the two scales are generally unrelated (i.e., people who score highly on the intrinsic scale are just as likely to score highly on the extrinsic scale as they are to score low) seemed unfathomable. Allport tried to resolve this puzzle by describing those who endorsed both intrinsic and extrinsic positions as "muddleheads" (Allport, 1966).

Certainly, some people are indiscriminate in their approach to religion; however, I do not think that everyone who endorses the two approaches is confused (Pargament, Brannick, et al., 1987). An individual could, without much muddleheadedness, endorse several of the items on the intrinsic and extrinsic scales. After all, what is inconsistent about the extrinsic item "The purpose of prayer is to secure a happy and peaceful life" and the intrinsic item "It is important to me to spend periods of time in private religious thought and meditation?" Part of the problem here may be that Allport's measure of extrinsic religiousness does not carry the full weight of his concept. The items on this scale do not depict an individual selfishly pursuing his or her goals at all costs. Instead, they describe someone who looks to religion primarily for help in satisfying personal and social needs.

In his conception of intrinsic and extrinsic religiousness, Allport forces the individual's hand. You must make a decision, he says. Choose the faith or choose yourself. But are the two necessarily incompatible particularly when the antisocial elements of the extrinsic orientation are removed from the measure? Recall from the Project on Religion and Coping that spiritual religious purposes were positively associated with many other personal and social religious goals: meaning, hope, intimacy, comfort, and esteem, to name a few. In another study (Echemendia & Pargament, 1982), items reflecting the search for personal support, comfort, and solace through religion emerged as a part of the *intrinsic* factor, once again underscoring the point that religious and at least some personal ends are far from inconsistent. A forced-choice between the sacred and the secular overlooks the capacity of religions to spiritualize humanity and humanize God. The lack of correlation among the intrinsic and extrinsic scales then may suggest that many people do not feel a need to choose between themselves and God. Their refusal to conform to a forced-choice logic does not make them all muddleheads. Rather, it suggests that, for some, there is room for both God and self at the center of religious experience.[3]

Are There Only Three Religious Orientations?

There are empirical and theoretical reasons to suspect that there may be more than three religious orientations. Some empirical study indicates that these three orientations oversimplify the intricacies of religious means and ends. Several years ago, Ruben Echemendia and I found that when religious orientations are measured by a more diverse set of questions, a richer picture is revealed (Echemendia & Pargament, 1982). In addition to the intrinsic–personal support factor just noted, our factor analysis revealed three distinct extrinsic factors: Social Support—the search for a sense of community and fellowship through religious life, Obligation—religious involvement out of a sense of duty or guilt, and Social Gain—the use of religion to raise one's social standing and self-image. Kirkpatrick (1989) reported similar results. His factor analysis of the intrinsic and extrinsic religious scales yielded an intrinsic factor and two extrinsic factors: one dealing with religion as a means to social gain, and the other involving religion as a means to personal comfort and protection. Others have found some signs of multidimensionality within the intrinsic and quest scales as well (Batson & Schoenrade, 1991b; King & Hunt, 1969; Watson, Morris, & Hood, 1989).

Important as studies of intrinsic, extrinsic, and quest orientations are, our theoretical review of the varieties of religious means and ends points to some limitations in these three orientations and encourages us to look beyond them. For instance, none of these orientations speaks to the wide-ranging content of religious beliefs, practices, or feelings. In the process some critical distinctions may be obscured: The believer in a benevolent, loving God is grouped with the believer in a capricious, judging God; the evangelist is not distinguished from the advocate for human rights; and the individual who feels God's presence in his or her life may appear to be the same as the individual who experiences God as only an abstraction.

As notable is the omission of the diverse forms of religious social experience, so central in one way or another to personal religious expression. Although we have spoken of religious orientations as embedded in a social world, they are typically studied as if they exist apart from a larger social context (Barton, 1971). A full accounting of religious orientations must attend to the social dimension of religion as well as the cognitive, behavioral, and emotional. And what about other religious destinations—the desire for physical health, the search for intimacy and connectedness, the yearning for a radically improved world? These are simply a few of the ends that are not an explicit part of the three major orientations to religion. When measured more comprehensively, I suspect we will find that there are more configurations of religious means and ends than we have, as yet, imagined (see Weinborn, 1995).

Religious Disorientation

In this chapter, I have considered many religious means and ends, and some of the ways they come together to form religious orientations. The focus here has been largely descriptive. Yet religious orientations can be evaluated as well as described. I will take up this sensitive, value-laden task later in the book. Here let me simply note that religious orientations are not equally worthwhile. This is not to say that there is one orientation best for all. But some religious pathways are better constructed than others, some religious destinations are more viable than others, and some pathways are better suited to some destinations than others. At their best, religious orientations offer well-integrated, coherent frameworks for living. At their worst, they are fundamentally disorienting, consisting of religious bits and pieces that leave people lost, confused, and headed toward dead ends.

BEYOND RELIGIOUS ORIENTATIONS

Where do I want to go, and how do I get there? Few questions have more important implications for the general course of our lives. Religion offers answers to both of these questions. Studying the full range of religious orientations to the search for significance represents an important next step for the psychology of religion. It is not, however, the only important step.

Even if we were able to identify religious orientations more sharply, we would still be left with a critical question. How do these religious orientations translate into concrete life situations? Religious orientations are dispositional phenomena, generalized tendencies to use particular religious means and seek particular religious ends. They are abstractions, on the same level as other abstract dispositions such as mental health, personality, and social attitudes. They are also one step removed from particular situations of living. Knowing someone's religious orientation alone tells us relatively little about how it is actually involved in the person' thoughts, actions, and hopes in a specific encounter. This is a key reason why the coping process is so important to the psychological study of religion. It forces us to ask when, why, and how religion comes to life. Only in specific situations can we witness the actual workings of religion. Having explored the first central concept of the book, religion, we turn now to the second, coping.

Part Two

A PERSPECTIVE
ON COPING

Chapter Four

———⟨⟩———

AN INTRODUCTION
TO THE CONCEPT
OF COPING

Over the last 30 years, scientific interest in the coping process has increased dramatically and the literature on the topic is now quite extensive. In this chapter and the one to follow, the concept of coping will be introduced. I will consider some of the historical forces that led to the study of coping, and I will show that the concept of coping is itself rooted in a certain view of the world, one that sees people as both shapers and products of their circumstances. Finally, some of the essential qualities of coping will be discussed. This introduction will set the stage for subsequent chapters on the interface between religion and coping.

THE HISTORICAL CONTEXT OF COPING

For thousands of years, philosophers and artists have been interested in the ways people approach the critical times in life. Plato depicts Socrates as a model of composure and integrity when his life is threatened. The plays of William Shakespeare represent a veritable catalogue of human response to the most significant moments of life. Artists of the atrocities of the 20th century, from Picasso and Shostakovich to Wiesel and Sartre, have depicted how people can respond to stress by destroying and

71

deforming the things they care about most deeply. There is no shortage of language or art to describe the human character under siege. Grief, vengeance, heroism, suffering, renewal, anxiety, courage, surrender, forbearance, resilience, cowardice, despair, triumph—some of the most powerful words in our vocabulary speak to the stance of the individual toward conflict, crisis, and loss.

Only in relatively recent years, however, have scientists become interested in studying people as they go through critical points in life. The emerging interest in coping is no accident. Psychologist Forrest Tyler (1970) has described how forces both external and internal to the field have shaped the peculiar character of modern science. The same point appears to hold true for the scientific interest in coping. We turn first to some of the sociocultural forces that have made coping a common part of our vocabulary.

External Historical Forces

Several years ago I recall speaking to a student from India after he had finished participating in a study on the reasons why there is injustice in the world. Asked about his reactions to the study, he replied in a very nice way: "You Americans are so concerned about the reasons why things happen. Why this? Why that? This is very hard for me. People in India do not think like that." His remark reminded me of my own cultural biases. More generally, it illustrated how the questions we ask, the language we use, and the ways we think about the world are embedded, subtly but profoundly, in culture. The concept of coping is, itself, tied to a particular time and place.

Over the past several hundred years, cultures have undergone dramatic changes. Western culture in particular has become increasingly complex, differentiated, and technologically oriented. With these changes, life for the individual has become more unstable and unpredictable. Mead (1968) describes what is it like for the child growing up in the midst of cultural flux:

> Instead of being able to develop more and more automatic behavior, he must learn to be increasingly on the alert for lights that turn off differently, lavatories with a different flushing system, games which have the same names but are played with different rules, etc. Far more important, on the social level, he meets ever-changing standards of manners and morals, shifting criteria of refusal and acceptance. There is no chance for relaxation, for, even as he becomes adept and in part accustomed to the ways of his adult contemporaries, his own children begin to display new forms of behavior to which he has no clues. By

the time grandchildren arrive, the gap is so great that many grandparents are refusing even to try to bridge it. (Mead, 1968, p. 836)

Rules, roles, standards, and morals—the fabric of culture once a part of the background of life, rarely noticed, or questioned—have moved to the foreground as objects requiring definition and redefinition. Culture, which once "completed" people, now leaves many with "empty selves" (Cushman, 1990).

The acceleration in the pace of cultural change has also disrupted the traditional institutions of society, particularly the institution most responsible for the construction and transmission of worldviews—religion. For most of history, religion legitimated the character of reality by investing virtually all aspects of life—artistic, economic, social, physical—with sacred status (Berger, 1967). (Only Woody Allen might imagine the members of an earlier culture anxiously discussing whether there *really* is a life after death.) Since the time of the Protestant Reformation and the advent of nonreligious explanations of the world, however, the sphere of the religious institution has shrunken from this all-encompassing involvement to the realm of the family and the individual. As it has diminished in scope, religion has increased in its pluralism, offering people more and more selections from a menu of definitions of reality. There are, for instance, more than 200 religious denominations reported in the United States alone (Jacquet, 1989).

Berger (1967) argues that it is increasingly difficult to develop an overarching, universally convincing view of reality, a "plausibility structure." After all, if one's conception of the world is so evident and convincing, why doesn't everyone see the world in the same way? With the loss of plausibility, Berger says, the character of reality has become more of a private affair. In the marketplace of "alternate visions," people looking for a product engage in a transaction with religious institutions looking for customers. What was once a matter of cosmos and culture is now a matter of individual psychology.

While the rapidity of cultural change has been associated with significant technological advances, it has been associated with major disruptions as well. Life expectancy has increased; however, the prevalence of chronic debilitating illness has also increased. Communication throughout the world has become more rapid, but along with it has come the rapid transmission of diseases such as HIV/AIDS. Industry has become more efficient, but efficiency has been accompanied by layoffs, unemployment, poverty, and family dislocation. Technology has advanced, but it has brought with it the problems of environmental contamination, weaponry development, and terrorism that threaten civilization itself.

Thus, in spite of the advances of technology, the individual continues to face critical problems, some of which are completely new to life. Adding to the burden is the loss of some of the cushion of culture, the plausibility structure for interpreting and dealing with crisis. Without this cushion the individual, family, and local community must assume greater responsibility for the coping process. Illustrating this point, anthropologist William Caudill (1958) notes that among many societies, the system of kinship provided a formalized structure to assist the husband or wife facing the premature death of a spouse. Close relatives such as a husband's brother or a wife's sister were offered as a substitute to replace the lost person. In contrast, our culture does not provide a great deal of formalized assistance to the grieving widow or widower. The strain of dealing with the loss shifts more to the smaller social unit, the nuclear family and, in particular, the individual.

Undoubtedly, for many people, culture has been less of a cushion than a yoke, and cultural change has been more freeing than alienating. But the point remains, without the aura of factuality (cf. Geertz, 1966) provided by culture, the responsibility for grappling with the world falls more heavily on the shoulders of the individual.

Changes in culture have set the stage for a psychology of coping. Among cultures that envelop their members within a compelling prescriptive approach to the world, the word "coping," filled with connotations of personal choice and individualized constructions of reality, seems to be part of a foreign language. Among more industrialized societies, those providing less of a cultural defense while at the same time raising a whole new set of difficult problems for the individual, the language of coping begins to make more sense.

Internal Historical Forces

Science, too, is wrapped in a larger cultural context, and its interests reflect this world (Tyler, 1970). Perhaps it is no accident then that many of the thinkers pivotal to the 20th century (e.g., Freud, Darwin, and Marx) described life as a process of conflict and struggle. But thinkers such as these did more than reflect the culture; they shaped it as well. They spawned significant lines of research, each distinct in some ways, but each reflective of a common, underlying, deterministic vision—people caught up within a swirl of colliding forces.

The Intrapsychic Response to Stress

Psychodynamically oriented theorists and researchers placed much of their attention on the intrapsychic response of the individual to conflict (e.g., A. Freud, 1966). Freud (1923/1961) was particularly interested in anxiety, the hallmark of conflict between the instinctual desires of the id and the constraints of society. The ego, he said, is armed with mechanisms for dealing with this conflict. Denial, repression, projection, regression, sublimation, and reaction formation are some of the defensive tools the ego has to reduce tension. Although the defenses were defined as mechanisms of the ego, their source of power was located ultimately in the instinctual energy of the id. The defenses, Freud felt, are methods for achieving the greatest instinctual gratification with the least pain from conscience and society. But they also protect people from confronting their own instinctual natures. Moreover, they distort perceptions of reality. The son who discourages his widowed mother from remarrying may defend his stance by rationalizing that he has his mother's best interests at heart. In doing so, he is able to maintain a close relationship with his mother. At the same time he does not have to face his unconscious longings for her. Neither does he have to face the reality of his mother's loneliness and desires for a new fulfilling life. By sheltering people from undesirable wishes, feelings, and impulses, the defenses make some gratification possible. But they also make it impossible for people to see more than a part of themselves and the world. To add one final note to this pretty grim portrayal of the human condition, Freud believed that human activity is *constantly defensive* because instinct is constantly in conflict with social reality. As Maddi (1989) concludes his critique of Freudian theory: "We are forced, in his frame of reference, to accept a view of humans as controlled by forces from within and pressures from without and furthermore, as ignorant of that damning fact" (p. 56).

The Physiological Response to Stress

Physiologically oriented researchers shifted the focus from the intrapsychic to the biological response of the organism to traumatic experience. Through his experimental studies, Cannon (1939) was able to document how the body, in spite of its extreme natural instability, attempts to maintain a level of physiological homeostasis when disturbed by factors such as hunger, thirst, or cold. The sympathetic nervous system, he believed, plays a crucial role in this process of stabilization by preparing the organism for fight with or flight from the trauma. Building on this tradition of research, Selye (1976) identified a common pattern of physiological response to toxic substances. "Adrenal enlargement, gastrointestinal ulcers, and thymicolymphatic shrinkage," Selye reported "were constant and invariable signs of damage to a body faced with the demand of meeting the attack of any disease" (Selye, 1982, p. 10). These effects, Selye proposed, were part of a broader pattern of change over time, what he called the General Adaptation Syndrome, consisting of three stages of physiological response: the alarm reaction, the stage of resistance, and the stage of exhaustion. Selye believed that these stages represent universal responses to a wide range of intrusive circumstances, from allergens, germs, and physical trauma to overcrowding, demanding jobs, and changes in climate. Although he recognized individual differences in the responses of organisms to crisis, his work focused more on the commonalities of response. Physiology, according to Selye, constrains the reactions of the organism to difficulties in life. It sets the parameters for how the organism will respond and it limits the amount of energy available to the organism for adaptation.

Selye's work was and continues to be influential in efforts to understand the physiological struggle with difficult conditions. It is important to note that Selye is credited for popularizing the concept of stress, a concept we will say more about later. It is also important to note that physiology, for Selye, parallels intrapsychic history for Freud; both fix strict limits on the person's ability to deal with crisis and conflict.

The Psychological Response to Stress

Responding to the social unrest and upheavals of the 20th century, other mental health researchers and professionals extended the interest in the stress response from the physiological to the psychological arena. Prior to World War II, the symptoms reported by soldiers in combat were generally attributed to physical rather than psychological or social factors. For instance, the label *shellshock* reflected the belief that exploding shells led to cerebral concussions and the rupture of small blood vessels. Similarly, combat-related symptoms of fear, tremor, and nightmares were viewed as signs of brain damage (Marmar & Horowitz, 1988). However, it soon became clear that the symptoms of combat-related stress were far too prevalent to be explained by physical illness or injury alone. In their inquiry into the reactions of American flight crews to combat, Grinker and Spiegel (1945) noted: "The psychological deficiency resulting from combat stress is of the greatest practical concern because no one is immune. If the stress is severe enough, if it strikes an exposed 'Achilles' heel' and if the exposure to it is sufficiently prolonged, adverse psychological symptoms may develop in anyone" (p. 53).

Many researchers then began to take a closer look at the psychological response to critical situations. Wars, fires, floods, tornadoes, prison camps, illnesses, deaths, injuries—each of these experiences became a laboratory for the study of the psychological response to crisis. Although much of this research was conducted by psychodynamically oriented researchers who tended to emphasize the individual's predisposition to the stress response, others grew more interested in delineating the generalized pattern of psychological reaction to crisis. Grinker and Spiegel (1945), for instance, identified an array of common symptoms associated with the stress of combat, such as irritability, sleep-related problems, anxiety, depression, alcoholism, and psychosomatic complaints. Similarly, psychiatrist Erich Lindemann (1944) studied the grief reactions of several groups, including the relatives of those who had died in the fire at the Cocoanut Grove nightclub in Boston, in the armed forces, and in a hospital. He described a "remarkably uniform" syndrome of acute grief common to these groups: "Sensations of somatic distress occurring in waves lasting from twenty minutes to an hour at a time, a feeling of tightness in the throat, choking with shortness of breath, need for sighing, and an empty feeling in the abdomen, lack of muscular power, and an intense subjective distress described as tension or mental pain" (p. 141). The interest in pinpointing fixed and common responses to crisis continues today in the large body of study on acute stress and posttraumatic stress disorders.

Social Stressors

Other researchers were less interested in the nature of the individual's response to conflict and trauma (be it intrapsychic, physiological, or psychological), and more interested in identifying those conditions that precipitate problems in life. In a classic study of the late 19th century, sociologist Emile Durkheim (1951) found a significant set of ties between rates of suicide and the social conditions of Europe. For example, suicide was more likely among Protestants and Catholics than Jews, and more likely among single, divorced, separated, and widowed people than married people. Durkheim concluded that suicide is associated with lower levels of social integration. Jews, and to a lesser extent Catholics, and married people, he maintained, are more intimately connected to a social group that protects them from the trials of life. Without the benefits of intimate ties, the individual is left more to his or her own resources and is far more vulnerable to suicide. But the social conditions rather than the lack of individual resources were identified by Durkheim as the crucial contributor to suicide.

Many sociologists and epidemiologists followed in the Durkheim tradition, offering socioenvironmental explanations for the relationships they observed between social deterioration and higher rates of crime, poor health, and mental disorders. The research of Holmes and Rahe represents one of the more recent examples of this line of study (Holmes, 1979; Holmes & Rahe, 1967). Working with tuberculosis patients, they observed that prior to their admission to the hospital, many had experienced major changes in life: jail, financial change, health change, moves, changes in employment. They went on to compare hospital employees who developed tuberculosis through their work in the hospital with a matched set of employees who remained free of the disease. Those who developed the disease had had a significantly greater number of changes in their lives over the previous 2 years than those who did not. Similar effects were found for patients suffering from other diseases—significant life changes were associated with a greater risk of illness. The nature of any specific event was less significant to Holmes and Rahe than the cumulative weight of these events on the individual. Building on this model, they developed the Social Adjustment Rating Scale (Holmes & Rahe, 1967) to measure recent life changes. It has since become one of the most heavily used instruments in the social science literature. Study after study has explored the relationship of life changes to measures of mental health, physical health, and illness. Further, the notion that life change leads to illness has become an important part of popular culture.

Regardless of whether the focus was on the intrapsychic, physiological, or psychological response to traumatic events or on the nature of the critical situations themselves, this research painted a similar portrait: people battered, buffeted, shaped, and molded by crisis, conflict, and culture in transition. This body of work also set the stage for the study of coping.

FIRST STEPS IN THE STUDY OF COPING

Some theorists and researchers took issue with the portrait of people implicit in much of the previous research. They did not dispute the notion that life is often a struggle. They disputed the deterministic flavor to the research, the view that individuals are products of their circumstances. Several strands of evidence suggested that people are not simply ensnared by their intrapsychic, biological, psychological, and social conditions. These were the first steps in the study of the coping construct.

Robert White (1963) seriously questioned the psychodynamic position that behavior is exclusively motivated by sexual instinct. From infancy onward, he noted, longer and longer periods of time are spent "as an explorer," inspecting strange sights, practicing new motions, experimenting with vocalizations, playing with food, and manipulating new objects. Since none of these activities is associated with the satisfaction of a primary drive, it is difficult to view them as erotically driven. But the behavior certainly appears to be motivated, for (as any parent knows) young children show signs of persistence and frustration if their exploratory activities are thwarted. White proposed the term "effectance" to describe the motivation underlying this kind of exploratory behavior. Children, he said, are motivated to produce effects on their environments, to act on the world, to create consequences. But it is the activity itself, not its consequences, that is so satisfying. Instinctual drives, White maintained, cannot account for the full range of human behavior. He raised the question:

> A dangerous enemy enters the territory; which resident will survive, the one that has learned only where to satisfy instinctual need or the one that has explored the territory out of curiosity? An intruding rival comes on the scene; which animal will survive, the one that has fought only when angered or the one that has playfully practiced the art of fighting with its litter mates? Effectance, through the additional learning it brings about, makes the difference between life and death. (p. 37)

Effectance motivation and the sense of competence that grows out of it, White maintained, are also needed to explain how we have managed to deal successfully with our environments.

White's work was representative of a larger body of theory that challenged the view of the individual driven by psychosexual forces and that pointed to other core human tendencies. Object relations theorists emphasized the efforts of the individual to develop a self through interpersonal encounters. Alfred Adler saw the individual striving for perfection and superiority. Gordon Allport distinguished the proactive, future-directed efforts of the self, or proprium, from the more "opportunistic" biologically tied reactions of the organism to environment. Erik Erikson emphasized the human potential to forge a meaningful existence at every stage of the life cycle. Abraham Maslow proposed that, once his or her more basic needs are satisfied, the person can pursue higher needs, such as those for belonging, love, and self-actualization. In perhaps the sharpest break from psychoanalytic thought, Carl Rogers asserted that the most inherent of all human forces is the tendency toward growth, actualization, and fulfillment of the individual's intrinsic potential.

Research investigations have provided some support for these alternative visions. A number of studies have raised serious questions about the invariability of the human response to stressful situations. Hinkle

(1974) noted that the organism is equipped with a vast range of potential physiological reactions to the environment:

> During the course of their adaptations to their social environment, direct neural regulatory effects upon their organs can produce such pronounced phenomena as . . . variations in bowel function, ranging from complete constipation to continuous hypermotile diarrhea; variations in the heart rate ranging from a transient sinus arrest to a sinus tachycardia greater than 180 per minute; and changes in blood pressure, ranging from transient hypotension without detectable blood pressure, to systolic pressures greater than 200 millimeters of mercury. (p. 346)

Hinkle maintained that the physiological response of the organism to difficult conditions is less universal and more finely differentiated than Selye proposed in his General Adaptation Syndrome (e.g., Lacey, 1967). Similarly, research on the epidemiology of mental disorders failed to support the single-factor etiology model adapted from the study of infectious diseases. Few disorders can be traced to a microbe, vitamin deficiency, or other single agent. Instead, they result from a more complex interplay of genetic, environmental, situational, social, and psychological factors (Schwab & Schwab, 1978).

Evidence from the life events literature has also pointed to considerable diversity in how people respond to critical life situations. Although an association has repeatedly emerged between cumulative life events and psychological distress, the size of this relationship is not very large (Rabkin & Streuning, 1976). Apparently, many people who have experienced a number of life events do not feel distressed; on the other hand, many people in distress have been spared critical life events.

These findings are consistent with studies which have revealed that people are not always shattered as a result of severe problems. For example, Goertzel and Goertzel (1962) examined the childhoods of 400 renowned men and women of the 20th century (e.g., Samuel Clemens, Theodore Dreiser, Anton Chekhov, Leo Tolstoy, Eleanor Roosevelt, Clara Barton). More than three-fourths of them experienced major traumas as children, including poverty, abuse, broken homes, physical handicaps, estranged or dominating parents, and illness. Similarly, studies of children growing up in a variety of destructive environments have identified a small but significant proportion who did not appear to show any of the expected detrimental effects (e.g., Garmezy, 1975; Murphy & Moriarty, 1976). In fact, some of these children were thriving. They appeared to be resilient or invulnerable to the effects of stress. These findings have suggested that the maxim "stressful life events cause distress" is too simple. Somehow, some of the people, some of the time, are able to manage and even master exceptionally difficult circumstances.

Several researchers have attempted to identify the characteristics of people who seem to be able to handle the ups and downs of their lives more effectively than others. The point of comparison here is not between "normal" and "abnormal," but between competent and less competent. For example, building on studies of Peace Corps volunteers (Smith, 1966), mentally healthy young males (Grinker, 1962), and effective high school and college students (Silber et al., 1961), Tyler (1978) developed a tridimensional model of the competent self. Effective people, he said, have a favorable set of attitudes toward themselves. They see themselves as worthwhile and efficacious in their lives whether things go well or poorly. Effective people also have a favorable set of attitudes toward the world, a sense of moderately optimistic trust in others. Finally, effective people are characterized by an active problem-solving orientation. Tyler and his colleagues have found that this model is useful in distinguishing more competent from less competent people within a variety of groups: high school and college students (Tyler, 1978), the poor (Evans & Tyler, 1976), parents and their children (Mondell & Tyler, 1981), church and synagogue members (Pargament, Steele, & Tyler, 1979), and the elderly (Tyler, Moran, Gatz, & Gease, 1982).

In their responses to deterministic visions, few theorists and re searchers have denied the power of internal and external forces. However, they have drawn the line at the assumption that people are simply products of these forces. The evidence of people curious about and actively engaged in mastering their circumstances, of individual differences in response to stress, of resilience in the face of terrible conditions, and of people living effectively in a topsy-turvy world has led to a different conclusion—that people are engaged in *transactions* with the environment around them. If it is true that we are affected by impulses we are not aware of, it is also true that we have enough awareness of ourselves to recognize this to be the case. If it is true that we are socialized by a myriad of external forces, then it is also true that we are part of these socializing forces. And if it is true that we are shaped by the situations we encounter, it is true that we avoid, select, construct, define, and redefine these situations as well. This transactional perspective was and continues to be an important part of several general developments in the field of psychology, such as social learning theory (Bandura, 1978), human ecology (Bronfenbrenner, 1979), general systems theory (von Bertalanffy, 1968), and community psychology (Rappaport, 1977).

The construct of coping grows out of this historical context of

external and internal forces, theory and research, argument and coun-
terargument, but most immediately, it is rooted in a transactional
perspective that assumes a reciprocal and evolving relationship between
the individual and the world.

THE CENTRAL QUALITIES OF COPING

Consider the following three case examples:

The Housewife Turned Reluctant Social Activist

Lois Gibbs does not fit the stereotypical view of the grassroots
activist. She dresses conservatively, speaks quietly, and can laugh
about life. She described herself as a "typical housewife," until her
children began to develop a number of rashes, fevers, and peculiar
symptoms. She questioned others in her community, Love Canal,
and discovered that she was not alone. Might there be some
connection between these symptoms and the chemical dump located
adjacent to the town? When she contacted the local government,
they reassured her that there was no problem. As reports of illness
in the community mounted, Lois Gibbs grew more alarmed. Naturally a shy person, she forced herself to challenge official positions
and act as a mobilizer of other people in the community. Her work
led to the development of a powerful national advocacy organization for safe environments, the Citizen's Clearinghouse for Hazardous Wastes. Looking back on her experiences, she feels she learned
that citizens cannot put blind faith in their government, that
government often must be forced to change by pressure from the
grassroots, and that problems can be solved when local people come
together to work on shared concerns. Listening to her describe her
experience, it seemed clear that Lois Gibbs also changed personally
through this process. Standing confidently in front of a few hundred
psychologists, there were no signs of the shyness she reported before
her experience at Love Canal.

The Worker Trapped by High Expectations

Greg came to psychotherapy because he had punched his fist
through a wall at work after his boss had been verbally abusive.
Greg's response was puzzling. Why hadn't he confronted his boss,
spoken to his supervisor, or, if things were so bad, simply left? In
talking about his life outside of work, I learned that Greg had faced
hardship since he was a child. His parents were both heavy drinkers
who managed to keep their alcoholism a secret from the community.

Greg had been the "pride of the family," a good boy who caused few people any trouble. The well-being of his family, he felt, was his responsibility. In the intervening years, things had not changed much for Greg. He continued to feel trapped by his feelings of responsibility to people who expected too much of him no matter how competently he performed. When asked why he put his fist through the wall after his conflict with his boss, Greg said: "I had to do something and there was nothing else I could do." Through therapy Greg learned how the wounds he had suffered continue to affect him, and how he might approach the critical problems of his life differently. Greg was able to apply these insights to the troubles he faced at work, but his boss was not receptive. When the abuse continued at work, Greg decided to quit. Unfortunately, there were few jobs available in the area, and Greg ultimately moved his family to another community at considerable emotional and financial cost.

The Running Rabbi Hobbled by Illness

Rabbi Hirshel Jaffe had been blessed with good health and abundant energy (Jaffe, Rudin, & Rudin, 1986). Known as "the Running Rabbi," he ran 6 or 7 miles a day, never smoked or drank, and treated his body like a finely tuned instrument. Rabbi Jaffe said, "I guess I thought if I jogged I'd live forever" (p. 8). He applied this same energetic style to his rabbinical work, throwing himself into efforts to help others and asking little for himself in return. So it was his entire way of life that was threatened when he discovered he had leukemia. The battle he describes with this disease was as much a fight to maintain a sense of mastery as it was a struggle with the leukemia itself. As he faced a variety of situations beyond his control, his reactions ranged from "We'll lick this" to "I might as well just give up" (p. 54). The disease posed a different kind of challenge to his family and congregation who were used to receiving comfort, not offering it. Ultimately Rabbi Jaffe loses his battle, not with the disease, but with the effort to maintain his way of life. However, the lost way of life is replaced with one he sees as more rewarding. The Rabbi's relationships with others become reciprocal rather than one-sided. And through his struggle, he develops a greater appreciation of his limits: "I've yielded something to eternity, which is my medical fate. You can't change that. But, strangely, somehow I feel more alive" (p. 143).

In these brief case studies we hear some very different stories. The characters are unique, the plots develop in different directions, and the endings are not all the same. But they share the drama of people grappling with situations that have put them to test. As the audience to this drama we can witness the full range of human expressions: fear and hope, loss and gain, threat and challenge, passivity and forceful action, love and hate. The drama is not a one-person show. Nor is it a one act play. It is a series of acts on a stage filled with other people silhouetted against a larger background of time and place. These stories capture some of the flavor of coping.

How do we begin to describe the nature of this concept more systematically? Perhaps the first place to start is by distinguishing some of the important qualities of coping that appear in each of the three vignettes.

Coping as an Encounter between Person and Situation

Central to coping is a picture of people struggling, as best they can, with difficult situations in life. Lois Gibbs confronts a chemical dump in her town that threatens the health of her family and community. Greg encounters conflict with his boss who, like other people, expects too much of him. Rabbi Jaffe battles for survival with leukemia. This theme of individual-confronted-with-difficulty runs consistently through the many definitions of coping that have been introduced over the past 30 years. (See Table 4.1.) For example, Friedman et al. (1963) describe coping in terms of mechanisms for meeting threat. Menninger (1963) sees it as devices for regulating everyday emergencies. Pearlin and Schooler (1978) and Silver and Wortman (1980) speak of responses to strains or potentially harmful outcomes. Lazarus and Folkman (1984) talk about efforts to manage taxing internal and/or external demands. Although the language is varied, each description focuses on the place where the individual meets a situation. This is where coping is found. At its core, coping is a transactional process, a process of exchange and encounter between the individual and a situation within a larger milieu.

Coping as Multidimensional

Coping is not restricted to one dimension of functioning. All three of the people above began to think differently about their situations and themselves. Greg came to realize that he could no longer take responsibility for other people. Rabbi Jaffe developed more understanding of the limits of personal control in his life. Lois Gibbs grew increasingly mistrustful of the government and increasingly knowledgeable about how to fight it. These were not abstract intellectualized changes. They were associated with strong feelings and physiological reactions: frustration, fear, anger, relief, happiness, and sadness. They were also accompanied by action. Rabbi Jaffe began to spend more time listening to people, Lois Gibbs built a grassroots coalition of people to advocate for a safer environment, and Greg protected himself when he was abused at work. The coping process involves virtually every dimension of human functioning: cognitive, affective, behavioral, and physiological. But it is not limited to what goes on within the individual; it occurs within a larger context of relationships and settings.

Coping as a Multilayered Contextual Phenomenon

No one copes alone, in spite of the fact that he or she may feel alone. It is impossible to remove the individual completely from layers of social relationships—family, organizational, institutional, community, societal, cultural. The individual carries these systems along in coping, and these

TABLE 4.1. Some Definitions of Coping

"All of the mechanisms utilized by an individual to meet a significant threat to his psychological stability and to enable him to function effectively" (Friedman, Chodoff, Mason, & Hamburg, 1963, p. 616).

"Normal regulatory devices for the emergencies of everyday life" (Menninger, 1963, p. 146).

"An array of covert and overt behavior patterns by which the organism can prevent, alleviate, or respond to stress-inducing circumstances" (McGrath, 1970, p. 33).

"A process, involving effort, on the way toward solution of a problem, as contrasted on the one hand with ready-made adaptational devices such as reflexes, or on the other hand, with complete and automatized mastery and resulting competence" (Murphy, 1974, p. 76).

"Coping involves purpose, choice, and flexible shift, adheres to intersubjective reality and logic, and allows and enhances proportionate affective expression" (Haan, 1977, p. 34).

"Any response to external life strains that serves to prevent, avoid, or control emotional distress" (Pearlin & Schooler, 1978, p. 3).

"Any and all responses made by an individual who encounters a potentially harmful outcome. In addition to overt behaviors we would include cognitions . . . emotional reactions . . . and physiological responses (Silver & Wortman, 1980, p. 281).

"Constantly changing cognitive and behavioral efforts to manage specific external and/or internal demands that are appraised as taxing or exceeding the resources of the person" (Lazarus & Folkman, 1984, p. 141).

"The cognitions and behaviors that people use to modify adverse aspects of their environments as well as to minimize the potential threats arising from such aspects" (Mitchell, Cronkite, & Moos, 1983, p. 435).

"Behaviors that are employed for the purpose of reducing strain in the face of stressors" (Hobfoll, 1988, p. 16).

"The use of strategies for dealing with actual or anticipated problems and their attendant negative emotions" (Aldwin, 1994, p. 107).

systems may assist in the coping process or create obstacles and impediments of their own (Thoits, 1986). Lois Gibbs coped as a mother and wife deeply concerned about her family, with neighbors who supported her work, and with institutions and larger social structures that attempted to block and frustrate her efforts. Greg coped as a member of a family that supported and encouraged his need to please others. When he changed his behavior at work, he was extruded from the setting and larger community. Prior to his illness Rabbi Jaffe coped as a son and rabbi within a family and congregation that allowed him to take care of them. After he became ill he coped as a patient who had to experience what it was like to be taken care of, within a congregation that was willing to support his change in status. Although these social contextual factors may seem merely background factors in the coping process, imagine how the lives of these three people would have been changed had the local government of Love Canal responded immediately and favorably to Lois Gibbs, had Greg's boss supported his newly developed assertiveness, or had Rabbi Jaffe's congregation fired him after his illness because of his inability to care for them. Social relationships are completely intertwined in coping.

Coping as Possibilities and Choices

Does it follow that coping is *determined* by social and contextual forces? No. The most central of all qualities of coping is possibility: the possibility that the person can rebound from difficult circumstances, that a problem can be anticipated, prevented, or solved, that something good can be found in hardship, or that a devastating loss can be met with some integrity. Of course, not all possibilities are positive. If hardship can be met with equanimity, it can also lead to despair. Risky situations can result in failure as well as success. Cowardice under fire is as real a possibility as heroism. If adversity can harden some people, it can destroy others. But the key point is that, in coping, the individual can choose. Lois Gibbs could have responded to her situation by acquiescing to it, by moving quietly out of the community, or by developing psychosomatic problems. Greg could have dealt with his boss by quitting his job, knuckling under, or hitting his boss rather than the wall. Rabbi Jaffe could have faced his disease by depression and suicide, anger and social isolation, or denial that his illness was serious. They did not do so because they chose different ways of handling their circumstances.

Certainly choice and possibility are more restricted in some situations than others. Some stimuli elicit reflexive or automatic responses: When a piece of food gets caught in the throat, we instinctively cough; when a light turns red we automatically slow down, with little thought to the matter. But situations and responses such as these are generally excluded from discussions of coping. Murphy (1974), for example, defines coping as "a process, involving effort, on the way toward solution of a problem, as contrasted on the one hand with ready-made adaptational devices such as reflexes or, on the other hand, with complete and automatized mastery and resulting competence" (p. 76). Coping is reserved for those times that allow for possibility and choice.

There is no shortage of these times, however, for the individual is rarely in a position without some options. Yalom (1980) puts it well:

> All of us face natural adversities that influence our lives . . . but that does not mean that we have no responsibility (or choice) in the situation. We are responsible for what we make of our handicaps; for our attitudes toward them; for the bitterness, anger, or depression that act synergistically with the original "coefficient of adversity" to ensure that a handicap will defeat the individual. . . . When all else fails, when the coefficient of adversity is formidable, still one is responsible for the attitude one adopts toward the adversity—whether to live a life of bitter regret or to find a way to transcend the handicap and to fashion a meaningful life despite it. (p. 272)

Coping rejects the notion of psychic determinism as well as social determinism. The assumption that the response to crisis is not fully determined, but rather at least partially *chosen*, sets coping apart from defense mechanisms. This is not to say that people are always aware of their choices. Not all coping is fully conscious. Some ways of dealing with stressors may be so well learned that they require very little conscious processing. Similarly, the reasons why people do what they do or their goals in coping may not be altogether conscious (Martin & Tesser, 1989). Nevertheless, the concept of coping embodies a greater appreciation of the capacity for proactive decision making and conscious awareness in stressful situations than the concept of defense, which is said to be instinctually driven and largely unconscious.

In short, possibilities and choices are hallmarks of coping. The individual, it is assumed, *cannot not chose*. Even if a passive, avoidant, or reactive stance is taken toward problems, this does not erase the fact that, at some level, the stance was chosen. In this very basic sense, coping is an active process involving difficult choices in times of trouble.

Diversity as a Hallmark of Coping

Putting these qualities together, it should come as no surprise that coping can take so many different forms. Unique scripts are played out in the vignettes of Lois Gibbs, Greg, and Rabbi Jaffe These people came from different backgrounds. They brought different resources and burdens to the coping process. They faced different problems and approached them in different ways. Through their coping, they and those around them evolved in different directions.

These examples are not unique. Throughout the lifespan, the response to stressful circumstances is rarely uniform. In her observations of infants, Murphy (1974) describes individual differences among babies in a variety of situations. For example, when an adult leaves the room, some cope by "turning to visual stimuli, others turn to tactual stimuli such as toys, or they rub the blanket, scratch the side of the crib, and so on, or induce sensory experience by banging bouncing, rocking themselves" (p. 86).

Children are similarly diverse in their response to difficulties. In his work with vulnerable and resilient children under stress, Anthony (1987) draws the analogy between children and three dolls made of different material. When hit by a hammer the doll made of glass will shatter, the doll made of plastic will be permanently dented, and the doll made of steel will give out a "fine metallic sound."

The same point holds true for adolescents. Adams and Lindemann (1974) compare two late adolescent males with similar backgrounds who suffered virtually identical paralyzing fractures of the spine. One drops out of college, lives unhappily at home dependent on his family, criticizes those who try to help him, and overdoses on medication. The other completes college, lives independently, takes a job teaching history, and coaches a basketball team from his wheelchair.

Uniformity of response is also uncommon among adults, even in the midst of the most stressful events. Listen to Hamburg's (Hamburg, Hamburg, & DeGoza, 1953, cited in Silver & Wortman, 1980) observations of patients who had been severely burned:

> One patient is crying, moaning, complaining, demanding that more be done for him; another appears completely comfortable and unconcerned; another appears intensely preoccupied and seems to make very little contact with the observer; still another appears sad and troubled but friendly, responding with a weak smile to any approach made to him; and so it goes from one bed to the next. (p. 300)

Reviewing the literature dealing with responses of adults to crises such as these, Silver and Wortman (1980) find evidence of diverse attitudes and feelings. The death of a terminally ill child may lead to anger or hysteria, but it may also result in denial or relief and sorrow. The death of a spouse may be followed by shock, but it may also be tied to hostility toward the spouse or hope that the spouse will return. Victims of rape may experience tension, crying, and restlessness, but they may also show a more subdued reaction. Further, while changes do take place in the coping responses of people over time, Silver and Wortman find little evidence that these changes occur in uniform and predictable stages or that "time heals all wounds." In fact, these authors suggest beliefs in a generic response to crises may be harmful, leading to unrealistic expectations and pressures on the victim to respond "by the book."

CONCLUSIONS

In this chapter, I have explored the historical roots of the construct of coping. Changes in culture and discontent with the determinism embedded in major theories of the human condition laid the foundation for interest in a concept that suggests people are not necessarily passive victims of their circumstances. Coping, we have seen, has several basic qualities: It involves an encounter between an individual and a situation; it is multidimensional; it is multilayered and contextual; it involves possibilities and choices; and it is diverse.

There is, however, one more important quality of coping, and this quality is probably the most difficult to describe. *Coping is a process*, one that evolves and changes over time. The question is how to capture a process so varied and so fluid. Static definitions and invariant stage models will not do. Neither will linear models of the form Variable x leads to Variable y which leads to Variable z. These approaches may simplify complex processes, making them more easily understood and tested, but they lose some of the essence of the process itself. What seems needed is a more dynamic approach. In the following chapter, I try to convey something of the "flow" of coping. We will see that coping is, like religion, a search for significance. It is, however, a search of a different kind.

Chapter Five

Chapter Five

THE FLOW OF COPING

Coping, like religion, is a process, a search for significance. Unlike religion, however, coping does not necessarily involve the sacred. What makes coping distinctive is that it takes place at a particular time, in particular circumstances. *Coping is a search for significance in times of stress.* This search is anything but static. It is a process that unfolds over time. This chapter offers some sense of the rhythm and flow of coping. It begins with a very succinct overview of the coping process.

Virtually everyone is involved in a search for some sort of significance in life. Coping is the process that people engage in to attain significance in stressful circumstances. Stressful events do not simply happen. People actively approach, avoid, anticipate, and appraise situations in life according to their implications for significance. In the face of negative events, people are not helpless. They bring an orienting system, a general frame of reference for viewing and dealing with the world that helps ground and direct them through difficult times. A key task of coping is to translate this general orienting system into methods of coping specifically suited to the distinctive demands and challenges of the particular situation. These methods of coping are designed to conserve whatever people find of greatest significance and, if that is no longer possible, to transform it. People search for the most compelling ways to cope, that is, those methods that will result in the greatest gain to significance at the least cost. The entire process of coping is inextricably bound to a larger cultural context. Evaluating the coping process is not a simple task. There is no single best way to cope for all people and all situations. Good coping is instead defined by what works well for particular people in particular situations and by the degree to which the coping process is well integrated.

Implicit in this dense summary are eight assumptions about the coping process (see Table 5.1). In the remainder of this chapter, I try to "unpack" this summary by taking a closer look at these assumptions.

ASSUMPTION 1: PEOPLE SEEK SIGNIFICANCE

Much of human behavior is intentional. We are almost constantly deciding how to spend our time and energy. Of course, some of these decisions are made routinely or mindlessly. And the act of decision making may be obscured by the feeling that outside forces have made our decisions for us. Yet there is little doubt that we are volitional, goal-directed beings. Psychologists Martin Fishbein and Icek Ajzen (1975) have documented the power of intentions through a series of very straightforward studies. They questioned people about their intentions to behave in particular ways in particular situations immediately before the event. For example, students were asked whether they planned to attend a basketball game or go home for Christmas. Adults were asked who they planned to vote for prior to the 1964 presidential election. They then looked at the relationship between the intentions of their participants and their subsequent behavior. As it turned out, intentions were highly predictive of actual behavior (correlations from 0.70 to 0.90), as long as the individual had the resources to perform the activity and the behavior was not constrained by external forces. Fishbein and Ajzen conclude that behavior can often be predicted most efficiently and most strongly by simply asking people what they intend to do. Their

TABLE 5.1. Eight Assumptions about the Coping Process

Assumption 1:	People seek significance.
Assumption 2:	Events are constructed in terms of their significance to people.
Assumption 3:	People bring an orienting system to the coping process.
Assumption 4:	People translate the orienting system into specific methods of coping.
Assumption 5:	People seek significance in coping through the mechanisms of conservation and transformation.
Assumption 6:	People cope in ways that are compelling to them.
Assumption 7:	Coping is embedded in culture.
Assumption 8:	The keys to good coping lie in the outcomes and the process.

research and other investigations (see Sappington, 1990) underline the basic point—*people strive.*

Earlier, we noted that people strive toward significance. Let's elaborate a bit more on this concept. There are three properties of significance: subjective, objective, and motivational.

The Sense of Significance

I recall a young man who had been struggling with depression for several months. One day he came to my office fairly beaming with happiness. His wife had given birth to their first child and he had witnessed the whole drama. "You know," he said, "I've been trying to find something that matters for a long time, with no results. But it hit me watching my son being born—this really matters! A new life. It's something momentous."

Significance is, in part, a phenomenological construct involving feelings and beliefs associated with worth, importance, and value. It embodies the experience of caring, attraction, or attachment. We can speak of feelings of significance or the sense of significance, as in the case of the young father who had discovered something in life that mattered a great deal. Significance is, in the words of William James (1902), "the hot place in a man's consciousness" (p. 193).

But significance is more than a phenomenological experience. This "hot place in consciousness" is object oriented; we care *for,* we are attracted *to* something. We might call these somethings, whatever they are, objects of significance or even "significants." The concept of significance calls our attention not only to the *sense* of significance, but to the *objects* of significance as well.

The Objects of Significance

Shaped by culture and experience, or generated through a more creative process, people can come to value a virtually limitless set of significant objects (Klinger, 1977; Rychlak, 1981). They may be material (e.g., money, food, cars, houses, drugs, or weapons), physical (e.g., health, fitness, or appearance), psychological (e.g., comfort, meaning, growth), social (e.g., intimacy, social justice), and/or spiritual (e.g., closeness with God, religious experience).

Although many writers have explicitly avowed or implicitly assumed that we are all guided by one particular significant force (see Chapter 3), there has been little agreement on what this critical force is. It may be simpler to conclude that we have more than one object of significance in life. After all, don't most of us look for a bit of material possession, good health, close relation, and psychological and spiritual well-being at the same time? Along these lines, some theorists have proposed multiple objects of significance. Maslow (1970) believed that people pursue a hierarchy of needs, including physiological ones, safety, belongingness and love, esteem, and self-actualization. In one of the most comprehensive classification systems, Murray (1938) delineated 20 needs that direct behavior, including the need for achievement, the need for autonomy, the need for affiliation, the need for order, and the need for deference. Erikson (1980) saw the issues of greatest significance changing as identity developed through the stages of the lifespan.

This literature suggests there is no single generic object of significance. It may be more accurate to say that the significance people seek is made up of a system of objects, an organization of values. Perhaps what differentiates individuals and groups from each other most sharply are their patterns or configurations of valued objects (Carver & Scheier, 1991). Rokeach (1968) offers a nice empirical illustration. He sampled the political writings of socialists, Hitler, Barry Goldwater, and Lenin for the number of times they mentioned different values. Rokeach then ranked these values in terms of their frequency of use. Two terminal values, freedom and equality, were ranked first and second for the socialists out of 18 possible values. For Hitler they were ranked 16th and 17th. For Goldwater, freedom was ranked first and equality was ranked 16th. And for Lenin, freedom was ranked 17th and equality was ranked first. When we speak of significance, Rokeach's work suggests, we are speaking in the plural rather than in the singular—a *system* of objects of greater and lesser value.

There is another point that needs to be made about the objects of significance. Although the search for significance is necessary for a productive life, not all of the things we search for are necessarily good for us, at least according to normative standards. We may be guided by the desire for a good meal or for an addictive drug. Self-esteem can be sought as one part of a broader system of significance or as the only thing that matters in life. Through relationships we may seek intimacy and warmth or someone to blame and control. In short, there are important differences in patterns of significance; some are better than others.[1] As James (1902) said, "It makes a great deal of difference to a man whether one set of his ideas, or another, be the centre of his energy" (p. 193).

The Motivation to Attain Significance

Significance, be it constructive or destructive, has motivational properties—people are drawn to it. There are, of course, times when significance is blocked or when a significant object is lost. The frustration, pain, and, in some cases, psychopathology that results might be seen as signs that the search for significance has come to an end. But we have to be careful here, for searches take many forms. In the apparent vegetativeness and hopelessness of depression, we can find people longing for the return of a lost loved object. In the social withdrawal of the agoraphobic, we can witness someone going to great lengths to avoid anxiety. In the bitterness of the victim of a crime, we can find an individual struggling to redress an injustice. Even suicidality can be interpreted as a search—in this case, a search for an end to pain or an end to ordinary consciousness.

Kotarba (1983) describes the case of T. Q., a 28-year-old suffering from rheumatoid arthritis and cartilage degeneration in his knees that left him in almost constant pain. Medications did little to alleviate his suffering. Psychological and pastoral counseling were rejected as viable alternatives. Ending the pain became the focus of T. Q.'s life. Even his dreams focused on that goal:

> I saw myself getting out of bed in the middle of the night and grabbing this big meat cleaver we keep in the kitchen, and cutting off my legs. I saw my body shrinking as I took off parts to reduce the pain. . . . But I remember that the pain never went away during the dreams. . . . It felt as if I had to cut away my whole body to get rid of all the pain, but that's suicide, I guess. (p. 686)

The "last straw" for T. Q. was the failure of a new medication that had offered some promise for reducing his pain. Suicide then became "the *real* last resort" (p. 686). T. Q. attached his sense of significance to a life-negating act. He spent much of his awake time trying to decide how to kill himself, and a few months later he succeeded by overdosing himself with medication. The search for significance does not have to be life promoting. Searches that negate life can be every bit as tenacious as the quest for more affirming forms of significance.

A case could be made that people strive for significance no matter what. There are, however, some convincing accounts of people who have lost all hope for *any* kind of significance, constructive or destructive. They simply stop caring about anything, including an end to pain, including death (see Frankl, 1984; Spitz, 1945). To paraphrase the philosopher Schopenhauer, nothing matters, but even more importantly, it does not matter that nothing matters. Death may come in these instances not because it is sought, but because the individual has simply shutdown (see Engel, 1971).

Tragic and striking as they are, I believe these cases of complete shutdown are relatively rare. Among people who claim no interest in life, we can often find evidence otherwise in their actions. Beneath their unhappiness may be an unconscious refusal to give up something that mattered a great deal or a desperate attempt to put an end to pain. But (as any clinician can attest) some people cling as doggedly to nullifying searches as others do to positive ones. Total shutdown in the search for significance is only a last resort, and an uncommon one at that.

To summarize the first assumption about coping, the search for significance is the overarching guiding force in life, one that directs people along very different paths. Unlike many guiding forces proposed by psychologists, this search has no universal object; it subsumes anything people care about—be it material, physical, psychological, social, or spiritual, be it good or bad. As will be discussed later, the pursuit of significance is a necessary condition for a productive life, but it is not a sufficient condition. Many elements will contribute to the ultimate success of this quest.

It may seem a bit paradoxical that this first assumption about the coping process makes no mention of coping, but the search for significance is not limited to times of stress. Even so, coping is our particular interest here. In the remaining assumptions we will see how this most basic characteristic of human experience underlies the process of coping.

ASSUMPTION II: EVENTS ARE CONSTRUCTED IN TERMS OF THEIR SIGNIFICANCE TO PEOPLE

Discussions of life events, stress, and coping often begin with the nature of the event—what a life event is and what makes it stressful. This is as logical a place to start as any, but it can leave the impression that events simply appear out of nowhere, and we must then cope *with* them. This impression is misleading. *Events do not simply happen.* People create, anticipate, and plan for events in ways to enhance significance. We look forward to talking with a friend, relaxing after work, going to a party, or reading a book, and we arrange to do the things we most care about.

Negative events are no less constructed than positive events. People do what they can to avoid those situations that detract from significance. They also take on difficult tasks, challenges, and hardships, in fact, create stress, in an effort to achieve the things they value. For example, a couple may take in an aging parent in declining health who requires continual care because they love her too much to see her live with strangers in a nursing home. A painful disruptive event? Yes, but it has not simply happened. It has occurred as the result of some forethought, some decision making that the significant benefits are worth the cost of the burden and disruption. Viewed from this vantage point, stress can be a necessary if not desirable part of life.

Certainly some events cannot be easily foreseen, avoided, or planned for—a sudden death, an accident, war, an illness, or a natural disaster. In some of these instances, however, we may have an inkling of what is to come. For example, in their observations of parents of children with leukemia, Friedman et al. (1963) noted that many parents suspected their child had the illness before they received word from their physician. They started to construct the situation *before* it occurred, anticipating what was to come and preparing themselves for the loss of their loved one. Coping, in this sense, can be said to begin before the actual event takes place.

Even events that come as a complete surprise do not simply happen. They too are constructed. A large body of psychological study has focused on the cognitive construction of major life events.

Primary Appraisals

Psychologists Richard Lazarus and Susan Folkman (1984) have provided a meaningful way of categorizing different kinds of cognitive constructions. They use the term "primary appraisals" to describe evaluations of life events in terms of their implications for the individual's well-being.[2] An event may be defined as benign or irrelevant, having little to do with what matters to the individual. Some events, though, have different implications. They harm, threaten, and/or challenge personal well-being. Harm is defined as "some damage to the person that has already been sustained," threat as "harms or losses that have not yet taken place but are anticipated," and challenge as "the potential for gain or growth" (pp. 32–33). Events with these particular implications are called stressful.

To put it in the language of significance, the stressfulness of an event lies in its ability to reach out and shake the things that people care about. The more our significance is threatened, challenged, or harmed, the more, it can be said, we are stressed. Take, for example, the fearful questions voiced by many elderly people when they face blindness: "Will I be dependent upon others? Will I have to give up my home? Will my family and friends still want to spend time with me" (Jacobs, 1984, p. 161)? Listen to the losses of value perceived by people upon hearing that they have cancer: "I'm an old woman now," "I have not long to live," or "My wife who has multiple sclerosis still needs me" (Kesselring, Dodd, Lindsey, & Strauss, 1986, p. 80).

Events become stressful when they cut to the core of our values. Yet because values differ, people can respond quite differently to the same event. A powerful case in point comes from the response of eminent physicist Stephen Hawking to his encounter with amyotrophic lateral sclerosis ("Lou Gehrig's disease"), a progressive motor neuron illness leading to complete paralysis and, eventually, death. Most of us would experience this disease as a terrible loss and threat to our well-being. Hawking, though, viewed his illness differently: "In a curious way I am fortunate," he said to a reporter. "My disease has left me with the one piece of equipment central to my work—my brain." Devastating as it was, the illness did not destroy the object of significance most important to this theoretical physicist; he is still able to continue his investigations into the origins of the universe.

Obviously, perception plays an important role in the assessment of whether an event will become stressful. No matter how real the threat, harm, or loss is, unless the event is at some level appraised as important, it will not be experienced as stressful. This appraisal does not have to be fully conscious or deliberate (Aldwin, 1994). It may grow out of a vague sense of uneasiness that something seems out of kilter. Or the appraisal may be automatic, as in the case of the soldier who dives for cover at the sound of gunfire. But regardless of whether the appraisal is fully conscious, perception is critical to the determination of an event's stressfulness. As Aldwin (1994) notes: "a person must be aware of a problem before he or she begins to cope with it—however that awareness is defined, or comes about" (p. 42).

Of course, our perceptions of stress do not always correspond with the objective risks. For example, on November 10, 1965, the headline of *The New York Times* read: "Power Failure Snarls Northeast" (*Page One*, 1986). At the bottom of the same page was a small story describing one of the first immolations in the United States in protest of the Vietnam War, an early warning of the terrible conflict to come.

Appraisals of danger, harm, and loss can also grow out of seemingly benign situations. Yalom (1980) notes how luxury, leisure, and freedom from the basic concerns of everyday life can generate crises of their own. In spite of his great wealth, Leo Tolstoy experienced a crisis of meaning that led him close to suicide. "What for? I now have six thousand desyatins in the province of Samara, and three hundred horses—what then?" (cited in Yalom, 1980, p. 420).

If the most serious of events can be viewed with equanimity and if seemingly positive situations can be appraised as stressful, then stressful experience must involve something more than the nature of the event itself. That "something more" is, in part, the primary appraisal of the situation for its significance to the individual.

Secondary Appraisals

That "something more" involves another perception as well—the appraisals of the resources and burdens the individual brings to the coping process. Does the individual believe he or she has the ability to handle the problem? Does the person feel it is his or her responsibility to solve the problem? Does the individual perceive that there are external resources—social, financial, material—available to deal with the situation? Does the individual feel weighed down by burdens that make it virtually impossible to master the crisis? Lazarus and Folkman (1984) label these kinds of evaluations, *secondary appraisals.*

Secondary appraisals interact with primary appraisals to determine the stressfulness of a situation. Take the example of a car breakdown. For most of us, a car breakdown leads to fearful primary appraisals: worries about how to get the car fixed, fears about repair costs, and threats to our security and safety. But secondary appraisals can affect the perceived stressfulness of the situation. A breakdown in front of an open service station will be evaluated quite differently from a breakdown late at night in the middle of the country. A breakdown encountered by a car mechanic with a full set of tools in her trunk and a lot of time on her hands will be experienced very differently from the one faced by the harried executive, unsure whether the engine is located in the front or back of his car. The evaluation of an event for its significance to the individual is, in short, tied to perceptions of the resources and burdens for dealing with the event. We are most vulnerable to events that affect the things we care about for which we perceive the fewest resources and the greatest burdens. I will examine these resources and burdens a little later in this chapter.

The Power of Appraisals

Numerous empirical studies have documented the important role of appraisals in the coping process. Lazarus and his colleagues pioneered much of this study through a classic series of investigations (e.g., see Lazarus, 1968, for a review). In one study, they presented their participants with a silent film showing adolescent Australian aborigine boys going through crude operations on the penis and scrotum as a rite of passage (Speisman, Lazarus, Mordkoff, & Davison, 1964). Cognitive appraisals were manipulated by presenting groups with sound tracks involving different interpretations of the film: In one sound track the traumatic nature of the event was emphasized; in another the rite of passage was described as a harmless experience for the adolescents; and a third described the film in an emotionally detached manner. The trauma sound track elicited greater subjective reports of stress and autonomic reactions than did the other two sound tracks or a control condition.

Drawing on this research, Frijda (1988) has proposed as a first basic rule of emotions, the "Law of Situational Meaning: Emotions arise in response to the meaning structures of given situations; different emotions arise in response to different meaning structures" (p. 349). More recently, Lazarus (1991) has elaborated on the connection between appraisals and emotions. Distinct emotional reactions, he proposes, can be traced to several factors, such as the particular goal that is endangered or lost and attributions of cause and responsibility for the situation. Anger, for example, grows out of the appraisal that an important part of one's ego identity has been unfairly threatened or damaged by people who should be held accountable for their actions. Sadness, on the other hand, develops from the appraisal of a significant irrevocable loss that cannot be attributed to an external agent. Guilt is tied to appraisals that the individual is responsible for a transgression of an important moral value. Thus, the appraisal process has important implications for emotions. Other researchers also point to the important connections between appraisals and subsequent coping efforts (Folkman, Chesney, Pollack, & Coates, 1993; Folkman, Lazarus, Dunkel-Schetter, DeLongis, & Gruen, 1986; McCrae, 1984).

This discussion has emphasized the important role of perception in the determination of stressfulness. I have suggested that events, in and of themselves, are not *sufficient* conditions for stress. This is not to say that the character of the event is unimportant. Few people can avoid the perception of terrorism, debilitating illness, or untimely death as a threat or a loss. And different events have defining qualities of their own that press and shape the coping process into certain forms, even if they do not completely dictate their shape completely (see Cook & Oltjenbruns, 1989; Mattlin, Wethington, & Kessler, 1990).[3]

Efforts to identify the qualities of situations that make them stressful or nonstressful are important. It remains the case, however, that people have considerable latitude in how they construct their events, creating and anticipating some, while preventing and sidestepping others. Even unavoidable events can be cognitively constructed in different ways. What makes a life experience stressful is not only the event itself, but primary appraisals of the threat, harm, or challenge the event poses to the search for significance, and secondary appraisals of the resources and burdens the individual brings to the coping process.

ASSUMPTION III: PEOPLE BRING AN ORIENTING SYSTEM TO THE COPING PROCESS

We do not live totally at the mercy of stressful life events. In the face of crisis, we are guided and grounded by an orienting system. The orienting system is a general way of viewing and dealing with the world. It consists of habits, values, relationships, generalized beliefs, and personality. The orienting system is a frame of reference, a blueprint of oneself and the world that is used to anticipate and come to terms with life's events. The orienting system directs us to some life events and away from others (e.g., Bolger & Zuckerman, 1995). The orienting system is also the reservoir we draw on during hard times. Depending on the character of this system, it may be a help or hindrance in the coping process, for orienting systems are made up not only of resources but of burdens as well. Resources are attributes that are generally helpful in many situations. Burdens are attributes that are generally unhelpful. The orienting system also contains qualities whose value varies from situation to situation. Below we focus on some of the resources and burdens people bring to coping as a part of their orienting systems.

The Resources of Coping

Psychologists have identified a number of resources and highlighted their value in the face of stress (see Antonovsky, 1987; Hobfoll, 1988; Lazarus & Folkman, 1984). Prior experience with a stressor illustrates one such resource. This is how Norris and Murrell (1988) accounted for the greater resilience of the elderly to natural disasters. Because of their more extensive experience with tragedy, they suggested, the elderly are able to come to terms with the reexperience of trauma more easily than younger people. To test their hypothesis, Norris and Murrell studied the effects of flooding in 1981 and in 1984 on over 200 older adults in southeastern Kentucky. The results supported their hypothesis. Adults who reported experience with flooding before 1981 showed no increase in anxiety from 1981 to 1985. In contrast, the levels of anxiety increased over this time period among the less experienced older adults. Interestingly, prior encounters with tragedies other than floods, such as combat experience, a fire, or a serious car accident were also helpful in reducing the impact of the floods.

Other valuable coping resources have been identified. Bandura (1989) concludes from his own research and literature review that an optimistic sense of personal efficacy in life is associated with many positive consequences, including the ability to persevere under difficult conditions, the capacity to keep oneself together emotionally in coping, and the knack for avoiding situations that cannot be handled. Cohen and Wills (1985) conducted an extensive analysis of the empirical literature on the role of social support as a resource in times of stress, and conclude that "having access to persons to talk to about one's problem promotes well-being in the face of stress but not necessarily under nonstressful conditions" (p. 349). Dubow and Tisak (1989) reported that, among children who had experienced a number of important life events, those with more highly developed problem solving skills had fewer behavior problems and higher grade-point averages than those with less developed problem-solving abilities. Brandstädter and Renner (1990) found that the general tendencies to pursue goals tenaciously and adjust goals flexibly when necessary were both associated with lower levels of depression and higher levels of personal well-being.

These are only a few of the resources people bring to coping. Like significant objects, resources come in many shapes and sizes: material (e.g., transportation, food, shelter, money); physical (e.g., vitality, health); psychological (e.g., competence, a coherent view of the world); social (e.g., interpersonal skills, supportive social systems); and spiritual (e.g., feeling of closeness with God, congregational involvement). These are the tools people carry along with them in the coping process. But to focus solely on the resources people bring to coping would be one-sided, for people bring not only resources to coping, but burdens as well.

The Burdens of Coping

To different degrees, we all carry burdens that interfere with the search for significance. Burdens, like resources, may be material, physical, psychological, social, or spiritual; they can take a variety of forms, such as a history of failure, a physical handicap, a destructive family, a personality problem, financial debt, or dysfunctional beliefs about oneself or others.

Although theorists and researchers generally prefer to speak of a lack of resources rather than burdens, burdens are something more than the absence of resources. Being in debt is a different condition than not having any money, divorce is a different status than not being married, the feeling that people are dangerous and hostile is different than the feeling that people are not supportive. Burdens involve real liabilities and deficits.

Just as resources are generally helpful in coping, burdens are generally unhelpful. Peterson, Seligman, and Vaillant (1988) conducted a longitudinal study of the relationship between the pessimism of Harvard University students at the age of 25 and their physical health status later in life. Pessimism was defined by the tendency to see bad events as stable (i.e., "it's never going to go away"), global (i.e., "it's going to ruin everything"), and internally caused (i.e., "it's me") (p. 23). Even after controlling for their initial level of physical and emotional health, a pessimistic explanatory style was predictive of poorer physician-rated health of the men from ages 45–60.

Researchers have identified other burdens. Working with a group of Mexicans and Americans, Wheaton (1983) reported that fatalistic beliefs and inflexibility in coping exacerbated the effects of stress, albeit differentially, on symptoms of anxiety and schizophrenia. The burden of caring for a loved one with dementia has also been associated with poorer physical and mental health (Schulz & Williamson, 1994) and declines in immunological functioning (Kiecolt-Glaser & Glaser, 1994), though the scope and severity of these changes have not been determined.

In sum, people bring both resources and burdens to coping. Together they contribute to an orienting system (cf. Kohn, 1972), a material, biological, psychological, social, and spiritual frame of reference for thinking about and dealing with life situations. Certainly, some orienting systems are stronger and more comprehensive than others, but any system will have its points of weakness and limitations.

I do not mean to imply here that the orienting system is static. Like the other elements of coping, it changes over time. Some have compared resources to a bank account that is drawn upon during times of stress (e.g., Benner, Roskies, & Lazarus, 1980; Hobfoll, 1988).

The Bank Account of Resources and Burdens

The metaphor highlights the finite and precarious nature of our resources and burdens. In coping with stressful events, people must take care not to diminish their assets too quickly or incur too great a liability.

This leads to another reason why coping can be so difficult. While stressful life events are threatening, challenging, or harming the things we care about, they can also be attacking our resources and adding to our burdens, making the effort to attain significance all the more difficult. For example, people with AIDS must face the depletion of physical, emotional, and financial resources while struggling with the added burdens of medical treatment, career disruption, and stigma from family, friends, and community. In any crisis, those who experience a greater loss of resources are more likely to encounter more distress (Freedy, Shaw, Jarrell, & Masters, 1992). How people tap into their remaining resources and work around their accumulating burdens to attain significance in the face of this crisis is one of the key tasks for coping.

This example speaks only to the "withdrawal of assets" and "accumulation of liabilities" from the bank account of coping. Some theorists have stated that this is all we can expect when we face stress—a drain on our reserves until we reach exhaustion. Selye (1976) wrote: "It is though at birth each individual inherited a certain amount of adaptation energy . . . he can draw upon this capital thriftily for a long but monotonously uneventful existence, or he can spend it lavishly in the course of a stressful, intense, but perhaps more colorful and exciting life. In any case there is just so much of it, and he must budget accordingly" (p. 82).

The possibility of development and growth through coping has only begun to be examined (see Aldwin, 1994; Tedeschi & Calhoun, 1995). But, our banking metaphor suggests that resource development *is* a possibility. After all, most people do more than inherit their wealth and make withdrawals from it. They find ways to deposit and withdraw their resources and burdens from their accounts.

The investigation of veterans from World War II and the Korean War by Elder and Clipp (1989) provides a nice case in point. They introduce their study by describing two commonly acknowledged legacies of war for the veterans: the "No Legacy: The War is Over" involves a denial of any feelings or reactions to the wartime experience, and the "Pathogenic Legacy" involves the experience of stress-related symptomatology some time after the return to civilian life when circumstances trigger unresolved war-related conflicts. The researchers do not deny the power of these legacies, but they assert that a third possibility has been overlooked, the "Developmental Legacy." They write:

> Combat exposed men to conditions that stretched survival skills to the limit, as in the control of emotions during excruciating pain or fear. Managerial skills were learned through the demands of leadership and combat experience. Among men who survived war's traumatic experiences, this past and present can be tapped as a resource whenever life becomes exceedingly difficult. (p. 317)

Elder and Clipp put their premise to test through interviews with three groups of veterans: those who had not experienced combat, those who had experienced light combat, and those who had experienced heavy combat. In their interviews they asked the veterans to describe the positive and negative influences of their military involvement. Veterans who had experienced heavy combat reported greater deprivation and trauma from war, including combat anxieties, misery, bad memories, death or destruction, and the loss of friends. Even though combat involvement was associated with greater pain and loss, it was also tied to greater gain. In comparison with those less involved in combat, the heavy combat veterans were more likely to say that they had learned to cope with adversity and had grown to value human life more. Of course, these self-reports could be dismissed as the distorted recollections of those trying to minimize the painfulness of their experiences.

Fortunately, these veterans were also part of a longitudinal study of personality from 1928 to the present. Data from the California Personality Q-sort were available to confirm or disconfirm the interview findings. The analyses revealed that the heavy combat veterans did indeed become more goal oriented, less helpless, and considerably more resilient from adolescence to midlife than veterans with less combat involvement. The legacy of war, Elder and Clipp conclude, goes beyond denial and pathology. It encompasses growth as well.

The study by Elder and Clipp (1989) has been buttressed by more recent studies that show that people in crisis can find ways not only to avoid exhaustion, but to strengthen themselves psychologically, socially, and physically (Aldwin, Levenson, & Spiro, 1994; Dienstbier, 1989; Park, Cohen, & Murch, 1996). Through coping, resources are not only used, they are developed; burdens are not only taken on, they are lightened. Like a bank account, the resources and burdens people bring to coping accumulate and dwindle in the marketplace of transactions between individual and situation.

ASSUMPTION IV: PEOPLE TRANSLATE THE ORIENTING SYSTEM INTO SPECIFIC METHODS OF COPING

The orienting system has the *potential* to advance, shape, and limit the coping process in many ways. I stress the word potential because the orienting system is a system of only possibilities. All of the general support, knowledge, or abilities in the world are fine, but when new challenging situations come up we still have to ask, "What do I do now?" The answer is revealed in the activities of coping. Coping methods are the *actualized* means to attaining significance in the face of stressful events. They consist of the concrete thoughts, feelings, behaviors, and interactions that take place in specific difficult situations. In the coping process, the orienting system must be translated into specific methods of coping.

The account of Natan Sharansky (1988) provides a nice case in point. Intimidated, arrested, and imprisoned in the Soviet Union for his pro-Jewish activism, Sharansky struggled to find a way to maintain his identity. In the midst of horrific circumstances, he had to move from his general beliefs and principles to specific applications. Using his experience as a chess player, Sharansky devised a game plan. He delineated a set of specific methods of coping with the stress of his ordeal that would allow him to preserve his integrity and commitment to human rights. For example, he sought every opportunity to communicate with the outside world and spoke guardedly, but not dishonestly, with the KGB.

Sharansky's game plan helped him survive his years of imprisonment with his identity intact.

Carver et al. (1993) conducted an empirical study that illustrated how one element of the orienting system, an optimistic personality, was translated into specific methods of coping and, in turn, psychological adaptation. They studied women with breast cancer before surgery and at four time periods after surgery. An overall sense of optimism in life, they found, was related to less distress before surgery and at each time after surgery. Optimism was also associated with three methods of coping with breast cancer: greater acceptance of the disease, less denial, and less behavioral disengagement. These coping methods were, in turn, predictive of lower levels of distress over time. Thus, the specific methods of coping with cancer appeared to bridge the relationship between an optimistic personality and psychological outcomes. Other researchers have found comparable results (e.g., Bolger & Zuckerman, 1995). These findings make an important point: A knowledge of personality or other aspects of the orienting system is not sufficient to understand the encounter of a person with a particular event. Attention must be paid to the specific forms of coping in that situation.

The task of translation and transition from an orienting system to specific coping activities is not necessarily simple or straightforward. Not everyone will be as analytical as Natan Sharansky. Before it can be translated into action, the orienting system must be accessed. However, access can be blocked by a number of barriers (see Lazarus & Folkman, 1984). A lack of awareness is one such barrier. This is, essentially, a problem of secondary appraisals. Most of us have resources (and burdens) we are unaware of. The failure to perceive resources can cause serious problems.

I remember one client who described himself as "a wimp." A midlevel bank manager, he felt pushed around, bullied, and generally ineffectual. In talking about his job, his eyes became glassy, his voice turned to a monotone, and his shoulders drooped. I found myself feeling very tired in therapy. In search of some spark in his life, I shifted the focus to his earlier years and discovered that not only had he put himself through school by working two jobs, he had been on the boxing team in college, and flew airplanes on weekends—hardly the behavior of a wimp. When he talked about flying, he fairly crackled with energy. He seemed surprised when I commented on the difference between his style at work and his style behind the controls of his airplane. The key moment in therapy came when he recognized that his problem was not a "chronically wimpy personality," but a failure to identify and tap into his resources. He pinpointed the solution when he said, "I guess I need to learn how to fly at work, huh?" My client illustrated an important point: People cannot cope with tools they do not believe they have. Accurate secondary appraisals of resources and burdens are necessary for the generation of successful methods of coping.

In sum, the transition from the general to the specific, from the orienting system to particular methods of coping with crisis, is another key part of the coping process. It is important to note that the orienting system does not fully determine how a person will handle a stressful situation. It makes some methods of coping more available to the individual than others. However, as we will see shortly, the person must still choose from among several possible ways of coping. If none of the available choices offers a compelling solution, then the individual can choose to cope in a fundamentally different way, one that transforms the orienting system itself.

ASSUMPTION V: PEOPLE SEEK SIGNIFICANCE IN COPING THROUGH THE MECHANISMS OF CONSERVATION AND TRANSFORMATION

In the search for significance people can say, do, or feel just about anything. Thoughts, emotions, behaviors, and interactions can all become methods of coping. Obviously, we need some way of ordering and understanding the tremendous range of coping activities. Traditionally, coping methods have been classified according to various structural characteristics.

One structural approach is *descriptive.* For instance, a computer search and literature review by one group of researchers pointed to twelve categories of coping methods: cognitive restructuring, problem solving, tension reduction, social skills, self-disclosure, structuring, seeking information, stress monitoring, assertiveness, avoidance/withdrawal, suppression/denial, and self-medication (Matheny, Aycock, Pugh, Curlette, & Cannella, 1986). Although descriptive approaches such as these bring some organization to a scattered body of literature, they lack a conceptual grounding. As a result, they offer little help in understanding how the different coping activities develop or how they are similar to and different from one other.

Another structural approach to classifying coping methods, one more conceptually based, is *sequential.* Psychologist Eric Klinger (1977) describes an incentive–disengagement cycle of coping activities initiated by the loss of something valued. Invigoration is the first phase of this sequence. Energized and challenged, the individual tries harder to attain the incentive, which may have taken on even greater value because it has become "hard to get." In the next phase, aggression, the individual turns to more primitive means of achieving goals. Hostility, vengeance, and sadism, Klinger maintains, can offer a way to reduce further threats and restore a sense of effectiveness and control. There is a time in this process, however, when the individual gives up. This third phase, depression, is characterized by grief, longing, and sadness for the lost incentive. Eventually, though, people rebound. In the final part of the cycle, recovery, the person successfully disengages from the lost value and forms new interests in life.

Klinger illustrates these phases of the incentive–disengagement cycle with an annoyance many of us can relate to, the soda machine that swallows money and gives nothing in return:

> You now take out your only other [change] and repeat the sequence. . . . You reread the instructions with concentrated care, pushing the appropriate buttons, your motions perhaps becoming stiffer and choppier, the beginning, perhaps of a flush on your face. The button pushes by now have become punches, and you whack the dispenser on its side once or twice. Eventually, perhaps after an additional attack on the machine, you depart, your irritation melting into disheartment, a lump rising in your throat. Your hope for refreshment has turned to disappointment mingled perhaps with some strains of self-pity and lingering irritation. After a while, however, the bad feelings fade as you produce other satisfactions and they are eventually forgotten. (p. 138)

Sequential approaches such as Klinger's provide ways to understand how coping activities may evolve over time. Even so, recalling the research cited earlier (e.g., Silver & Wortman, 1980), it is far from clear that people progress through a series of coping stages consistently and uniformly. The sequence of coping with the soda machine is familiar to many of us, but, as Klinger recognizes, it is not universal: Some walk away from the soda machine without a whimper of protest, some remain sad and disappointed for quite a while, and a few will go ahead and file a lawsuit.

A *typological* approach offers another way of placing the variety of coping activities into more manageable and theoretically relevant categories, such as approach or avoidance coping (Roth & Cohen, 1986). Critics, however, have argued that distinctions such as this one are too simplistic. Within any coping episode, both approach and avoidance coping efforts may be used at different points in time (e.g., Schneirla, 1959; Shontz, 1975). Moreover, there are important distinctions to be made within these broad categories of coping. For example, exercise and alcohol use are both ways to avoid problems, but they have very different implications for well-being.

In recognition of these concerns, several researchers have developed more finely differentiated classification systems that integrate typological with other coping approaches (e.g., Carver, Scheier, & Weintraub, 1989; Folkman et al., 1986; Moos, Brennan, Fondacaro, & Moos, 1990). Tyler (1978) for example, defines a continuum from active coping efforts in which the individual approaches problems in a forceful, self-directed, and planful way to passive coping efforts in which the person waits for events to unfold and relies on outside forces to deal with problems that arise. Tyler's approach to measuring coping activities blends the typological with the sequential. Active planfulness in coping is assessed across different phases of problem solving, from the definition to the resolution of the problem. Additionally, coping is measured within different spheres of living—personal, task, and social. The recognition given to the psychosocial nature of coping in this approach is particularly noteworthy.

Descriptive, sequential, and typological approaches offer different ways to organize and understand important dimensions of the structure of coping. Each has its own advantages and disadvantages, and in this book I will draw on the different approaches at different times. But none of these approaches speaks directly to the underlying function of coping as it has been defined here, namely, the search for significance. For that we must consider coping activities from a different perspective, the functional.

I have emphasized that when a stressful life experience is encountered, the search for significance does not end. We continue to look for significance in times of trouble. It is true that we cope *with* stressful events, yet it is just as true that we cope *toward* the values most important to us. But how? There are two functional mechanisms guiding the coping process: conservation and transformation. Conservational forms of coping attempt to protect significance; transformational forms of coping attempt to change it.

The Conservation of Significance

Conservation is often the initial tendency in coping. When a situation places a significant object at risk, the first response is to try to hold on to it. Take the process of denial in the face of crisis as an example. Why should the sound of a tornado be dismissed as the rumble of a passing train? Why is a persistent pain in the chest so often interpreted as only indigestion? Harmful as these forms of denial may be, they reflect the efforts of the person to cling to the things that matter to them. The sound of the tornado is dismissed to preserve the illusion of a home safe from the weather. Pains in the chest are overlooked to avoid the confrontation with mortality. In each case the event has been interpreted in a way designed to protect something of value to the person.

Conservation is not simply an initial tendency. People tenaciously try to conserve significance, even in the most threatening conditions. This is the conclusion reached by Allport, Bruner, and Jandorf (1956), after examining the written life histories of 96 anti-Nazis who suffered through World War II. These life histories contain striking illustrations of persistent attempts to hold on to what mattered most in the face of an emerging catastrophe. One writer, unsuccessful in selling his works abroad, returns to Germany in 1933 in spite of the imminent dangers. How does he explain this seemingly foolish act? "I had my mother, whom I had to care for; I had all my relatives, all my friends—many non-Jews among them—who were faithful to me; I had my comfortable home" (p. 441).

That we persist in attempts to protect our values even in the most desperate conditions can say something about the depth of our values and the tenacity of the human spirit. But, to inject a bit more pragmatic note, it also speaks to the fact that people are often drawn more to the reassuring lull of the familiar than to the new and the strange. This seems to be a very basic human characteristic. In describing the process of intellectual development, psychologist Jean Piaget (1954) has noted how the child's initial efforts are conservative—to assimilate or fit the environment into his or her way of looking at the world. The child "resists every new accommodation" (p. 353). Only when the efforts to assimilate have failed will the child accommodate by changing his or her mental structures to fit with the world.

The coping process reflects this basic human tendency to conserve. Much of coping can be characterized by the effort to maintain and preserve significance, whether it involves the management of problems and emotions as Lazarus and Folkman (1984) emphasize, or the conservation of other objects such as health, status, self-esteem, possessions, jobs, family, a way of looking at the world, or a familiar way of life. In fact, Hobfoll (1988) argues, conservation is the pivotal mechanism underlying the process of coping with stress.

The Transformation of Significance

Crucial as it is, there is more to coping than conservation. Recall White's (1963) observations of how infants and children seem to be motivated to explore new situations. He speaks to the human propensity to create newness, excitement, and change in life. The conservation mechanism cannot fully account for this characteristic, the tendency for people to "shake things up."

Of course, in many instances we are less "shakers" than "shaken." Through stressful life events, resources are attacked, burdens are assumed, and coping activities are restricted, blocking the means for achieving significance. In the more devastating cases, stressful life events shake and shatter not only the means for achieving significance but the nature of significance itself. I remember a woman in her early 20s who came to therapy after a car accident that killed members of her family, almost killed her, and left her with chronic and incapacitating pain. Before the accident she had been energetic, popular, and optimistic, looking forward to college, marriage, and a productive life. The accident threatened an end to all of her dreams. In fact, her injuries had resulted in the loss of many of the things she cared about most deeply—friends, family, jobs, vitality, and independence. She had, in short, lost her way.

Transformation is often painful. Attempts to create major life change can lead to anxiety and discontent, but there may be no better alternative, for when old objects of significance are no longer attainable, conservation cannot work. Indeed, efforts to conserve a way of life that is no longer feasible are a sign of trouble. The young woman in the previous example was compounding her problems by trying to take up the life she had had prior to the accident. Against the advice of her physician, she tried to dance with her friends, hold down a regular job, and live the life of a healthy 23-year-old. Unfortunately, she was not a healthy 23-year-old, and her attempts to conserve her way of life only made matters worse.

At times such as these, the search for significance requires transformation rather than conservation. Transformational forms of coping attempt to change the character of significance itself—to relinquish old values, to discover new ones, and to build a life around this new center. Efforts to transform can be creative, productive, even heroic. Indeed, what most heroic mythological adventures share is a story of an individual tried, tested, and changed through adversity (Campbell, 1988). But not all attempts at transformation are growthful. Some attempts result in no change at all, and others lead to defeat. The heroes of mythology and real life have their foils who face the same trials, but respond by destroying themselves and others. Transformational and conservational coping activities represent *efforts* to change or hold on to significance. These efforts may or may not meet with success.

Conservation and Transformation of Means and Ends in Coping

The nature of conservation and transformation can be elaborated a bit more. In coping, people try to conserve or transform not only their objects of greatest significance, but their usual ways of attaining significance as well; that is, their resources, burdens, and general ways of viewing and dealing with the world. To put it another way, the methods of conservation and transformation apply to both the destinations of significance (i.e., ends) and the pathways to significance (i.e., means). As Figure 5.1 shows, any approach to coping involves conservation or transformation of both means and ends. Let us take a closer look at the four possibilities in this matrix.

1. *Preservation.* Faced with life stress, our first route of action is almost automatic; we try to hold on to our world and the things we care about. To deny the reality of the threat, to call on others for emotional support, to persist in one's approach to living are some of the ways people try to preserve the means and ends of significance in hard times. As with the other functional mechanisms of coping, preservation can be helpful or harmful. Nelson Mandela's steadfast commitment to his beliefs and values during his long imprisonment was a model of courage and integrity. The National Aeronautic and Space Agency (NASA), however, ran into trouble because of their commitment to an old way of solving problems. Confronted with the challenge of protecting their huge space rockets from inclement weather, NASA simply magnified old designs for aircraft hangars by a factor of 10 or more (Watzlawick, 1988). The experts were surprised to discover that a hangar of this size creates its own climate, including clouds, rain, and static electricity, "and

| | Destinations of Significance | |
	Conservation of Ends	Transformation of Ends
Conservation of Means	Preservation	Re-Valuation
Transformation of Means	Reconstruction	Re-Creation

Pathways to Significance

FIGURE 5.1. Four methods of coping: the conservation and transformation of means and ends.

thus produces from within itself the very phenomena it was supposed to protect" (p. 29). This "more of the same" solution backfired.

2. *Reconstruction.* When the usual pathway to significance is blocked by an obstacle and old solutions do not work, we may back up and try to find another way around it. An unskilled worker, threatened with the loss of her job, returns to school to broaden her skills and increase her marketability. To find out why his relationships with women have ended in failure and how he might build a more lasting relationship, a man joins an assertiveness training group. Victimized by a crime, a woman who once believed that she was personally invulnerable to tragic events struggles to rebuild her "assumptive world" (cf. Janoff-Bulman, 1989); her task is to construct new beliefs about herself and the world that sustain her sense of efficacy and meaning in life. In each of these cases, old skills, habits, or beliefs are no longer sufficient to the search for significance. To reach the goal, the individual, instead, attempts to change aspects of the orienting system. New resources may be sought, old burdens lightened, or habitual ways of thinking and feeling changed. In any event, the goal remains the same, but a new path is taken to reach it. This is the essence of reconstructive coping.

3. *Re-valuation.* When it becomes too difficult to attain significance, ends may need to be transformed and means conserved. Re-valuation often occurs in times of transition, when old values are lost and the individual faces the twin tasks of sustaining him- or herself while struggling to find new sources of value. Re-valuation was an implicit part of the coping advice my brother, a physician, gave a dying patient who asked: "Why should I bother to live? What is there to live for?" My brother suggested to his patient that he now had new and different things to live for: a day with some time free of pain, a meaningful conversation with his wife, the opportunity to say good-bye to the people he cared about, and some time to reflect on his life. The suggestion here was not for wholesale changes in living, but rather to find new objects of significance. Studies of people faced with life-threatening situations indicate that many go through a "reckoning time" (cf. Tedeschi & Calhoun, 1995), a process of reprioritization in which they try to take more pleasure out of the present, develop a deeper appreciation of loving relationships, and focus more on enjoyable activities (e.g., Collins, Taylor, & Skokan, 1990). Re-valuation is generally a time-limited coping mechanism, for the attempt to find new goals is often followed by a change in the path to reach them. Had my brother's patient lived, his re-valuation might have been followed by an effort to reconstruct his life to fit with his new priorities.

4. *Re-creation.* When severe enough, the stresses of life can splinter both the pathways and destinations of significance. The young woman,

paralyzed by an accident, learns that her old dreams and established approach to her world have been shattered. She must cope to create virtually a new way of life. The alcoholic discovers that sobriety cannot be achieved by anything less than a radical change. He copes by joining Alcoholics Anonymous, a group that encourages not only abstinence from what has become his chief object of significance, liquor, but an entirely different approach to living. Members are asked to take stock of themselves and make a host of changes: form new and more supportive relationships, make amends for earlier mistakes, stay away from situations and old friends that led to drinking, take life one day at a time, admit their powerlessness over alcohol, and acknowledge the power of something greater than themselves (Robertson, 1988).

Coping mechanisms, like physical mechanisms, have purpose built into them. Just as an iron is designed with a certain function in mind, coping mechanisms have a design of their own. The functional approach focuses on the identification of these purposes. Some methods are conservational in nature; others are transformational. While resistance to substantive change is embedded in the act of denial, the insistence on radical change is an inherent part of the coping activities prescribed by 12-Step Programs. Even the customary introduction of members to the group challenges them to confront their condition: "Hi, my name is Bill and I'm an alcoholic."

Determining whether a coping activity is conservational or transformational is not always easy. Some coping methods have sufficient built-in flexibility that they can serve either purpose. Two college students may respond to failure in the freshman year by seeking out professional counseling. While the first may be looking for symptomatic relief without substantive change (i.e., conservation), the second may be trying to decide whether she really wants to be in college (i.e., transformation). As this example shows, the functions of coping are determined not only by the design of the mechanism, but by the intentions of the person doing the coping. Even a mechanism well designed for one purpose can be adapted to serve other ends. An iron may be best suited for pressing clothes, but it can also be used as a hammer, paperweight, or weapon.

Whether a coping method is conservational or transformational also depends on the individual's personal history. For the college student who has always taken pride in solving problems herself, seeking counseling would be transformational. For the student who has often sought out counseling in the past in times of trouble, the same method of coping would be conservational. In short, the functional analysis of coping can point to methods that are generally conservational and methods that are generally transformational. More precise determinations require an evaluation of not only the methods of coping, but the motivations behind the methods and the context of the individual's life. In subsequent chapters, I will return to these issues while examining religious coping methods of conservation and transformation.

This assumption about coping has highlighted the variety of shapes and sizes of coping activities. In an effort to bring some order to these activities, they have been described in terms of their multidimensional structure. They have also been described from a functional point of view. Conservation and transformation were delineated as the functional mechanisms guiding the search for significance. But we are still left with the question of what determines the form and function of coping activities. When and why do we turn to some ways of coping rather than others? How do we select particular forms of coping in particular situations?

ASSUMPTION VI: PEOPLE COPE IN WAYS THAT ARE COMPELLING TO THEM

The search for significance in times of stress can be hard. Options for coping are circumscribed by the press of events, by the character of the orienting system, and by internal and external constraints. They are further circumscribed by secondary appraisals, that is, our perceptions of what resources are available. There are, in short, a limited number of things we can do when confronted with stressful situations. Of course, it is not very often that we run out of options completely. New options can be created in coping. Nevertheless, even when choices are plentiful, coping can be difficult. Because we have to give up valued resources or accumulate undesirable burdens to gain valued ends, because we have to give up some ends to get others, and because there is a limit to how much significance we can attain in life, we are often faced with trade-offs in coping.

How do we deal with these potential tradeoffs, the pros and cons that accompany the choices we do have? To pick the best method, I believe we form one final type of appraisal.[4] Through a *tertiary appraisal process* we select the *most compelling option*, the strategy expected to bring the greatest gain and the least loss of significance through the use of the fewest resources and the accumulation of the least burden. There are two key points in this view of the tertiary appraisal process. The first is that we try to maximize significance, increasing the gains and reducing the losses to the things we care about. The second point is that in selecting a coping method, we weigh its implications not only for the goals we hope to reach, but for the route we must travel to get there.

Generally we try to save our energy and take on the lightest burdens in our travels. To put it another way, we prefer the path of least resistance. That does not mean coping is necessarily easy. When the path is blocked or the goal is lofty, the path of least resistance may still be steep and tortuous.

Other writers have described a similar process. Hobfoll (1988), for example, has described a "mini–max" decision-making strategy in response to stressful events, one of "minimizing loss, maximizing gain" (p. 26). Similarly, in his theory of emotions, Frijda (1988) puts forth the Laws of the Lightest Load and the Greatest Gain: "Whenever a situation can be viewed in alternative ways, a tendency exists to view it in a way that minimizes negative emotional load . . . [and] a tendency exists to view it in a way that maximizes emotional gain" (p. 356).

Let us take an example of tertiary appraisals. A married couple decides that they would like to have a child. Both spouses have looked forward to pregnancy and the challenges of parenting. Although their attempts to conceive are not successful in the first 6 months, they do not take much notice. Over the next 6 months, however, they become uneasier as their efforts continue to prove unsuccessful. They start to wonder whether they might not have a problem. But what will they do about it? Clearly, their choices will be limited by their system of resources, burdens, constraints, and secondary appraisals. They have not read much about infertility. Other members of the family "got pregnant the first time they tried." They do not have a great deal of money, and the closest medical center is 30 miles away. But they are people who do not give up easily when they run into trouble.

Which option will maximize significance? This is where the tertiary appraisal process enters the picture. In all likelihood, radical change will not be the first response. To give up trying to attain a goal so important would seem drastic, premature, and inconsistent with their view of themselves. Seeking out a medical specialist also seems too time-consuming and expensive at this point in the process. Although they know there is an infertility support group in their small community, they are reluctant to attend because they do not like to think of themselves as "infertile." Preservational coping methods might be appraised as the more compelling alternative. Initially, they make a few jokes about sex and try not to think too much about pregnancy. They do mention their uneasiness to a few close friends and family members, who reassure them not to worry. And they become conscious of having sex more regularly. All of these coping efforts are preservational strategies designed to sustain their goal of becoming parents at minimal cost to their resources and general orientation to the world.

If, however, their efforts at conception continue to fail, then preservational methods might no longer be appraised in the same way. To continue to downplay the threat of the situation might preserve one object of significance, their view of themselves as a "normal" couple, but place the other, their desire for a baby, at too great a risk. Reconstructive methods would be more likely—reorienting themselves and their way of life in an attempt to protect their dream of becoming parents. The couple talks to their family physician, who refers them to an infertility specialist. They decide to invest the time and money in a series of infertility tests and treatments, beginning with the least expensive and least intrusive treatments. When these treatments fail, they reluctantly decide to ask their families for a loan to pay for the more expensive infertility treatments. Over the course of time, they begin to think about themselves as truly infertile and start to attend the local infertility support group.

After 2 years of failure, frustration, and mounting debt, the couple enters a period of re-valuative coping. They still try to conceive, but, for the first time, they begin to seriously reappraise the goal of parenthood. Is it worth the financial strain, the loss of time, the emotional roller-coaster of hope and frustration every month? Can they imagine a life without children? Do they have other things to care about that would lend significance to their lives? Out of this period of re-valuation, the couple may decide that they are willing to pay virtually any price to have a child, and return to a new form of reconstructive coping. Perhaps they participate in a new and experimental method of treating infertility or perhaps they decide to go on an adoption list.

On the other hand, what was once unthinkable, a life without children, may become more compelling than the alternative when that alternative takes such a terrible financial, psychological, and interpersonal toll. The couple might decide that the effort to have children has slim hope of success and is no longer worth the cost. Re-creation, a complete transformation of the couple's life, one involving new pathways and destinations, becomes more attractive. Together the couple grieve the loss of their dream of being parents, and gradually shift their attention to new directions. Perhaps the wife returns to college for a degree in music. Perhaps the husband becomes active in volunteer work in the community. And perhaps they decide that it is time to make changes in their network of friends, moving away from those who have shared the problems of infertility to those with shared educational and communal interests.

In presenting these bare-bones of the tertiary appraisal process, it may appear to be cold, calculating, even mechanical. Yet few of us sit down with a piece of paper and systematically and dispassionately weigh and compare our coping options in times of stress. What makes a choice compelling has as much to do with feeling as it does with thinking. Most decisions in coping are reached with some measure of analysis and intuition, logic and emotion, and conscious as well as unconscious processing. Tertiary appraisals are matters of both heart and mind.

In sum, tertiary appraisals guide the selection of particular coping methods. They involve comparative assessments of those coping activities most likely to maximize gains and minimize losses to significance at minimal cost in terms of resources and burdens. To understand how a person will deal with a difficult situation then, we must know not only something about the situation, but about the individual's system of significance and system of resources and burdens. Like each of the critical elements in the coping process, tertiary appraisals evolve through the interplay of many forces.

ASSUMPTION VII: COPING IS EMBEDDED IN CULTURE

In this description of the flow of coping, individuals have taken center stage. How they construct, confront, and come to terms with life's trials and tribulations represents the drama of coping. What may be easy to overlook as we watch this drama unfold is the background. Coping plays itself out against the backdrop of larger cultural forces. This background is important in its own right. Depending on the "lighting" provided by culture, the coping process will take on very different hues. By culture I am referring to forces that go beyond the individual's immediate microsocial system (Bronfenbrenner, 1979). Culture has to do with the underlying blueprints of a society, blueprints that influence and pattern the "complex whole" of social life—its institutions, laws, knowledge, customs, morals, and lifestyles (Tylor, 1968). In the language of coping, culture shapes events, appraisals, orienting systems, coping activities, outcomes, and objects of significance. Let me give a few examples.

Sociologist Leonard Pearlin (1982) calls attention to the fact that cultures and societies themselves create stress. One way they do so is through conflicts among values, beliefs, and opportunities for achievement. Using the work of Robert Merton as an example, he notes that our society encourages socioeconomic success, yet limits the structures for attaining success: "The system of values stimulates motivation toward the attainment of monetary and honorific success among more people than could possibly be accommodated by the opportunity structure. Consequently, many of us who internalize the culturally prized success goals are doomed to failure" (p. 371). Pearlin goes on to note that times of rapid cultural change are often stressful because they create discontinuities between goals, aspirations, and values and the institutional structures that can accommodate them. Here we have a conflict between the ends of significance, culturally defined, and the means to attaining significance, culturally limited.

Major cultural changes also contribute to more immediate events. In the last quarter of the 20th century, a major collision of cultures has taken place between the world's oil producers and its oil consumers. In the 1970s, the oil producers formed a cartel that effectively limited the supply of oil. At first, this megacultural event seemed far removed from our day-to-day lives, but it soon created very immediate problems in the form of long gasoline lines and daily disruptions. The shortage also resulted in higher prices for almost all consumer goods and services, triggering, in turn, inflation and an economic recession. The economic hardship may have increased the incidence of many more immediate critical life events, such as unemployment, divorce, crime, suicide, and mortality (e.g., Dooley & Catalano, 1980). As far removed as it seems to be, cultural change reaches directly into individual lives.

Resources, burdens, and coping activities are also a part of a larger culture. Breznitz (1980), for example, discusses how children in Israel, exposed to death, violence, and war at any early age, suffer from the burden of greater preoccupation with terrorism than children in other cultures. He recounts the story of a child who participated in a study of creativity. Asked "What can you do with a shoe?" the child immediately replied: "I can throw it at a terrorist." Breznitz also notes evidence of more advanced death concepts among Israeli children than American children.

Caudill (1958) describes how individual, immediate microsystems, and larger cultural macrosystems are linked in the face of stress. In some situations, the effects of a crisis are limited largely to the individual and his or her immediate system; in these instances, the microsystem can support the individual and sustain itself. In other situations, such as community disasters, the crisis disrupts both individual and immediate social system; here much of the onus for coping falls back on the larger cultural system. And in the 20th century we have witnessed events that have attacked not only the lives of individuals and their immediate family, friends, and communities, but their cultures as well. The catastrophic nature of these events is tied to this total loss of the personal, the social, and the cultural. Commenting on the genocide of World War II, Benner et al. (1980) write:

> Our cultures give us ways of thinking about and dealing with the death of a child or even our own incapacitation or untimely impending death. But no cultural framework provides a way to encompass

genocide. Thus the individual who has experienced these traumatic events is faced not only with a loss of individual values and beliefs but also with the failure of the total culture to provide a meaningful explanation for these events. (p. 253)

Without the benefit of cultural support, we fall back on ourselves in coping. But to "go it alone" may be a nearly insurmountable challenge, for our visions of the future, our sense of the past, our ability to interpret and learn from experience, our definitions of ourselves, and the meanings we make of life are all embedded in a larger culture. Culture, in short, provides the grounding in the search for significance.

This assumption about coping has underscored the importance of this "ground" when we consider the "figure" of the individual moving through the coping process. The examples that have been presented illustrate some of the ways culture shapes coping. But it is just as true that culture is shaped *by* coping. Through coping efforts, we can support the cultural fabric. Occasionally, however, we tear and reweave this fabric into new patterns. History has been punctuated by people who, coping with stress, changed the blueprints of social life for good or bad. There is, in short, a give-and-take between the individual and the larger culture in coping.

ASSUMPTION VIII: THE KEYS TO GOOD COPING LIE IN THE OUTCOMES AND THE PROCESS

Psychologists and other helpers are interested not only in understanding coping, but in evaluating it as well. Many of the issues people bring to counseling can be conceptualized as problems in coping: depression over the death of a loved one, posttraumatic stress associated with a natural disaster, family conflict as a child moves into adolescence, and so on. How do we evaluate a process as rich, contextual, and fluid as coping? Two evaluative approaches can be articulated: the outcomes approach and the process approach (see Folkman, 1992).

The Outcomes Approach

The outcomes approach is unabashedly pragmatic. The "good" and "bad" of coping are defined by whatever produces positive and negative end-results. Identifying what works and what does not, however, is not an easy task. For one thing, what do we mean by "works?" Defining the outcomes of coping can be a tricky business. The evaluation of the outcomes of coping is made even more difficult by the nature of coping itself, a process that offers no single keys to success. Let us take a closer look at these issues.

Assessing the Outcomes of Coping

Ideally, evaluations of the outcomes of coping should meet several criteria. First, they should be relevant to the demands and challenges raised by the particular stressful situation. Second, they should be tailored to the individual's objects of significance. Third, they should be sensitive to the possibilities for failure and success in coping. Fourth, they should be alert to the fact that coping may have different effects over time. Finally, they should be sensitive to the trade-offs that take place in coping and the potential for unexpected results.

1. To appreciate the effects of coping, Folkman (1992) has pointed out, it is important to identify outcomes that are relevant to the demands of particular stressful situations. For example, the regulation of anxiety may be especially important in uncontrollable and threatening situations, such as awaiting the results of a biopsy. However, in situations that involve a loss, it may be more relevant to consider whether the individual has been able to restore his or her morale and develop new objects of significance.

2. Even when we focus on a particular situation, however, it is important to remember that people may strive toward different ends. For some bereaved spouses, the search for meaning in the loss may be the main concern. Others may be most interested in reestablishing new relationships as soon as possible. Still others may be preoccupied by the desire for tangible and emotional support. The success of the coping enterprise should be evaluated, in part, according to the individual's own goals. This highly individualized evaluation may be difficult to do. It is easier to ask how well the individual feels he or she coped with the situation (coping efficacy) or whether the situation was resolved (prob-lem resolution) (Menaghan, 1983). Researchers often look for signs of success in the coping process by measures of mood. If the individual has attained some degree of significance without depleting his or her re-sources too greatly, it is assumed that improved mood will follow. However, these measures do not speak to *what* has been conserved or transformed (unless better mood is the goal of coping). They are, instead, *indicators* of how well things turned out.

3. The search for significance is not always successful. That people seek significance does not mean that they will find it, or hold on to it once found. In some instances, coping activities may be more harmful

than helpful. For example, in their study of the psychological impact of the nuclear incident at Three Mile Island on people who lived within 55 miles of the area, Cleary and Houts (1984) found that both avoidant and active strategies for dealing with the crisis were predictive of greater emotional upset 3 months later. What people tried to do seemed to make matters worse than better.

On the other hand, coping also presents opportunities for achievement. Unfortunately, the potential for success in coping may be somewhat underestimated by mood-related measures of outcome that focus, for the most part, on the negative side of the pole (e.g., emotional distress, state anxiety, state depression, negative affect). By evaluating outcomes exclusively according to these criteria, the best that can be hoped for in coping is the absence of distress or "mood neutrality." Others, however, have begun to assess the potential for benefits and growth in coping (e.g., Collins et al., 1990; Pargament, Ensing, et al., 1990; Tedeschi & Calhoun, 1995). For instance, Park and her colleagues (Park, Cohen, & Murch, 1996) have developed a measure of stress-related growth. Their scales assess growth in the interpersonal arena (e.g., "I started a deep meaningful relationship with another"), in the personal domain (e.g., "I rethought how I want to live my life"), and in the realm of coping skills (e.g., "I learned better ways to express my feelings"). These items are especially relevant here, for they speak to the possibilities of transformation as well as conservation in coping. It is important to appreciate the full range of potential outcomes in coping—failure and loss, success and growth, and no change at all.

4. The implications of various methods of coping may change over time. Some coping approaches may be helpful in the short-term, but problematic in the long run. For instance, one metaanalysis of coping research indicated that avoidant methods of coping are more effective in reducing distress than approach methods in the short-term, but less effective than approach methods in the long-term (Mullen & Suls, 1982). On the other hand, some methods of coping may be associated with immediate discomfort, but longer-term gains. For example, Pennebaker and Beall (1986) found that the act of writing about a traumatic event had the immediate effect of increased tension and distress; however, it was also associated with better physical health over the next six months.

5. Finally, it is important to note that the end-results of coping are not necessarily all good or all bad. Oftentimes, coping leads to a "mixed bag," one that simply mirrors the difficult choices that must be made when confronted with the realities and limitations of decision making.[5] Some trade-offs take place among various objects of significance. Faced with the decision of whether to undergo chemotherapy, a

man with cancer may opt to forgo it, recognizing that he will have a shorter life, albeit one of greater quality. Other trade-offs apply to the relationship between the individual and the social system. In a series of studies of the effects of a heart attack on patients and their wives, patients who denied the seriousness of their illness showed less evidence of anxiety/depression and disability and were more likely to resume work and sexual activity (Stern, Pascale, & Ackerman, 1977; Stern & Pascale, 1979). However, denial by the patient was also associated with depression by the wife. "Faced with the impossible situation of wanting support from a block of granite and not being able to hammer away to get it as in the past, she herself crumbles in a welter of anxiety, depression, and confusion" (Stern & Pascale, 1979, p. 86). These studies also alert us to the sometimes unexpected outcomes that can emerge from coping. The search for significance in stressful times may ultimately lead in directions that could not be easily predicted from the starting point.

No Single Key to Good Coping

Some have argued that the key to good coping lies in particular activities of coping, as we hear in popular coping advice, such as: "If you don't succeed, try, try again!" "Think it through!" "Don't get carried away by your emotions!" Some ways of dealing with problems may indeed be more helpful than others in many life situations. It does not follow, however, that certain ways of coping are *always* better than others. The helpfulness of any coping strategy may depend as much on the particular problem the individual is facing and the person doing the coping as the strategy itself.

For example, it is almost a truism in psychology that active coping methods that emphasize the role of personal control in dealing with stressful situations are preferable to passive efforts (e.g., Lefcourt, 1976). Several studies support this notion. For example, there is evidence that active coping may facilitate the immune functioning and long-term survival of cancer patients (Fawzy et al., 1993) and the long-term psychological adjustment of arthritis patients (e.g., Brown, Nicassio, & Wallston, 1989). Other evidence, however, suggests that active coping may have its potential downside. Researchers have found that active coping efforts in social and nonsocial situations lead to increases in blood pressure and heart rate (Smith, Allred, Morrison, & Carlson, 1989). Active vigilant methods have also been associated with harmful effects for people with hypertension and heart disease (Seeman, 1991). It should also be noted that the same coping method may also have different implications at different points in time. In the early stages of a heart attack, denial has devastating consequences. After the coronary, however, denial has been associated with lower anxiety, shorter hospitalization, and perhaps lower risk for morbidity and mortality (see Fowers, 1992). Thus, the picture is not so clear-cut.

The task of finding a coping method that will be helpful to all people, for all purposes, across all situations seems difficult, if not impossible. This is not to say that we cannot and should not evaluate coping activities. Nor does this mean that some coping methods are not generally more helpful to many people and across many situations than others. The central point here is that any evaluation of the impact of coping on outcomes should be sensitive to the particulars of the individual, the situation, and the social context. No single method of coping in and of itself is likely to hold the key to success.

The Limits of the Outcomes Approach

The outcomes approach is, by far, the most commonly used way of evaluating the effectiveness of coping. Pragmatism does have a great deal of appeal: The merits of coping are judged by its products. Unfortunately, though, judging coping by its outcomes can be misleading at times. What are we to make of people who struggle valiantly but unsuccessfully with injustice, or those who, try as they might, are unable to make any sense of the deaths of their loved ones? In certain situations, significance may be exceptionally hard to find, regardless of how well the individuals cope. Lehman, Wortman, and Williams (1987) interviewed people who had lost a spouse or a child in a motor vehicle crash 4–7 years earlier. It was clear that most of the respondents were still trying to find some significance in their loss. A majority of the spouses and parents reported thinking: "If only I had done something differently, my [spouse/child] would still be alive" (p. 226); 32% of the bereaved spouses and 52% of the bereaved parents said they had tried to make sense of the death of their loved one in the last month. Unfortunately, for many, the search for significance was unsuccessful. Several years after their loss, 68% of the spouses and 59% of the parents reported they had not been able to make any sense at all of the death. Does it follow, however, that this bereaved group was coping ineffectively?

On the other hand, how do we evaluate the coping of those who achieve positive outcomes through no effort of their own or through undesirable but successful means, as in the case of the student who resolves his fears of failing by hiring someone to write his term paper? If outcomes are the criteria of good coping, then those who struggle unsuccessfully to find meaning in the death of a loved one have coped poorly, and the student who achieves a good grade dishonestly has coped well. Clearly, something is wrong here.

As coping has been described in this chapter, outcomes are only one part of the process. The link between what people do and what they achieve in coping can be tenuous. This notion contradicts the view, perhaps the positive illusion, that our lives are under our complete control. But, recall the stark fact of concentration camp life in World War II; only 1 out of 600 survived. Survival was determined by factors largely out of the victims' control; how people coped had relatively little bearing on this most basic of all outcomes (Benner et al., 1980). Because many forces come into play besides individual ones, there are no guarantees that "good" coping efforts will lead to good outcomes, nor, for that matter, are there any guarantees that poor coping will result in poor outcomes. Outcomes in themselves are not the only key to good coping. Evaluations of coping must also attend to the process.

The Process Approach

Stressful life experience, significance, appraisals, the orienting system, resources, burdens, coping methods, outcomes, and cultures are all elements of the coping process, but none determines its flow alone. The key to good coping from the process perspective can be found in the workings of the "body of coping" as a whole. This still leaves us with the difficult question of what makes a good or bad coping *process*. We will take this question up in more detail later in the book (Chapter 11), where the process of coping is evaluated in the religious realm.

Here let me briefly note that an effective coping process is well integrated. Each of the parts meshes appropriately with the others, and the system operates in a coordinated fashion. The ineffective coping process is poorly integrated. The elements of coping become disentangled or out-of-alignment, and the system itself loses its balance. The problem here lies in the system rather than any single element of coping.

Any encounter between a person and a stressful situation can be evaluated according to three process dimensions: means, ends, and individual–system fit. With respect to the means of coping, it is important to evaluate the extent to which the various appraisals and methods of coping in a particular situation are appropriate to the demands of the situation and the goals of the individual. In the effective coping encounter, the individual's appraisals are well attuned to the realities of the situation (primary appraisals) and to the individual's own resources and burdens in coping (secondary appraisals) (Folkman, 1992). The choice of methods of coping (tertiary appraisals) is also appropriately tailored to the situation, the individual's capabilities and limitations, and the individual's objects of significance. For example, from a process point of view, the failure to take appropriate action in a situation that calls for direct action is problematic. The woman who decides to ignore a lump in her breast is coping poorly, regardless of whether the lump turns out to be malignant. The individual who persists in efforts to solve an insolvable problem is engaged in a very different, but equally dysfunctional, form of coping.

An evaluation of coping should also consider the ends of significance the individual is striving toward. It is not the case that one destination is better or worse for all people. Problems in coping can arise, however, when there is a loss of balance in the various goals that contribute to an individual's pattern of significance. The single-minded devotion to any end can become problematic when that end is defined narrowly or when it is unbalanced by other objects of significance (James, 1902; May, 1970). The desire for intimacy unopposed by the need for autonomy can lead to the most desperate kind of dependency. Dedication to the pain-free life can ultimately paralyze because the only way to avoid pain completely is to avoid living. The search for meaning alone can turn into obsession.

Finally, it is important to consider the degree of fit between individual and social system in coping. Social systems, like individuals, have their own viewpoints about the most appropriate goals in life and the best ways to reach them. When coping is going well, people may be unaware that they are in fact being supported and nurtured by their families, friends, and institutions. There are times, however, when individual and system experience "coping conflict," when the person's needs clash with what the social system is willing to provide, as in the case of the abused wife who receives little support from her family when she talks about leaving. These problems of individual–systems fit can be all the more troubling when neither individual nor system is willing to tolerate or work through their differences with each other.

The process approach does not suggest that there is a single best way for everyone to cope. But it does not assume that all ways of coping are equally worthwhile either. Instead, effective coping is defined by the degree to which the various elements of the coping process are well integrated and flow smoothly. There are, from this perspective, many effective ways of coping (and many ineffective ways as well).

Although I have reviewed the outcomes and process approach to evaluating coping separately, the two are not rivals. Each adds an important perspective, and in many instances the two approaches will converge. After all, effective processes of coping should lead to better outcomes. Indeed, several studies have shown that coping strategies better suited to the demands of a stressful situation are more likely to result in positive outcomes (e.g., Vitaliano, DeWolfe, Maiuro, Russo, & Katon, 1990). In short, both outcomes and process approaches offer important insights into the coping process. We will draw on both of these traditions in our evaluation of the roles of religion in coping later in the book.

CONCLUSIONS

This chapter has focused on the nature of coping as a process. Rather than picking apart the pieces of this process, I have tried to capture something of its flow through a discussion of several underlying assumptions about coping. Along the way, I have drawn on the impressive contributions of many theorists and researchers. But even though it is rooted in a tradition of thought and study, this description of the coping process has some distinctive points of emphasis:

1. The notion that coping is directed rather than simply driven underscores the proactive as well as reactive character of coping. People cope not only *with* stressful events, but *to* significance.

2. The view that people bring an orienting system to coping, one that includes resources and burdens, is another special emphasis.

3. The assumption that people struggle to maximize not only the ends of significance, but the means to significance, helps explain some of the subtleties and give-and-take that are so much a part of coping.

4. The idea that people have the potential not only to conserve the things they care about through coping, but to transform them as well, is another distinctive feature of this perspective. It accounts for the fundamental, sometimes dramatic, changes in values and way of life that can materialize through coping.

5. The recognition of the imperfect link between the methods and outcomes of coping underscores the need to evaluate coping processes as well as products. This process approach is especially relevant to mental health professionals and other helpers who are regularly involved in efforts to facilitate the flow of coping.

6. Finally, the emphasis on coping itself represents a shift from the large body of literature that has focused more on the character of stressful events than on how critical experiences

are constructed and handled. The process of interpreting and struggling with adversity, of whatever kind, may offer one of the clearest windows into human character—strengths, frailties, and all.

The distinctive features of this perspective on coping, I believe, make it particularly well suited to the study of religion. You will be able to judge this for yourself as we move along.

Having introduced the two key constructs of this book, religion and coping, I will now begin to put the two together.

Part Three

THE RELIGION AND COPING CONNECTION

Chapter Six

WHEN PEOPLE TURN TO RELIGION; WHEN THEY TURN AWAY

Although little was said about coping in the introduction to religion and little mention was made of religion in the introduction to coping, this is a book about the psychology of religion *and* coping. Why was so much time spent defining the two apart from each other? I do not believe that the relationship between religion and coping can be appreciated unless each concept is understood in its own right. By delineating the boundaries of the two concepts carefully, we reduce the risk of distorting either phenomenon or confusing one with the other.

Interestingly, one meaning of the term "cope" is an ecclesiastical garb. This definition hints at some important parallels between religion and coping. Neither religion nor coping is trivial. Each deals with matters of great value and importance in life. And each is concerned with the paths people take to reach significance as well as the nature of significance itself.

Though there are important similarities between religion and coping, they differ in a critical respect—their point of reference. The coping process is oriented to stressful life experiences; it may involve religious thoughts, practices, feelings, relationships, and objects of significance, but not necessarily. Religion, on the other hand, is oriented to the sacred; religion may be a part of those times when people are put to test, but it is not restricted to these times.

131

It must be emphasized that religion is not simply a way of coping. Mental health professionals and social scientists are particularly vulnerable to this misconception, for when notions of personality, mental health, and adjustment loom so large in one's worldview, religion is easily reduced to a small part of this world—one among many tools in the human armamentarium for solving problems. However, this is an unfortunate caricaturization of religion that ignores its other distinctive features (Geertz, 1966). Of course, religion can be fully involved in coping. But, more than that, it can provide an overarching framework for living, applicable to the widest range of human experience.

To put it another way, not all coping is religious, and not all religion is coping; neither process completely subsumes the other. The paths of religion and coping may never touch; they may overlap a great deal; or they may converge and diverge at different points in life.

In this chapter, I begin this exploration of the religion and coping connection. First, I take a critical look at the old adage, "there are no atheists in foxholes," and consider the extent of religious coping in stressful circumstances. I then focus more closely on some of the factors that determine when religion and coping converge. Working from coping theory, I examine the reasons why religion is involved in coping. I conclude the chapter by taking a look at the flip side of the coin—why some people turn away from religion in hard times.

ARE THERE REALLY NO ATHEISTS IN FOXHOLES?

Religion, crisis, and coping seem to have a particular affinity for each other. We find this notion embedded in old sayings and aphorisms. "Man's extremity is God's opportunity" (James, 1902, p. 206). "There are no atheists in foxholes." Or one of my favorites: "Dear God, help me get up. I can fall down by myself" (Rosten, 1972, p. 250). How true is our folk wisdom?

Some Anecdotal Accounts

Support for these old sayings can be found in some striking accounts of critical moments in life. Listen to this description of the crisis of meaning experienced by Leo Tolstoy in midlife:

> During the whole course of this year, when I almost unceasingly kept asking myself how to end the business, whether by the rope or by the

bullet, during all that time, alongside of all those movements of my ideas and observations, my heart kept languishing with another pining emotion. I can call this by no other name than that of a thirst for God. This craving for God had nothing to do with the movement of my ideas—in fact, it was the direct contrary of that movement—but it came from my heart. (James, 1902, p. 153)

Consider the nation's mood and response on the day before the invasion of Normandy in World War II:

The whole country knew on June 6 that something dire, something that might fail, was taking place . . . in a Brooklyn shipyard, welders knelt on the decks of their Liberty ships and recited the Lord's prayer. At the opening, the New York Stock Exchange observed two minutes of silent prayer. All over America church bells tolled, and the Liberty Bell was rung in Philadelphia. In Columbus, Ohio at 7:30 in the evening, all traffic stopped for five minutes while people prayed in the streets. (Fussell, 1994, p. 37)

Crisis and coping play a critical role in the life stories of the most prominent religious figures themselves. Siddhartha Gautama embarks on the path to become world redeemer (and Buddha) rather than world conqueror after he encounters three shattering Sights: the sight of an old man bent and broken with old age (decrepitude), the sight of a disease-riddled body (sickness), and the sight of a corpse (death). The teachings of Confucius, with their emphasis on a social and cosmic order, develop out of a time of social anarchy when warring armies massacre populations in the tens of thousands. God's eternal covenant with Abraham and his children grows out of crisis and coping—the divine command to sacrifice Abraham's only son, Isaac, and Abraham's willingness to respond with faith and fidelity. It is an ultimate crisis, the Crucifixion of Jesus Christ, which sets the stage for his triumphant resurrection. The revelations of Muhammad take place against the backdrop of a brawling chaotic society as well as the tragic deaths of his parents in childhood. From Isaiah, Paul, Saint Augustine, and Luther to George Fox, John Wesley, Mary Baker Eddy, and Malcolm X, the experiences and insights of pivotal religious figures have been tied to periods of personal and social upheaval and oppression.

In short, vivid anecdotal reports and narrative accounts of the lives of religious leaders suggest a strong connection between religion and times of trouble (for other examples see Koenig, 1994). But just how strong is this relationship?

Some Contrasting Anecdotal Accounts

In spite of the common lore that religion is invariably a part of life's most difficult moments, it is not hard to find descriptions of people in crisis yet uninvolved in religion. Some come to crisis with little in the way of religious feeling and remain that way throughout their trials. In the midst of his struggle with leukemia, columnist Stewart Alsop wrote: "I wish I could say that this strange experience with leukemia has given me profound spiritual insights. But it hasn't. The big bearded reality of my childhood is no longer a reality to me. . . . I have been an agnostic since I was about eighteen. I am an agnostic still" (cited in Fichter, 1981, p. 56). A survivor of the concentration camp at Buchenwald states: "I never believed in God. Not before the Holocaust, not during my stay in the camps and not afterwards. I didn't need the Holocaust as proof of God's nonexistence. I was never in doubt that He didn't exist" (Brenner, 1980, p. 96).

Others may bring a background of religious beliefs, practices, and feelings to their difficult times, and yet, in the midst of trouble, turn to other resources or find that their faith is no longer there for them. Reviewing his 25 years of practice as a physician, Covalt (1960) notes: "I recall no person who called out to God or audibly prayed when he knew he was dying. Usually, these persons are exerting every bit of energy in a struggle to keep alive. I do not believe my experiences are different from those of other physicians" (p. 663). One survivor of several concentration camps recalls:

> I used to have a very personal intimate relationship with God. I thought everything I did and every move I made God knew and was right there. . . . He'd be there just above me, watching and admonishing and saying "tut-tut-tut" about those inner thoughts I might have. . . . Then the Nazis came, and where did He go? God was no longer near me. Disappeared. And I am no longer the person I was. (Brenner, 1980, pp. 67–68)

If there is a relation between religion, coping, and crisis, as the first set of anecdotal accounts imply, these latter vignettes suggest it is far from perfect. Apparently, for some, religion was never an important part of life and a crisis does not change this basic fact. For others, religion was a part of their orienting system, yet strangely, in times of stress, it was uninvolved in the process of coping.

Before we try to draw too many conclusions, it is important to note there are problems with these kinds of anecdotal accounts, powerful as they are. They are based on the individual experience, which may be atypical; they do not speak to the question of whether people generally turn to religion as a way of coping in crisis. Empirical studies become more relevant here.

Empirical Perspectives

How do we evaluate the extent of religious coping? On the face of it, this would seem to be a fairly straightforward question with a fairly easy answer. Simply look at the numbers of people who turn to religion to cope with crisis. Like so many seemingly simple questions, however, the answer becomes more complicated when we take a closer look. Studies of the prevalence of religious coping provide necessary baseline information, but they are difficult to *evaluate*. At what point would we say that religion is an *important* part of coping—if 30% turn to religion, 50%, 80%? Two additional points of comparison are needed. First, do people make more use of religion in difficult circumstances than they do other ways of coping? It would also be important to know whether people are more likely to turn to religion in times of crisis than in other times of life. Perhaps those who involve religion in more difficult times involve religion in the daily frustrations of living as well. To say that they turned to religion in crisis without saying that religion was a part of their lives more generally would paint a misleading picture of their faith. In this chapter, these strands of empirical study are reviewed: the prevalence of religious coping, comparisons of religious versus nonreligious approaches to coping, and comparisons of the extent of religious coping in more versus less stressful situations.

Four points should be kept in mind when reviewing this research literature. First, we are summarizing the findings of very different studies. They cover diverse populations, facing a variety of difficult situations. They also measure religious coping in various ways—from elaborate scales of different types of religious coping to a few brief items about the overall use of religious coping. To simplify our task here at least a bit, we will postpone a finer grain analysis of subtypes of religious coping methods until later.

Second, because much of religious coping is a private experience, it is almost always measured through individual *self-reports*. These self-reports can be biased (although some researchers have tried to control for these potential biases).

Third, these studies focus on the extent of religious coping, not the question of the outcomes of religious coping. Studies of the helpfulness of religion in coping will be considered in a later chapter. For example, even though often cited in the literature to underscore the religion and coping connection, the classic studies of American soldiers in combat in World War II by Stouffer and his colleagues (1965) have not been included in this section. Their results are based on a question that deals more with the efficacy of religious coping than the prevalence of religious coping. Stouffer et al. asked their participants: "When the going was tough, how much did prayer help you?" (p. 174) rather than "When the going was tough, did you pray?" Of course many, if not most, people who turn to religion in stressful situations may find it helpful. However, we will see in subsequent chapters that religious coping may have many outcomes, negative as well as positive.

Finally, it is also important to distinguish the central question here, the extent to which people involve religion in coping, from another important question: whether stressful situations produce profound, long-lasting changes in the individual's general religious approach to life. This latter question will also be considered in a later chapter. The studies that will be reviewed focus on measures of religious coping in stressful circumstances, not measures of religion as a dispositional process (e.g., average frequency of church attendance or prayer, religious orientation).

The Prevalence of Religious Coping

Several investigators have reported the proportions of people who involve religion in coping with stressful experiences. The results of these studies are summarized in Appendix A. Perhaps the most striking finding is the wide range in prevalence of religious coping reported across the different studies. Some investigators such as Conway (1985–1986), Gilbert (1989), Greil, Porter, Leitko, and Riscilli (1989), and Pargament, Ensing, et al. (1990) find that religion is used in coping by the large majority of their participants, with figures reaching as high as 91%. Others, such as Bowker (1988), Gurin, Veroff, and Feld (1960), and LaGrand (1985) indicate that only a minority of participants, from 4% to 35%, reportedly made use of religion in dealing with their stressful events.

How can these wide differences be explained? They may be partly attributable to the differences in methodologies of these studies. For instance, the relatively small percentage of people who report religious involvement in coping in the Gurin et al. (1960) study likely reflects their stringent method of measurement; they counted only those who mentioned religion as their first spontaneous response to the question of how they handle their worries. Higher percentages are reported in studies that assess religious coping by checklists or surveys than in studies that measure religious coping by open-ended questions. Which method of measurement provides the more accurate estimate is unclear. Surveys and checklists may elicit biased responses from their participants, who present themselves as more religious than they actually are. Open-ended approaches are subject to other problems, such as the willingness of people to talk spontaneously about topics as sensitive as religion.

Important as these methodological issues are, the wide range in prevalence of religious coping reported in these studies and samples may reflect a more basic point—that *religious coping is, in fact, variable.* Some of the studies in Appendix A hint that this may be the case. For example, whereas 78% of a sample of congregation members indicated that they turned to religion for understanding and/or dealing with a serious negative event (Pargament, Ensing, et al., 1990), only 58% of a community sample responded in the same way to the identical question (Wicks, 1990). Similarly, 92% of Egyptian patients with cancer voiced a belief that God will help them, in contrast to only 37% of the Swiss patients faced with the same disease (Kesselring et al., 1986). Furthermore, in scanning the Appendix, the prevalence of some kinds of religious coping appears to be lower than other kinds.

So what can we conclude from this literature? Two contrasting points stand out. There are substantial numbers of people who appear to involve religion in critical times of life. For some groups of people faced with some difficult situations, religion is commonly called on in coping. But the converse seems just as true. Many people apparently deal with crises in their lives without turning to religion. In sum, the data provide little support for the belief that religion is no longer an important part of contemporary life. However, they also provide as little support for the common lore that "there are no atheists in foxholes."

Religious versus Nonreligious Coping

"To find religion is only one out of many ways of reaching unity" (James, 1902, p. 172). Stressful situations may mobilize many coping responses, nonreligious as well as religious. In evaluating the religion and coping connection, it is only logical to ask whether religion takes on an especially prominent role in coping in comparison to other coping strategies or whether it is simply one of a number of approaches people use to grapple with difficult situations.

A number of studies have compared the frequencies of religious and nonreligious forms of coping and found that religion looms large. For example, McCrae (1984) studied the coping mechanisms reportedly used by a community sample of men and women faced with events categorized as losses, threats, or challenges. Of the 28 coping mechanisms, "faith" was the second most frequently used for dealing with threats (72%), and the third most frequently used for dealing with losses (75%). Faith was less frequently used in coping with challenges (43%). Conway (1985–1986) interviewed black and white urban elderly women who had experienced stressful medical problems in the past year. Asked how they coped with their medical problems, prayer was selected by 91% of the sample; it was the most frequently reported of all coping mechanisms including seeking information, resting, treatment, prescription drugs, and going to a doctor. Segall and Wykle (1988–1989) studied black primary caregivers of family members with dementia. They were asked, "If you had to identify one special way that you've used to deal with caring for your confused relative, what would that be?" By far the most common response was a religious one, involving prayer or faith in God. Religious responses were mentioned by 65% of the group. Bulman and Wortman (1977) asked people paralyzed in severe accidents how they explained their misfortune. The notion that God had a reason for the accident was the most common of all answers to the question "Why me?" Other researchers have also reported religious coping methods to be among the most common, if not the most common, ways of coping with the stresses of physical illness (Baldree, Murphy, & Powers, 1982; Jalowiec & Powers, 1981; Thompson, Sobolew-Shubin, Galbraith, Schwankovsky, & Cruzen, 1993), a disabled child (Leyser, 1994), and the incarceration of a spouse (Carlson & Cervera, 1991).

A few studies, however, have yielded different results. In their classic investigation of how Americans view their mental health, Gurin et al. (1960) found that prayer was cited less often as a first response to worries (16%) than "passive reactions," such as denial or doing nothing (34%), or "coping reactions," such as seeking help or doing something about the situation (44%). Compas, Forsythe, and Wagner (1988) studied the percentages of college students who made use of eight strategies for dealing with academic and interpersonal stressful events over a 4-week period. The religious coping strategy ("sought or found spiritual comfort and support") was the method least frequently reported by students for both the academic event (29%) and the interpersonal event (21%).

As with the studies on the prevalence of religious coping, there is some variability in the results of these comparative studies. Judged against the yardstick of other coping methods, religion, in some instances, seems to play a larger role in the coping process. In other cases, however, religious coping appears to recede in comparative importance.

Religious Coping in More Stressful versus Less Stressful Situations

Philosopher Abraham Joshua Heschel (1986) wrote: "To pray is to take notice of the wonder, to regain a sense of the mystery that animates all beings, the divine margin in all attainments" (p. 205). For Heschel and others, faith is not limited to those times of greatest pain and suffering; it is as applicable to the daily experience of living as it is to moments of upheaval. To the extent that people live by this all-encompassing faith, we would expect comparable levels of religious involvement across a wide range of situations, the everyday as well as the momentous, the less significant as well as the more serious, and the positive as well as the negative.

On the other hand, many have maintained that religion is mobilized in crisis. As psychologist Paul Johnson (1959) put it: "When the values of life are at stake, there is reason to be earnest. In times of crisis religion usually comes to the foreground. The more urgent the need the more men seek for a response" (p. 82). This latter perspective suggests that we will find more signs of religious life in crisis than in other circumstances. Once again we turn to the empirical literature for some clarification.

There is a great deal of evidence to show that religious involvement is not confined to stressful periods of life. For example, in a national survey of Americans, McReady and Greeley (1976) found that mystical experiences were relatively commonplace. When asked what triggered this type of mystical ecstasy, the participants noted many contributing factors: listening to music, prayer, the beauties of nature, a moment of quiet reflection, religious services, or watching little children. Missing from this list were stressful experiences.

Similarly, Bergin and his colleagues conducted an intensive study of the religious lives and experiences of 60 members of the Church of Jesus Christ of Latter-Day Saints at Brigham Young University (Bergin, Stinchfield, Gaskin, Masters, & Sullivan, 1988). Their research methods included interviews, group discussions, and questionnaires. Forty-four of the 60 participants described a "continuous" form of religious development, without sharp ups and downs or any apparent connection to difficult life experiences. Only seven participants reported a "discontinuous–compensating" pattern of religious development, that is, one characterized by fluctuations and a response to traumas and deficiencies in life.

It is difficult to imagine that the significant proportion of people who, for so many years, pray daily and attend their congregation weekly are responding to an unending series of crises in their lives (Gallup & Castelli, 1989). Data such as these suggest that many of the rituals, beliefs, interactions, and feelings that make up religious life have no immediate connection to stressful events. Religious experience is not reserved for the painful times of life alone; neither is religion simply a way of coping. But if it is not *exclusively* a way of dealing with stress, the question remains whether religion is expressed more in difficult moments than in less serious ones.

Several investigators have looked into this question. Welford (1947), for instance, was interested in whether people pray to release emotional tension or out of frustration with difficult situations. Protestant university or seminary students were presented with six vignettes describing unpleasant and pleasant scenarios such as a grave illness, the loss of a job, and a satisfying walk on a spring day. The participants ranked each of the vignettes according to the degree that it "stirred their emotions" (affective arousal), was beyond their ability to deal with (frustration), and elicited a desire for prayer. Welford found that both affective arousal and frustration were associated with a greater likelihood of prayer. One of his participants commented: "Things that are ordinary require less praying than situations when emergencies arise." Another noted: "I would feel most like praying in the hour of death because I believe that only prayer can carry you through such a time" (p. 317). Prayer, Welford concluded, is a response to both emotional tension and frustration, a response more common to unusual rather than everyday situations, particularly those in which human action is unlikely to be effective.

Welford's study pointed to the importance of arousal as well as frustration in prayer. However, he did not examine whether prayer was more likely in negative emotional than in positive emotional situations. Hahn and I (Pargament & Hahn, 1986) conducted a study that touched on this issue. We looked at religious coping in response to four types of health-related scenarios: (1) responsible behavior followed by a positive outcome (e.g., good personal health care leading to a positive physical examination); (2) responsible behavior followed by a negative outcome (e.g., a case of pneumonia in spite of good personal health care); (3) irresponsible behavior followed by a positive outcome (e.g., reckless driving after drinking at a party does not lead to an accident); and (4) irresponsible behavior followed by a negative outcome (e.g., reckless driving after drinking at a party leads to an accident). After reading samples of these scenarios, college students were asked several questions about how likely they would be to turn to God or their religious beliefs in dealing with each event. Several results were possible. The students could have involved religion more in unjust situations (responsible behavior–negative outcome, irresponsible behavior–positive outcome) than in just situations (responsible behavior–positive outcome, irresponsible behavior–negative outcome). The students could have looked to religion more in coping in response to their irresponsible behavior than in response to responsible behavior, regardless of whether the outcome of their behavior was positive or negative. The students could have turned to religion more in negative outcome than in positive outcome situations, irrespective of how they acted in the situations. Finally, they could have involved religion to the same degree across the four types of situations. Our analyses indicated that the students turned to religion more for the negative outcome events than for the positive outcome events, regardless of how responsibly they had behaved. For them religion generally served more as a source of support for difficult times than as an antidote to an unjust world, as a moral guide, or as an object of gratitude for happy occasions.

Bjorck and Cohen (1993) also found higher levels of anticipated religious coping by college students in response to hypothetical scenarios involving threat (e.g., getting caught in a storm at sea without a life jacket) and loss (e.g., getting laid off from a job) than in scenarios involving more positive challenge (e.g., an opportunity for a scholarship). In addition, religious coping was elicited more by the threat vignettes than by the loss vignettes, suggesting that fear and uncertainty are elements of stress with particularly important implications for religious coping. These results were largely replicated in a study of a more ethnoculturally diverse sample (Bjorck & Klewicki, in press).

An important question can be raised about studies of coping that involve hypothetical situations (including our own). How well do responses to imagined situations reflect what people *really do* in hard times? Some research has compared levels of religious coping among people actually faced with more stressful and less formidable circumstances. In a study of adults who had experienced a variety of life events over the past year, prayer was mentioned more often as a response to severe situations such as health crises and catastrophes than as a response to less serious problems such as job-related concerns (Lindenthal, Myers, Pepper, & Stern, 1970). Poggie, Pollnac, and Gersuny (1976) interviewed fisherman from southern New England about the role of rituals and taboos in their work. They found that fishermen engaged in more religious-like rituals and respected more taboos prior to longer fishing trips than shorter ones, and suggest that these behaviors are a response to the danger and anxiety surrounding the longer excursions. In the Project on Religion and Coping (Pargament, Olsen, et al., 1992a), my colleagues and I asked members of midwestern churches to describe the most significant negative event they had experienced over the past year. They then appraised this event along several dimensions, and noted the extent to which they turned to religion in an effort to understand and deal with the event. The members were more likely to turn to religion in coping when the event was appraised as harmful, unmanageable, a threat to their well-being, a threat to the well-being of others, and a challenge. Finally, Bearon and Koenig (1990) asked elderly adults living in the community what could be done to make their physical symptoms "go away or be less troublesome." The participants appeared to reserve their prayers for particular kinds of symptoms. One woman who prayed about pain and swelling in her joints, but not her bunions, said: "I don't think God wants to hear about my bunions. I think he's got more important things to think about like AIDS and the Persian Gulf" (p. 252). The most serious symptoms—heart palpitations, shortness of breath, and forgetfulness—were "universally prayed over."

Taken as a group, these studies provide clear signs of heightened religious activity in particularly difficult circumstances. This is not to say religion is uninvolved in less stressful times. Many people also report religious coping with daily hassles and frustrations (see Belavich & Pargament, 1995; Hathaway, 1992) In general, however, people appear to involve religion to a greater extent in more stressful than in less stressful moments of life. Does this signify a fundamental change in religious orientation? For some, but not most. We will see later in the book that the majority of people come through crisis with their basic religious beliefs and practices intact. The methods of religious coping that are mobilized in crisis are capable of conserving not only the individual's psychological and social world, but the religious world as well.

Conclusions

Anecdotes, life stories, and empirical studies alike underscore the connection between religion and life's greatest trials. But the connection is neither simple nor straightforward. Religion is more than a way of coping with stress. It is potentially relevant to the full range of human experience, not merely the negative. Yet we find unmistakable signs of religious coping as the seriousness of situations rises. Does this general finding apply equally to all people or all situations? Clearly it does not. For some groups and some encounters, religion is a common part of coping with crisis, one called into play as often or more often than many other approaches. For other people and other problems, religion seems relatively uninvolved, more a part of the background than the foreground of coping.

Old sayings about atheists and foxholes are inaccurate because they oversimplify the rich and varied ways people come to grips with critical events. The evidence reviewed here says that the story is more complicated. The answer to the question of whether people turn to religion in coping is both "yes" and "no," or, even better, "it depends." The better questions may be: Who turns to religion in coping, in what situations, and where?

WHEN RELIGION AND COPING CONVERGE

In an important theoretical paper in 1985, Spilka, Shaver, and Kirkpatrick made the point that religious attributions are far from random. Whether an event is understood and interpreted from a religious framework or a nonreligious framework, they said, will depend on three considerations: the nature of the person, the nature of the event, and the nature of the context surrounding both the person and the situation. The Spilka, Shaver, and Kirkpatrick framework seems very appropriate to coping.

Appendix B reviews empirical studies that attempt to describe the "who's, when's, and where's" of coping. Following Spilka et al. (1985) the studies are organized according to three broad dimensions: personal, situational, and contextual. Keep in mind that this literature focuses on predictors of religious coping rather than predictors of general religious beliefs, practices and orientations not explicitly related to stressful life experiences. Once again, studies that deal with the helpfulness of religious coping have been excluded from this table.

The studies in Appendix B cover a broad range of variables, populations, and methods. As a group, they indicate that religious coping is not a random affair. We are more likely to find it in some people, in some situations, and in some social contexts than in others:

1. At the *personal level*, a consistent finding is one of greater religious coping among those who are more religiously committed and involved. Studies also suggest that religious coping is more common among blacks, poorer people, the elderly, women, and those who are more troubled. (Many of these groups also show higher levels of general religious commitment).

2. At the *situational level*, Appendix B presents additional evidence in support of the point made in the previous section: Religious coping is more common in situations that are more threatening, serious, and harmful than in other situations. The exception to this general rule comes from studies of religious attribution; here we find that people are less likely to see God as the cause of negative events than positive events. Why this might be the case will be discussed later.

3. Finally, at the *contextual level* the evidence is a bit more meager. Relatively few studies have considered the impact of the social context on religious coping. What evidence is available, though, suggests that religious coping is greater within certain congregations, and cultures, and among those more involved in their religious contexts.

Of course, not all of these results are clear or consistent. Several findings need to be replicated. There may be many other potential predictors of religious coping, particularly at the contextual level, that have not been examined as yet. Further, I have glossed over potentially important distinctions among *kinds* of religious coping. Nevertheless, the evidence at hand makes an important point: In order to understand when the paths of religion and coping are most likely to converge, we have to know something about the person, the situation, and the social context.

This discussion of the who's, when's, and where's of religious coping has been largely descriptive. It leaves one further question, perhaps the most interesting one, unanswered. Why do some people turn to religion in coping in some times and in some places?

WHY RELIGION AND COPING CONVERGE

To answer this question and make more sense of the studies in Appendix B, let us go back to the theory of coping. This perspective points to two reasons why religion becomes involved in coping: because it is a *relatively available* part of the orienting system, and because it is a *relatively compelling* way of coping.

The Availability of Religion in the Orienting System

The notion of people "turning to religion" has come up several times in this chapter; it may be misleading to the extent it suggests that religion is merely a reaction to stressful events. Recall one of the key assumptions of coping: People bring an orienting system to the coping process. A religious orientation (e.g., religious beliefs, practices, feelings, and relationships) is one part of this larger orienting system. How large a part it is varies greatly from person to person. But as an element of the orienting system, religion can be said to *precede* crises, structuring the way critical situations are anticipated, interpreted, and handled.

Religion is more likely to be accessed in coping when it is more *available* to the individual, that is, when it is a larger part of the individual's orienting system for relating to the world. Several studies in Appendix B illustrate this point nicely. Let us take a closer look at a few examples.

Ritzema (1979) predicted that more religious people would be more likely to attribute the causes of the events in their lives to supernatural forces. Consistent with his prediction, people who attributed life events to divine intervention reported more orthodox religious beliefs, more frequent prayer, feelings of greater closeness to God, and greater importance of religious thoughts and feelings. We found similar results in the Project on Religion and Coping (Pargament, Olsen, et al., 1992a). Congregation members who involved religion in coping were more religious in several ways. They prayed and attended church more frequently; they reported closer feelings to God and more loving images of the deity; and they espoused greater religious commitment and orthodoxy. Johnson and Spilka (1991) illustrate the same point. They studied the role of religion in coping with breast cancer in a sample of women in the Reach to Recovery program. An intrinsic commitment to religion was associated with, among other variables, several specific religious coping activities, including praying with a minister, believing that God had a role in the cancer, and believing that God has control over the outcome of the cancer.

Generally, we cope with the tools that are most available to us. As these studies show, religion is a more accessible tool for those who make religious beliefs, feelings, practices, and relationships a part of their orienting system. These are the people who are most likely to translate their religious commitment into action in particular situations. Why? Perhaps, in part, because the more religion is embedded in the guiding framework for living, the more quickly and easily it can be accessed in coping. Spencer and McIntosh (1990) conducted a study relevant to this point, although it did not focus directly on the coping process. They presented their college students with a number of religious and nonreligious adjectives on a computer monitor, and asked them to indicate whether the adjectives were descriptive of themselves. They then compared the speed of response of those who defined religion as a central part of their lives with those whose religion was less extreme or important. While the groups did not differ in their processing speed for the nonreligious adjectives, the more religiously involved participants responded more quickly to the religious adjectives than the other participants. The Spencer and McIntosh study underscores how our orienting systems sensitize us to particular kinds of information (see also Hill, 1994). When religion becomes a part of that system, information relevant to the religious perspective is processed more efficiently.

Availability as a Relative Construct

Religion is only one part of the orienting system. Other resources may be more prominent and easier to access. To know when religion and coping will converge, the availability of religious resources must be compared to the availability of alternatives. For those with limited means and few alternatives, religion can take on even greater power as one of the few genuine resources for living. Perhaps this is one reason why we see religious involvement in coping more evident among members of less powerful groups in society—blacks, women, the elderly, the poor, and more troubled people.

Moore (1992), for example, details the emergence of the black church as one of the only resources available to black people in their fight against racism and their struggle for dignity. While Africans were separated from their culture, customs, and heritage of worship, their beliefs in the harmony of the physical and spiritual world could not be erased so quickly. The ambivalence of white society to religion among the slaves provided a "crack in the door" for the reemergence of an organized spiritual life. Meetings among slaves took place covertly in cabins or in open fields' "hush harbors" to avoid the retribution of slave owners who feared they were plotting for their freedom. Here, people could express their feelings, their solidarity and identity as a community, and their need for spiritual renewal. After the Civil War, organized religion continued to play a pivotal role in the black community. Independent black churches offered one of the only responses to oppression and one of the only avenues to greater power and control. For instance, the Sanctified Church developed an effective response to the patronizing custom by whites of calling black adults by their first names. In public forums and interracial situations, members of the church referred to each other only by their last name. Today, black churches, Moore maintains, remain among the most central resources for their members—symbols of strength and hope, launching pads for social change and political leadership, and sources of material, personal, and spiritual power.

On the other hand, religion may be less involved in coping for some with greater nonreligious resources, particularly those whose faith is only one compartmentalized element of their orienting systems. Virtually all religious groups at least implicitly recognize the "relative" nature of availability and do what they can to increase the prominence of religion within their members' orienting systems. Fundamental shifts from matters of day-to-day living to concerns of a spiritual nature are promoted. Religious faith and practice is encouraged as less a part of life than as a way of life. Relationships among people within the faith community are fostered, while involvement with "outsiders" can be discouraged. Religious interpretations of suffering, pain, and injustice are endorsed.

For example, Fazel (1987) describes how Shi'ah clergy and institutions in Iran strengthened the commitment of the Iranian people to the Iran–Iraq war in the 1980s by framing the conflict in the context of a religious narrative central to the Shi'ah tradition: the story of the unjust persecution and martyrdom of Hussain, grandson and rightful successor to the Prophet Muhammad. Saddam of Iraq and his army were likened to Yazid and his supporters, the much reviled forces that had destroyed Hussain and enslaved his family. The conflict between the two countries was defined as a "war of ideological revenge . . . to redress wrongs wrought against Hussain thirteen centuries ago" (p. 21). The Ayatollah Khomeini's rise to power in Iran was also compared to the return of the Mahdi, the Prophet's rightful successor, who, according to Shi'āh tradition, would reemerge, fight evil, and return the world to Islamic purity. Fazel (1987) argues that the success of the Iranian leaders in defining the war in religious terms helps account for the willingness of so many young Iranians to sacrifice and martyr themselves in this bitter, protracted conflict. Interestingly, Saddam of Iraq also tried to frame the conflict favorably to the Sunni tradition of Islam, but his effort was less successful (Ajami, 1990/1991).

The relative availability of religion is shaped by personal, situational, and social factors. To the extent that religion becomes a larger and more integrated part of the orienting system, it takes on a greater role in coping. To the extent that religion becomes less prominent in the orienting system, more disconnected from other resources, and less relevant to the range of life experiences, it recedes in importance in coping.

Religious Coping Does Not Come Out of Nowhere

I have reviewed some evidence here that people are more likely to turn to religion in coping as it becomes a larger part of their orienting system, one that is more available to them than other resources. I hope it is clear by this point that the phrase "turning to religion in coping" does not refer to a spontaneous generation of religion out of a vacuum. The theory of spontaneous generation fails as much in the religious case as it does in the biological. Even when religion seemingly comes out of nowhere, a closer analysis often reveals evidence of religious availability.

A case in point was Tim, a 40-year-old, divorced father of two (Pargament, Royster, et al., 1990, pp. 6–7). Tim looked like a throwback to the 1960s: He wore long hair, a buckskin vest, and handcrafted jewelry. He described a rough childhood. The son of alcoholic parents, he suffered abuse and neglect when he was young. His parents divorced when he was a teenager, and Tim began taking drugs. He was a heavy user of marijuana and LSD for 4 years, and led a "wild life." At the same time, he became increasingly depressed and tried to kill himself. Talking about this time, he said: "I couldn't handle it anymore, and I didn't want to get high anymore, but I couldn't function any other way. . . . Just to get through the week of work, I would be stoned all of the time, and any time I could, I would be tripping." The critical moment for Tim came 1 week after he had tried to commit suicide. He was partying with friends and taking LSD. This time, however, Tim reported a conversion experience—one that turned his life around and moved him out of the drug culture.

At first glance, this story seems to suggest that crisis alone *creates* religion. After all, here we have the case of a young man at the end of his rope, desperately looking for some way to change his life. Religion seemingly emerged out of nowhere to help him get his life back together. Through the interview, however, it became clear that Tim did not come to this critical moment empty-handed, and his conversion did not grow out of a void. He brought with him a set of religious resources, burdens, and predispositions, and these factors played an important role in his experience. When younger, Tim attended Sunday School classes and reported spiritual feelings: "I have always believed that there is something greater than just us," he said. Tim also recalled many conversations with relatives and family about religion: "All my life I had heard about God from my growing up experience. My brother and his family are—I guess you would call them born-again believers. They go to church three or four times a week, and they would talk to me, and I would talk to them, so the information about God and salvation I knew and heard."

Each of these earlier experiences comes to the foreground in Tim's religious conversion. In the midst of tripping with his friends, Tim went to the bathroom and had the following experience:

> I'm thinking this is pretty cool, bathroom, you know, commode, tub.
> . . . And then I was looking in the mirror. And as I'm looking there,
> just as we are sitting here talking, I hear . . . somebody talking to me
> that has a lot of influence, a lot of pack, a lot of punch behind him,
> cause I responded like, OK God, what do you want? I was looking in
> the mirror and it says "All your life you have believed in me." And I
> say "yeah, I've believed in God." There are just too many things . . .
> that justify it for me. (p. 7)

Later in his experience, Tim taps into his memories of church and religious instruction as a child. In the middle of his conversion he reports:

> This scripture started to filter through my head, and I couldn't
> remember what it was. I couldn't identify it, as I can now. It was John
> 3:16, and it's just that I remember parts of it from when I was kid
> . . . "God loved the world so much that if you believe you will have
> everlasting life. . . . [this is] a neon, I can see it . . . that means that,
> for right now, I am living forever." And I said, "Wow, that's pretty
> cool!" (p. 7)

Tim also calls on his religious conversations with his brother in his conversion. Talking to God through the mirror, Tim hears God saying: "All of your life you have believed in my son, Jesus." Tim responds "Yeah. And this was information that I remember my brother telling me about."

The central point here is that Tim's religious response to crisis did not occur in a vacuum. He brought a system of resources, burdens, and prior experiences that affected his coping. A religious solution to Tim's situation was available to him all along, although he had not made use of it. Tim was not an atheist in a foxhole—he was a conversion waiting to happen. This is not to say that Tim's response to crisis was not creative. I believe it was, but his creative solution emerged from an orienting system of potential and possibility that he himself had a hand in building.

People look for some grounding in coping. What they turn to is an orienting system to help them make sense of and deal with the world, an orienting system that includes, to a greater or lesser extent, religion. One reason why people involve religion in coping, then, is that it is available to them. But if we were to stop here this account would be incomplete, leaving the distorted impression that people cope through religion as simply a matter of convenience. Availability, convenience, and accessibility are important factors, but they are not the only reason why people cope in religious ways. The other reason is hinted at in the case of Tim. He did not respond to his encounter with God neutrally. It was an "a-ha" experience. Religion was more than available to Tim, it was compelling.

The Compelling Character of Religious Coping Methods

Geertz (1966) had this to say about religious experience: "It alters, often radically, the whole landscape presented to common sense, alters it in such a way that the moods and motivations induced by religious practice seem themselves supremely practical, the only sensible ones to adopt given the way things 'really' are" (p. 38). His words apply well to Tim whose newly found faith gave him not so much a new frame of reference, but a powerfully convincing experience of the world as it is. Not only that, it offered a compelling solution to the seemingly insolvable problems that blocked his search for significance. Tim had "hit bottom." Other efforts to build a more satisfying life had failed. Hopeless and depressed, he had little to lose and much to gain by attempting a radical change. However, Tim's transformation was not the result of a coldly analytical decision. His solution made sense, but it also felt right. This, in a nutshell, captures the meaning of a *compelling* solution. The term has an emotional as well as a cognitive connotation. It has as much to do with feelings as it does beliefs. Moreover, it embodies both the reactive and active characters so much a part of religious experience. To paraphrase Martin Buber (1951), Tim felt possessed by the power of God. He felt compelled. But at some level Tim also *chose* to give himself to this experience. He selected a way of coping he believed would maximize significance at minimal cost.

Not everyone in Tim's position would make the same decisions. Tertiary appraisals, the judgments that go into the determination of a compelling solution, are subjective and individualized. For this reason, while they may make sense and feel right to the individual, they are not always quite so compelling to the distant observer. Indeed, some religious choices may seem downright "crazy." They become more under-standable, however, when we move closer to the individual's world. One classic eyewitness account of a religious cult that predicted the end of the earth provides a vivid illustration of this point.

Compelling Coping in a Doomsday Cult

Festinger, Riecken, and Schachter (1956) describe a group of people who became convinced that the world was about to experience a physical cataclysm, a flood in which "Egypt would be remade and the desert would become a fertile valley . . . the 'uprising Atlantic bottom' would 'submerge the land of the Atlantic seaboard'; France would sink to the bottom of the Atlantic, as would England; and Russia would become one great sea" (p. 57). However, through the help of the Guardians, beings from outer space who try to foster the spiritual growth of humankind, the members of the group were to be spared.

> [Group members] would presumably survive the flood and remain on the earth until Christmas of the following year when they would be taken, bodily as well as spiritually, to Clarion, Venus or some other planet. There they would be spiritually indoctrinated, preparatory to being sent back to the earth, a cleansed and innocent earth, to repopulate it with good people who "walked in the Light." (p. 62)

Even after the date for the cataclysm came and went without incident, many group members remained strongly committed to the group and its beliefs.

From an external point of view, the behavior of the members appears to be difficult to decipher at best. After all, worldwide cata-clysms do not happen everyday. Why join a group that espouses such unusual beliefs? Why go out on a limb and make such a terrible prediction? Still more puzzling, why did group members cling so strongly to their beliefs after the prediction had been clearly disconfirmed?

First, it is important to understand something of the coping histories of the group members. The reasons the members became involved in the group were of less interest to Festinger et al. than the reasons they remained committed to it after its failed prediction, so the authors provide only brief descriptions of members' lives prior to their involvement in the cult. Apparently, however, many had tried other solutions to their problems, only to find them unsatisfying or ineffective. One woman, Daisy, had been troubled by terrifying nightmares and fantasies of loved ones stabbed, cut, and dismembered. Attempts to eliminate her obsessions through support from her husband, changes in her daily activities, a vacation, willpower, and prayer had failed. Another woman, Bertha, had struggled with infertility in her marriage of 20 years. She had become disillusioned with the Roman Catholic church, and had drifted from job to job until she became a beautician. For both of these women as well as their fellow group members, involvement in the beliefs and practices of the cult provided a way to achieve significance of various kinds: a sense of hope for the future, feelings of worth and importance, a sense of meaning in life, or feelings of spiritual connectedness. Daisy, for instance, came to believe that her nightmares and anxieties were the result of her "blindness and unreceptivity" to the efforts of the Guardians to "get light through to her" (p. 42). Bertha, in turn, experienced the joys of a pseudopregnancy through the group, proclaiming at one point that she was about to give birth to Christ.

To understand the group's coping behavior, it is also important to appreciate what it would have meant for the members to disavow their positions. Several had given up jobs, moved, and suffered the ridicule of family and friends to become a part of the group. To leave the group would have resulted in a heavy loss in their investment. As one member put it, "I have to believe the flood is coming on the 21st because I've spent nearly all my money. I quit my job, I quit comptometer school, and my apartment costs me $100 a month. I have to believe" (p. 80). A change of heart would have also meant a loss of support from the group, whose existence was dependent upon member commitment to their particular worldview. In fact, Festinger and his colleagues note that the members who were less integrated into the group were less likely than the others to maintain their beliefs after the prophecy failed.

But what about the costs of adherence to these unusual beliefs? The spaceship failed to appear on December 21, contrary to the group's prediction. That fact could not be denied, and clearly this failure was disturbing to many members of the group. However, they were able to partially reduce the dissonance it created through rationalizations—the group had misinterpreted the plan, the cataclysm had been postponed to a new date, or God had delivered the Earth from disaster because of the activities of the group. The costs were further reduced through their efforts to convince others of the truth of their beliefs. "If more and more people can be persuaded that the system of beliefs is correct, then clearly it must, after all, be correct" (p. 28). Thus, after December 21, the group lifted the veil of secrecy that had covered much of its activities, sought out publicity, and began efforts to personally proselytize others.

One member of the group, a physician, was exceptionally articulate in the description of his own tertiary appraisal process—his weighing of the pros and cons of continued commitment to the tenets of the group after its prophecies failed:

> I've given up just about everything. I've cut every tie: I've burned every bridge. I've turned my back on the world. I can't afford to doubt. I have to believe. And there isn't any other truth. The preachers and priests don't have it and you have to look closely to find it even in the Bible. I've taken an awful beating in the last few months, just an awful beating. But I do know who I am and I know what I've got to do. . . . These arc tough times and the way is not easy. We all have to take a beating. I've taken a terrific one, but I have no doubt. (p. 168)

What appears to be incomprehensible, even ludicrous, from the outside takes on a different character at closer range. Deemphasis of the empirical became part of a strategy designed to maximize significance. From an external perspective the cost of becoming part of such an outlandish group may seem inordinately high when compared to more "reasonable" ways of coping. But keep in mind that many of the members had gained little in the past from the so-called "tried and true" methods of problem solving. Moreover, the price of involvement in the group was diminished by the member's efforts to proselytize others and rationalize their beliefs to themselves. From their vantage point, the cost of a radical change back to more mainstream beliefs, relations, and practices was not worth the gain in realism and conformity. In this sense, the actions the members took were not irrational at all; they were steps taken to protect the ends of greatest significance to them. From their perspective, these steps were eminently reasonable. More than that, they were compelling.

As the Festinger et al. (1995) study suggests, the notion of a compelling activity is, like its twin contributor to religious coping, availability, a relative concept (also see Ritzema & Young, 1983). Through the tertiary appraisal process the most compelling solution is selected from the various possibilities. People cope religiously, in part, because religion offers more compelling solutions than the alternatives.

Admittedly, the example of the doomsday cult is not your everyday form of religious coping. But if seemingly incomprehensible religious experiences can be understood as attempts to maximize significance at minimal cost, the same point is likely to hold true for the more common methods of religious coping to be explored later. Some mental health professionals and social scientists have been too quick to dismiss religious beliefs and practices as "crazy" (also see Iannaccone, 1994). Viewed from the perspective of the individual, even "outlandish" forms of religious coping are not irrational at all; they are quite sensible.

It is important to add that compelling choices are not necessarily effective choices. Decisions that are completely reasonable within the individual's frame of reference can grow out of personal and social misconceptions. Moreover, these choices can have devastating consequences, as illustrated by the terrible loss of life in the Iran–Iraq war. To evaluate its effectiveness more completely, coping has to be gauged against both internal and external frames of reference. I will have more to say on this important issue in Chapters 10 and 11.

The Awareness of Human Limitations

What makes religion compelling as a way of coping with crisis? Let me suggest that religion is more compelling to those who are more acutely aware of the limitations of the human condition. Two groups are particularly sensitive to human frailties and limitations: people confronting the boundary conditions of existence and people who have integrated religion more fully in their lives.

Boundary Conditions

Philosopher and theologian John E. Smith (1968) presented a lucid account of the relationship between crisis and the holy. In all cultures, he notes, the major transitions and turning points of life—birth, puberty, choosing a vocation, marriage, death—are set apart from ordinary events. Marked off and celebrated through ritual and custom, they are extraordinary times—not simply holidays, but "holy days." What gives these moments their sacred quality? Two things, according to Smith. First, they touch matters most basic to existence. "Crisis times . . . direct our thoughts away from the banality of ordinary life to dwell, with awe and proper seriousness, upon the mystery of life itself. . . . It is as if the times of crisis were so many openings into the depth of life, into its ground, its purpose, its finite character" (p. 59). Second, they reveal the vulnerability of the individual to larger and more powerful forces. "The crisis times fill us with a sense of the finitude and frailty of man, of our creatureliness, of our dependence upon resources beyond our own, and of our need to find a supremely worshipful reality to whom we can devote ourselves without reserve" (p. 59).

The sense of the holy comes to the foreground for most people when they are disturbed, when issues of greatest significance are confronted and challenged in ways that push people beyond their personal and social resources. Beyond this threshold religious approaches to problems become particularly compelling to many people. Little and Twiss (1973) describe these circumstances as *boundary situations*, occasions in which people are confronted with the inexplicable, the irresolvable, and the limits of their world.

Hood (1977, 1978) was able to examine boundary situations in a fascinating set of studies. He proposed that mystical religious experiences—experiences in which the person feels a sense of union with God—are triggered by an incongruity between the individual and the situation. This incongruity may take two forms: when a stressful situation is anticipated and, instead, an unstressful one is encountered, and when a stressful situation is encountered unexpectedly. Either case, Hood (1977) says, "forces an acute awareness of self" and "of limits" (p. 156). But it is this awareness of personal limitations that makes the mystical experience more compelling, for personal limitations are transcended through the mystical connection with an ultimate reality. Hood (1978) asked high school students who were about to spend a solitary night in the woods to rate how stressful they expected the night to be. The actual stressfulness of the night was manipulated, fortuitously, by the weather—some nights it rained heavily and other nights it was dry. Upon their return to camp the next day, Hood asked the students whether they had had a religious mystical experience over the night. Consistent with his predictions, mystical experiences were reported most often by the students who anticipated a stressful night, but encountered no rain, and by the students who did not anticipate a stressful event, yet ran into a stormy evening. Both types of encounter were incongruous, highlighting the gap between the student's orientation to the situation and the situation as it unfolded. The mystical experience, Hood maintains, provided a resolution to the incongruity: "limits are transcended and the person is relatively suddenly made aware of particular aspects of self in a classic spiritual manner" (p. 285).

Why does religion comes to prominence more commonly in situations that shake us up? These are the situations that push us close to or beyond our limits. Here, at the edge of efficacy, the judgment of what is the most compelling solution to a problem can change sharply.

Personal, social, and technological strategies no longer provide effective solutions to critical problems, yet we continue to look for some kind of significance in life. This is the borderline beyond which religious solutions become particularly compelling. Psychiatrist Anton Boisen (1955), no stranger to boundary situations in his own life, writes:

> As one stands face to face with the ultimate realities of life and death, religion and theology tend to come alive. Meaning tends to outstrip symbol and we have to seek for new words to express the new ideas which come surging in. Among these ideas we frequently find the sense of contact with that ultimate reality to which we give the name of "God." (p. 3)

From the Boundary to the Center of Life

The notion that people find religion compelling in boundary conditions may leave the religiously committed reader with a bad taste in the mouth. It may suggest that religion is only a stopgap, a last resort of use only after all other resources for coping have been exhausted. The empirical evidence we have reviewed in this chapter indicates that people are indeed more likely to turn to religion in the face of more difficult situations. But these studies do not tell the full story.

The research also shows that more religious people are more likely to cope through religion. Earlier we noted that this finding can be explained by the greater availability and accessibility of religious coping methods to the religious committed. But this is only part of the explanation. Religious coping methods are also more compelling to the religious. Perhaps most central to religiousness is the spiritual belief or feeling that there are larger forces at play in the universe, forces that transcend human powers, even the human capacity to understand. Religious minds are keenly aware of the limits of selves disconnected from the sacred. Those who are most deeply committed live lives dedicated to the spiritual search, the effort to seek and sustain a relationship with the sacred. Not surprisingly, they often appraise religious coping methods as the most compelling routes to this end in times of stress. But for the deeply religious, virtually every encounter, ordinary and extraordinary, stressful and nonstressful, is to be understood and experienced with the sacred in mind. Religion, for them, moves from the boundary to the center of life.

Protestant theologian Dietrich Bonhoeffer (1971) expressed this sentiment 1 year before his death in a concentration camp where he had been imprisoned for more than 2 years for his opposition to the Nazis:

> I've come to be doubtful of talking about any human boundaries. . . .
> It always seems to me that we are trying anxiously in this way to
> reserve some space for God; I should like to speak of God not on the
> boundaries but at the centre, not in weaknesses but in strength; and
> therefore not in death and guilt but in man's life and goodness. . . .
> God is beyond in the midst of our life. The church stands not at the
> boundaries where human powers give out, but in the middle of the
> village. (p. 282)

For Bonhoeffer and others who have devoted themselves to the sacred, religion becomes a compelling part of most of life's encounters.

In sum, two groups are particularly sensitive to the limited nature of the human condition: those who face the boundary conditions of existence and those who see themselves and others in a larger field of spiritual forces. Who are these people? While they are not restricted to any group, they are more likely to be found among the less powerful in society—the poor, elderly, minorities, women, and disenfranchised. Many of these groups encounter a disproportionate share of major life crises, events such as serious illnesses, premature deaths of loved ones, and injustices that confront them with human limitations. These groups also tend to be more generally committed than others to a life oriented around the sacred (see Spilka, Hood, et al., 1985). Perhaps then it should not be surprising to find higher levels of religious coping among members of less powerful groups. For them, religion offers a particularly compelling source of solutions to life's greatest problems.

The Relationship between the Availability of Religion and the Compelling Character of Religious Coping Methods

It may be difficult to distinguish between the two reasons why religion becomes involved in coping. Most often both the availability and the compelling character of religion contribute to religious coping. Further, they often contribute to each other. As religious solutions become more compelling, the individual may take steps to make religion a more available part of the orienting system. Recall for a moment the case of Tim, the man with a drug addiction who encountered God in the mirror of a bathroom. Not only did his experience help him withdraw from drugs, it led to a complete change of lifestyle. Religion became a central focus of Tim's life. He became actively involved in church Bible study and evangelism; eventually he entered a seminary. His newly elaborated religious orienting system served as the foundation for additional religious coping activities, which, in turn, led to further changes in his religious orientation.

It also seems the case that as religion becomes a larger part of the orienting system, religious coping can become increasingly compelling. Proudfoot and Shaver (1975) illustrate this point through the American Nichiren Shoshu, a rapidly growing Buddhist sect that expresses its belief in salvation by repeatedly chanting a sutra before a black box containing a mandala, a Buddhist symbol of the universe. The sutra itself *"Nam myoho renge kyo"* ("Adoration to the Lotus of the Wonderful Law"), has little meaning to Americans or Japanese. But potential converts are steered away from attempts to understand the sect's beliefs and instead are encouraged to engage in the chanting ritual. Leaders invite newcomers to chant an hour in the morning and in the evening for 100 days. "Try it," they say, "it will change your life" (p. 326). From the perspective of self-perception theory, the leaders are correct; having committed themselves to a way of acting, some justification must be found by the newcomers for their behaviors. "It is likely after a hundred days the potential convert will be attracted by a set of beliefs which give meaning to the 'meaningless' activity in which he has been engaged and around which he has reordered his life" (p. 326). In the language of coping, the beliefs and rituals of the Nichiren Shoshu take on a potentially compelling character in coping only after they have been established as an available part of the individual's orienting system.

There are times when religion fails to provide compelling solutions to problems, yet remains involved in coping because there are few if any alternatives. For example, people may participate in religious rituals after the death of a loved one without a commitment to the rituals or their underlying system of belief because the culture does not provide other mechanisms for handling bereavement (Loveland, 1968). Before one way of coping is forsaken, a successor must be nearby (Toch, 1955). But the successor does not have to be awaited passively. The lack of compelling solutions can stimulate a push for better solutions and for improvements to an orienting system that has become "dis-oriented." It is in this process, as we will see, that the individual can play an active part in seeking out or creating a new kind of religious system that will serve as the foundation for more compelling solutions. However, these are not the only possibilities in coping. The individual can also turn away from religion.

WHY RELIGION AND COPING DIVERGE

Much of the focus of this chapter has centered on when and why religion becomes involved in coping. But no discussion of the interface between the two concepts would be complete without a look at the other side of the coin. Why, in particular, do some people turn away from religion in difficult times? Perhaps the same factors that contribute to religious coping contribute to the lack of religious involvement in coping. If it is true that religion takes on a larger role in coping because it is the more available resource and offers the more compelling alternative, it may be just as true that religion recedes in importance in coping because it is the less available and less compelling option. Let us consider a few examples.

Leaving the Convent

In the 1960s, the phenomenon of Catholic nuns leaving the convent, once a rare event, became increasingly commonplace. Helen Rose Fuchs Ebaugh (1988), a sociologist and former nun herself, spent several years studying the process of disengagement of Catholic nuns—why they left and how they dealt with their transition. Ebaugh provides some important background to her study. Completely committed to the service of God, nuns were, for centuries, physically, socially, and psychologically isolated from the world beyond the convent walls. Contacts with outsiders, including family and friends, were forbidden except under special circumstances. When the nuns ventured out beyond the convent, they went in pairs and not alone. This process limited the availability of nonreligious experiences.

The Second Vatican Council had dramatic implications for the church in general and the convent in particular. Religious orders were required to reexamine their way of life and dedicate themselves to the larger personal and social community. "The stress on cloister and isolation from the world gave way to emphasis upon availability and witness in the world" (Ebaugh, 1988, p. 104). Yet, in opening its doors to self-scrutiny and the larger world, the convent also opened itself up to doubts about the efficacy of the cloistered life. Many nuns began to examine nonreligious alternatives in more depth—building relationships with lay people, imagining themselves in secular roles, and developing more of an interest in fashion and physical appearance. Social support encouraged further exploration of alternatives. At the same time, the nuns were forming and reforming tertiary appraisals of the costs and benefits of leaving the convent.

> For most nuns, this consisted in realizing that religious life provides security and a network of friends and camaraderie that takes quite little effort to maintain. Nuns are assured of a job and being taken care of financially. On the other side of the coin, to remain in the order means, in many instances, denying one's needs, desires, and

sense of self-fulfillment. In other words, to stay means not being faithful to oneself. (p. 113)

The final decision to leave the convent often followed a critical moment, a symbolic turning point in which the relative advantages of disengagement became clear and compelling. One woman, a nationally respected Ph.D., left her order after a final conflict with her religious superior who would not let her negotiate her own salary increase on the job:

> I objected to the whole system and felt it perpetuated dependence and immaturity. But the real issue was broader than that. I was questioning celibacy and the whole value of religious life. The salary issue just came up at a point where I had pretty much decided to leave at some point anyway. It just focused things for me like a very ripe pimple. (p. 112)

Leaving the convent did not mean a complete break from the church for most of these nuns. Ebaugh reports only 3% also left the Catholic church entirely. Yet they turned away from an all-involving role and a unique way of life. Why? The convent became less an unchallengeable mode of living, and more one choice among many available lifestyles. In their evaluations of these options, the cloistered way of life emerged as less compelling than the worldly alternative.

Where Is God in Hell?

Times of war are often described in terms of their devastating physical, psychological, and social effects. Yet war can pose as great a threat spiritually. William Mahedy (1986), an Episcopal priest who served as a chaplain in Vietnam, argues that this war represented as much a moral crisis as a psychological crisis. The soldier who asked him, "Hey Chaplain, how come it's a sin to hop into bed with a mama-san but it's okay to blow away gooks out in the bush?" was raising questions about guilt, innocence, and, more broadly, his religious frame of reference. Many tried to accommodate both the war and their actions within their religious orienting systems. One " 'stalked the perimeter' after the battle in which he killed dying enemy soldiers, reciting the Act of Contrition and Hail Marys . . . begging God's forgiveness" (p. 84). Another commanding officer of an infantry company "asked God not to let him be a coward" (p. 109). Some were successful in their efforts, particularly those who were able to see the war as religiously just and God as on their side. But most, Mahedy feels, were not.

The Christian tradition, he notes, provides some measure of justification for war if it meets certain standards: if there is no other way to protect oneself and society from an unjust aggressor, and if the means used to achieve the military goals are commensurate with the ends. The Vietnam war, however, failed to meet these standards. Who was the unjust aggressor here? With many local villagers supporting the Vietcong, the answer was not plainly visible. And as civilians became increasingly caught up in the war and as the numbers of casualties rose and the level of destructiveness intensified, it became less and less clear that the means being used to fight the war were indeed proportionate to the ends. The notion that "it was necessary to destroy the village in order to save it" (p. 93) was far from convincing to many soldiers.

The belief in the unjust nature of the war had tremendous personal consequences for the soldiers ensnared in this conflict. Many felt a sense of personal sinfulness, immorality, and evil. "Night," Mahedy says, "closes in on the spirit" and in this "spiritual darkness" religion became unavailable (p. 98). God, they were convinced, was no longer with them, and efforts to prove otherwise only pushed them further from religious life. "[Soldiers] talked about chaplains with great anger and resentment as having blessed the troops, their mission, their guns and their killing: 'Whatever we were doing—murder, atrocities—God was always on our side' " (Lifton, 1973, cited in Mahedy, 1986, p. 117). In Vietnam the belief that God would make everything turn out was shattered. The chaplains, who were themselves struggling to come to terms with a war of such new and terrible dimension, were often unable to provide the soldiers with viable religious alternatives.

Religious belief and practice no longer offered these combatants a compelling path to significance. As Mahedy puts it, God went A.W.O.L. ("Absent without leave"). Their departure from religion was rarely passive or coolly considered: "On the contrary, the veteran's rejection of God is active, passionate, almost physical, and rooted in the best of reasons. They have been betrayed. On some level they had believed that God had promised something and then didn't or couldn't deliver" (p. 106). One soldier summarized it this way, "Before I went to Vietnam I believed in Jesus Christ and John Wayne, but in Vietnam both went down the tubes" (p. 118). The almost overwhelming task for them became one of constructing new sources of value and new routes to achieving them in the storm of war and its aftermath.

The Making of Atheists

Over 50 years ago, Vetter and Green (1932–1933) conducted an investigation entitled "Personality and Group Factors in the Making of

Atheists." Surveying 350 members of the American Association for the Advancement of Atheism, they discovered that among the younger atheists, half had lost one parent or both parents before the age of 20, far above what would be expected by the average parental mortality rates of this age group. Perhaps not surprisingly in light of this finding, a large number of their group also reported that they were unhappy in childhood and adolescence.

The Vetter and Green study, as well as the other accounts from firsthand experience, observation, and empirical research may seem to contradict the point made earlier in this chapter, that religion generally comes more to the fore under stressful circumstances. Here, instead, we see religious disenchantment and religious detachment after crises and transitions. How are we to make sense of this puzzle? The pieces of the puzzle begin to fall in place when we recall from the coping literature that events, in and of themselves, are not particularly strong predictors of behavior. This point holds true for religious behavior. While the crises of life can tip a person toward or away from religion, the direction will depend not on the nature of the event alone, but on the relationship between the event and what the person brings to it. Generally, the most disruptive problems in living underscore the precariousness of existence and the limits of the individuals' personal and social worlds. During these times, religious resources may be more available and provide more compelling solutions than the nonreligious alternative. Thus, we find religion to be a prominent part of the most disruptive conditions for people in general. However, for a smaller number, the religious response to the boundary conditions of life may be inadequate. For the atheists, the belief in a personal, loving God may have been impossible to square with the death of a parent at so young an age. Their losses called into question not the natural world, but the religious frame of reference, and it was the secular system that took on the larger, more compelling role in the search for significance.

CONCLUSIONS

Religion and coping are separable concepts, not to be mistaken for each other. But they are also related phenomena. I began the analysis of this relationship in this chapter by focusing on some of the first and most basic questions: What is the extent of the religion and coping connection? When do they meet, and why? When do the paths of religion and coping separate, and why? As we have seen, religion does not always play a key part in life's dramas, but neither has its role been eliminated or reduced to a bit part. In fact, religion often comes to center stage in critical situations. It does not materialize out of nowhere; its entrances (and exits) are, at least in part, predictable and understandable. People cope religiously because religion is relatively available and accessible to them and because religion offers a more compelling route to significance than nonreligious alternatives. The religious path is likely to be particularly compelling in boundary conditions when the limits of human resources come to the foreground. But those more consistently aware of their own limitations and more committed to the search for a connection with the forces that transcend their immediate worlds may find the spiritual a compelling part of virtually any situation, ordinary as well as unusual. Finally, it is important to note that there are times when it is the religious solution to the problems of life rather than the secular that is found wanting; in these times the religious approach to coping is likely to face challenge. Clearly, a complex of forces is operating here. The religion and coping connection cannot be understood through the person, the situation, or the context alone. It is the interplay of these forces that determines when the paths of religion and coping will come together and when they will go their separate ways.

Having considered when religion and coping meet and why, we can now ask what happens when the two processes come together. What kinds of roles does religion play in coping? We now take a closer look at the nature of this relationship.

Chapter Seven

THE MANY FACES OF
RELIGION IN COPING

This chapter examines how people involve religion in the search for significance in the face of pain and hardship. I will begin by noting how and why it can be so difficult to apply religious beliefs and practices to the concrete problems of living. Next, I will examine how religion expresses itself in many ways in coping, ways that belie popular stereotypes about religion. Finally, I will consider some of the individual, situational, and cultural forces that shape the many faces of religious coping.

FROM HEAVEN TO EARTH

"The prince of darkness may be a gentleman, as we are told he is, but whatever the god of earth and heaven is, he can surely be no gentleman. His menial services are needed in the dust of our human trials, even more than his dignity is needed in the empyrean" (James, 1975, p. 40). James's turn-of-the-century observations seem just as appropriate today. We have seen that many people look to their faith for support and solace in difficult times. Yet many also find it hard to translate the often abstract, seemingly removed historical accounts of the religious world into concrete forms that are meaningful to their current predicaments. Listen to this description of a couple having marital difficulties:

During one argument, the husband confronted the wife and asked what she thought they should do about the marriage, what direction they should take. She reached for her Bible and turned to Ephesians. "I know what Paul says and I know what Jesus says about marriage," he told her. "What do you say about our marriage?" Dumbfounded, she could not say anything. Like so many of us, she could recite the scriptures, but could not apply them to everyday living. Before the year was out, the husband filed for divorce. (Jones, 1991, p. 4)

This is not an isolated case. One of the most common complaints about churches and synagogues is the irrelevance of the religious services and educational programs to the problems of daily life (Pargament et al., 1991). Even the most devout may have trouble applying the abstractions of religion to life's hardships. In psychotherapy with clergy it is not at all unusual to find ministers, priests, or rabbis who fail to connect their faith to their specific problems.

When religion is disconnected from matters of practical importance it is unlikely to have much practical effect. In one study of homilies within Roman Catholic parishes, we found that the relevance of the sermons to daily life was by far the best predictor of the impact of the message on the members (Pargament & Silverman, 1982).

I recall one clergyman who came to therapy in a great deal of distress after suffering an accident that had left him paralyzed. The accident raised many fundamental questions for this man. Why had it happened? Could he have done anything to prevent it? How could he continue to function with his disability? Could he ever find enjoyment in living now that he truly knew how fragile life is? Yet in all his talk about these very basic issues of meaning, responsibility, and finitude he never mentioned a word about religious faith. Perhaps he was reluctant to bring up religious concerns to a psychologist. But when I raised the question of where his religion fit into his struggle, he drew a blank. In spite of the fact that he often worked as a religious counselor to people in dire straits not unlike his own, he himself was unable to move from the generalities of his faith to the specifics of his situation.

Why is it so hard to bring religion down to earth? The problem is, in part, built into religious systems. The religions of the world are vitally concerned with the most important of the human transitions and crises. Every major religious tradition has something to say about birth, the coming of age, the forming of new families, illness, accident, injustice, tragedy, and death. Most of the world's religions offer theologies and rituals for these general classes of events. However, no organized religion can provide a theology for every kind of death that could be experienced.

None is able to offer rituals predesigned and tailored to every kind of loss.

But, if no religion is fully elaborated, it is with good reason. A faith too tied to the specifics of a particular time, context, or situation would grow extinct as circumstances evolve. The symbols, rituals, and metaphors so central to religious life all lend it flexibility—an ability to bend, stretch, and generate new forms of expression with changing times and conditions. Moreover, the incomplete character of religion can add freshness and vitality to the spiritual search (Bakan, 1968).

The religion of any particular time and place is faced with a difficult dilemma. If made too concrete, it will lose much of its flexibility, mystery and vitality. Yet if left too abstract it will have little to say to the person confronted with very immediate and very real problems. Theologians are quite aware of this dilemma. The essential function of theology, Tillich (1951) says, is to create a balance between two poles, "the eternal truth of its foundation and the temporal situation in which the eternal truth must be received" (p. 3). A theology that confuses the truth of the moment with eternal truth is as untenable as a theology that is disconnected from present circumstances.

The leaders of religious communities also deal with this dilemma in the more concrete practice of religious life. In fact, perhaps their major task is to bridge the mysteries of the heavens with the realities of earth. In sermons, religious stories, inspirational literature, and pastoral work of many kinds we find the fundamental truths of a religious tradition linked to the situation of the day. Take a few examples.

A minister responds to an abused woman who wonders whether she deserves the treatment she has received:

> You are valued in God's eyes; your whole self is regarded by God as a temple, a sacred place. Just as God does not want a temple defiled by violence, neither does God want you to be harmed. God's spirit dwells in you and makes you holy. You do deserve to live without fear and without abuse. (Fortune, 1987, p. 7)

A rabbi likens the Ten Plagues inflicted on ancient Egypt to the plagues facing the world today.

> The final and ultimate (of the Ten Plagues) was the loss of Egypt's first-born children and thus the calling into question of its future. As the Jewish community grapples with the issues of a low birth rate, intermarriage, alienation and assimilation and Jewish illiteracy, it must

remember that the ultimate plague is that which destroys our future as a community. (Berkowitz, 1989, p. 14)

In any age and in any community, we find the basic teachings of a religious tradition confronting the unique demands of a particular time, place, and people. The challenge for the religious community is to respond to ever-changing circumstances while remaining within the boundaries of its world. This is the "cutting edge of religious life" (Paden, 1988, p. 89).

Psychologists of religion have had less to say about this cutting edge of religion. As we noted earlier, the tendency among social scientists has been to view religion as a general orientation. Typically, religion has been assessed macroanalytically by global, dispositional, distal indicators: how often the person generally attends religious services or prays, how important religion is to the individual. The applications of religion to concrete life situations have gone largely unstudied. Unfortunately, this has left a gap in our understanding.

Take, for example, a study of caregivers to people with Alzheimer's disease and recurrent metastatic cancer (Rabins, Fitting, Eastham, & Zabora, 1990). Recognizing that caregivers of the chronically ill are vulnerable to emotional and physical problems of their own, these researchers were interested in identifying the factors that affect long-term adaptation to the caregiving process. Religion emerged as one of the most important and helpful variables. More specifically, the strength of religious faith reported by the caregivers was related to a more positive emotional state 2 years later, as measured by indices of positive and negative affect. Although this study points to the beneficial role of religious faith for these caregivers, it leaves some very important questions unanswered. What is it about religious faith that is helpful? Does it reassure them that their relative will recover? Does it help them view the illness in a more positive light? Does it provide them with direction and guidance in their struggles? Does it enable them to find meaning in what may seem to be a senseless disease? It is not enough to find that general measures of religious faith or practice relate to general measures of adjustment or well-being. The central question remains: How does religion come to life in the immediate situation?

The coping framework provides one window into this transitional process, this movement from heaven to earth. When we turn our attention to coping, we can see people moving from the generalities of their faith to the specifics of religious action in difficult moments. We now consider some of the ways religion expresses itself "in the dust of our trials."

BEYOND STEREOTYPES

When psychologists talk about coping, the topic of religion does not usually come up. What discussion it has received has often been over-simplified and negative. The view that religion is simply a defense against the confrontation with reality, argued by Freud (1927/1961) many years ago, still holds wide acceptance among social scientists and mental health professionals. For example, one text on stress devotes one page to religion, and focuses exclusively on its defensive role in the appraisals of situations:

> Religion actively offers distortions of perception as "acceptable" ways of dealing with problems, and in many ways the comments made about the use of drugs in altering cognitive appraisal are appropriate here. Although emotional gains obviously accrue from being religious, there is a distinct possibility that the psychological defense strategies recommended by the religion may impair realistic behaviour, and may only be maintained at a cost to physical and psychological health. (Cox, 1980, p. 120)

What does it mean to say that religion is a defense? The term "defense" refers to a particular set of means for attaining a particular set of ends (A. Freud, 1966). By distorting the nature of the real threat or by steering clear of it (i.e., the means or methods of defense), the individual attempts to allay fears and apprehensions (i.e., the ends or goals of defense). Avoidance in the service of tension reduction is the essence of this concept. Defenses are said to be partially successful and partially maladaptive. They may reduce anxiety, but in failing to face the real issue head on, the problem remains unresolved.

Implicit in the view of religion-as-defense are three assumptions: (1) in terms of ends, the basic goal of religion is tension reduction; (2) in terms of the way situations are constructed, religion is a form of denial; and (3) in terms of the way situations are handled, religion is passive and avoidant. Elsewhere Park and I (Pargament & Park, 1995) have argued that these assumptions and the general notion of religion-as-defense are stereotypical. Like other stereotypes, there is a grain of truth to these beliefs, but only that. Religion can serve the purpose of tension reduction, it can distort reality, and it can be passive and avoidant, but it can also be more. In the introductory chapters, I defined religion as a complex multidimensional phenomena. Religion is no less complex or multidimensional when it comes to coping. In the following sections I challenge common religious stereotypes by presenting pictures of some of the many faces of religion in coping: in the ends we strive toward, in the ways we construct situations, and in the specific forms of coping we use in the search for significance.

Merely Tension Reduction? The Many Ends of Religious Coping

In the eyes of many mental health professionals, comfort, solace, and relief are the basic functions of religion. Similarly, some coping researchers have described religion exclusively as a form of emotion-focused coping. It is not too hard to marshal support for this argument. As we saw in the last chapter, people are more likely to turn to God for help in stressful times. And, as we will see in Chapter 10, religious involvement can allay feelings of anxiety and distress among groups in crisis. However, to say that people look to religion for emotional comfort in times of stress is one thing; to say that this is the sole purpose of religion is quite another.

Earlier we described some of the general destinations often associated with religion. We spoke of religion and the search not only for comfort, but for other ends as well: the sacred, meaning, the self, physical health, intimacy, and a better world. In the process of coping with stress, each of these general destinations turns into specific purposes.

People may strive toward something of a spiritual nature.

One of our interviewees in the Project on Religion and Coping (Pargament, Royster, et al., 1990), Jane a 41-year-old woman, described a lifelong search for God in the midst of exceptional hardship and struggle. As a child she had a deep spiritual feeling: "I can remember one instance in particular when I was about four or five when I was sitting in a field behind our house, and the sun was going down, and I just felt like God had his arms around me. I can see him in the sunset, and I can remember seeing him in that field." As an adolescent, Jane had a born-again experience. However, it was a "reverse success story." "I thought that when I became a Christian, when I asked the Lord into my heart, that I just [would never] do anything wrong again. That somehow I'd be transformed into this perfect little person. . . . And so, the first time I screwed up, I thought, that's it, I blew it, and had nobody to tell me any different." Jane's life went into a downward spiral. She became addicted to heroin, was involved in a series of unsuccessful marriages, and participated in witchcraft and the occult. All of these actions she viewed as misdirected attempts to recover the God she had lost.

The death of her mother was a turning point. At her funeral, Jane was profoundly affected by something a friend said to her:

> That when Jesus said, I will never leave you or forsake you, he meant it. That once you take this step, once you step over this line and ask me to come in, then I'm always there with you. . . . And boy, that hit me right between the eyes. I felt like that was written for me. And when she told me that, I just thought, my God, he's been there with me this whole time. He never left. From the moment I asked him into my life, in 1972, Jesus has been standing right by me. (Pargament, Royster, et al., 1990)

Although Jane now feels she has found God, she believes that her spiritual search continues through her efforts to experience God in her daily life. Toward this end she has dramatically changed her lifestyle. Jane reports that in the past 10 years she has returned to her hometown, quit her use of heroin, established a new network of friends, remarried successfully, and become active in personal religious devotions and her church.

Looking back over Jane's life, it is clear that she struggled with many crises. However, it would be misleading to say she simply coped *with* her problems, for her coping was quite active and purposeful. She coped with her situations to rediscover the spiritual presence she had once felt as a child.

Religion is also often involved in the search for very human ends of significance in coping. Comfort represents one of these ends, but it is not the only one. Consider, for instance, the varied accounts of survivors of the 1995 bomb blast in Oklahoma City that killed over 100 adults and children (see Table 7.1). In their words, we hear people faced with the same event looking for help in attaining diverse objects of significance.

It is important to recognize that the dividing line between the search for comfort and other human and spiritual ends is not necessarily sharp. Many personal, social, and spiritual goals can become intertwined. For example, in a Roman Catholic priest's description of his mother's funeral, it is hard to separate the spirituality of the moment from the feelings of intimacy, connectedness, and comfort with family and friends:

> The funeral was astounding. It was one of the highest moments of my life. It was incredible. The church was jammed. . . . The whole church, everybody was there. Many, many friends were there. Students from here, and the liturgy was a real experience of the resurrection. It was terrific. My blind niece played the piano. And I'll never forget those

TABLE 7.1. Objects of Religious Significance Described by Survivors of the Oklahoma City Bombing

Spirituality
"There has been so much loss that I'm holding on tighter than ever to my faith, my rituals, my God. For me, if I lose my faith, I lose everything."

Meaning
"We all have been paralyzed, dazed, wondering why, and there are a lot of unanswered questions that I'm not able to answer. But there's a God that knows all things and I'm convinced the Lord is not sitting up there in heaven trying to figure out how to handle things. He's already in control."

Comfort
"We don't know whether she's alive. We don't know what happened to her. We do know she's with God." (Parents of daughter missing in the blast)

Self
"You had to depend on a spiritual background to conquer the frontier, and in the tough times we faced in the Dust Bowl days, there was no strength but the Lord." (Commenting on the gritty, empowering Grapes of Wrath legacy passed on to Oklahoma City survivors)

Physical health
"The prayers here won't necessarily put this behind us, but it helps us to heal." (Man who attended a prayer service on behalf of a friend who lost his eye in the explosion)

Intimacy
"There's a spirit that bonds people together that's not a human spirit but the Holy Spirit."

Better world
"I'm working on forgiving those responsible [for the bombing]. Peace and justice is what we [parishioners] are fighting for. [I'm] vowing not to give in to hate."

Note. Accounts of Oklahoma City survivors from television interviews and newspapers.

psalms. And my best friend David gave the homily. Absolutely on the nose homily. . . . So there were so many powerful religious expressions and family expressions. (Pargament, Royster, et al., 1990, pp. 14–15)

The accounts we have reviewed here have been anecdotal and self-report. Some would say that people are unable to know or report accurately on their own motives in coping. Others would say that these reports are simply different ways of describing the same basic defensive motive. But if these personal accounts are to be believed, then we should be wary of reducing the ends of religious coping to any single universal object of significance. Instead, we should be alert to the many ends people seek through religion as they face their ups and downs of living. Tension reduction is an important end of religious coping, but it is not the only one. In the next chapters, we will bring more data to bear on the variety of religious ends and pathways people take toward them.

Merely Denial? The Many Religious Constructions of the Situation

One of the most common stereotypes is that religion is simply a form of denial, a way to reduce tension by repudiating reality. That is one way religion can be used to construct life situation, but it is not the only way. Religion can shape appraisals of critical events in other directions as well. Moreover, it can shape the events people actually encounter and avoid in their lives.

Appraising Life Events

Examples can always be found to support stereotypes. This holds true for the stereotype of religion-as-denial. Take the case of a 32-year-old man convicted and serving time for several theft and robbery offenses. Asked to describe his past, he says, "Since I got Jesus I don't have no memories of the past" (Peck, 1988, p. 207). Or consider the case of Baby Boy William, a premature neonate, who suffered from a variety of ailments (York, 1987). His condition deteriorated to the point where his kidneys stopped functioning and he could be kept alive only through artificial means at the cost of a great deal of physical suffering. The parents, however, refused to accept the bad news. "God will make William well and the Doctor will be proven wrong. . . . God is smarter than all doctors and will save our son" (p. 38). In the face of his evident decline, the parents refused to visit their son in the unit and came to the hospital only reluctantly when he was near death. Even then, however, they insisted that "William still has a chance and we expect a miracle" (p. 39). After he died, the parents left his body in the morgue for a few weeks before the arrangements for the funeral were made.

A few empirical studies have also reported a connection between religiousness and denial among some groups. In one study of fundamentalist patients suffering from terminal cancer, people who experienced higher levels of support from the church were more likely to deny the reality of their illness and the imminence of death (Gibbs & Achterberg-Lawlis, 1978).

Blatant examples of religiously based denial can be found. However, it is one thing to find instances of religious denial and quite another to conclude that religion is simply a form of denial. Evidence from other sources contradicts this unidimensional point of view. Some anecdotal accounts describe a God who helps people face the reality of their losses. One mother of a visually impaired child had this to say: "I wish my son could see, but he can't. God taught me to accept that fact, deal with it, and get on with life" (Erin, Rudin, & Njoroge, 1991, p. 161).

Empirical findings are also hard to reconcile with the stereotypical view of religion as denial. In a study of people who had reported at least one "consensually validated" life-threatening experience, Berman (1974) found that the religiously active group described as much initial anxiety, panic, or fear in reaction to the near-death experience as the religiously inactive group. Others have reported similar results (e.g., Acklin, Brown, & Mauger, 1983; Pargament, Olsen, et al., 1992b).

Certain religious beliefs may increase rather than decrease appraisals of threat and harm. For example, in one study of stressful reactions to the Persian Gulf war, religious faith was associated with more intrusive thoughts and dreams (Plante & Manuel, 1992).

> Neurologist Oliver Sacks (1988) illustrates the same point in his description of David Janzen who, at the age of 15, began to feel compulsions to hurt himself, break things, and shout out obscenities. This kind of behavior, particularly the cursing, did not sit well with his conservative Mennonite community. At a loss to explain his actions, David concluded that the Devil was at work in him. When he cursed he would say, "Devil! Why don't you get out of me and leave me alone?" (p. 97). David's symptoms grew more severe as he aged. Finally, at the age of 38, he met a physician who diagnosed his problem as Tourette's syndrome. Serious as this disease is, the diagnosis came as a relief to David: "It made me want to jump for joy. . . . It took away the terrible feeling of a curse. It was not the Devil working in me—which was my worst fear—and it was not medical doom. I had a simple disease, and it even had a name. A pretty name too—I kept on repeating it." (p. 98)

This account brings to mind once again the words of Clifford Geertz (1966): "Over its career religion has probably disturbed men as much as it has cheered them" (p. 18).

Studies of the religion–appraisal connection are few in number as yet. What we do know, however, suggests that religion does not always decrease perceptions of threat and harm. Denial is one way religion expresses itself in the appraisal of negative events, but it is not the only way.

Much of religion's power lies in its ability to appraise negative events from a different vantage point. Crises become an opportunity for closeness with God. Moments of terrible tension become a way to test and hone one's spiritual mettle. Suffering and failure become a chance to redress one's sins and achieve redemption. Even the most desperate situations can be appraised in a more benevolent light from the religious perspective. Consider the advice evangelist Billy Graham offers a man in constant pain who complains that his suffering makes it hard for him to think about God: "Throughout the ages there have been countless saints of God who have found that pain and sickness became a blessing instead of a barrier. They found it could actually help get life into its true perspective. . . . It may seem hard to thank God for your pain. But ask God to teach you whatever He wants of you during your lifetime" (cited in Kotarba, 1983, p. 683).

Empirical research also suggests a link between religiousness and positive appraisals of situations. Wright, Pratt, and Schmall (1985) studied the role of religion in the coping efforts of caregivers of people with Alzheimer's disease. One of their central findings was that caregivers who looked to religion for spiritual support in coping were more likely to define their demanding situation more positively. One of their participants put it this way: "It is the most rewarding and devastating experience of my life; I would not have given up this period to care for my parents for anything. There has been combativeness, wandering—lots of frustrations. But I'm learning for the first time to take each day at a time. This illness is teaching me to gain strength from the Lord" (p. 34). Other researchers have also reported relationships between measures of religiousness and appraisals of the "silver lining" in negative situations (e.g., Carver et al., 1989; Weisner, Belzer, & Stolze, 1991).

Of course, it could be argued that positive appraisals of difficult situations are simply more sophisticated, better camouflaged efforts to deny the pain of the negative. There is, however, some evidence that positive reconstructions of negative events are not tantamount to denial. In a study of cancer patients, Yates, Chalmer, St. James, Follansbee, and McKegney (1981) found that measures of religiousness were not related to reports of the *presence* of pain among patients. They were, however, related to reports of lower *levels* of pain. Similarly, in the Project on Religion and Coping, although global measures of religiousness were unassociated with appraisals of situations as a threat or as harmful, they were associated with appraisals of the events as an opportunity to grow (see Pargament, Olsen, et al., 1992b). More often than not, these findings suggest, religion places negative events in a positive sacred context without denying or distorting the fact that a fundamental change has taken place.

Creating and Avoiding Life Events

The stereotypical view of religion-as-denial also assumes that religion is largely reactive to problems. Religion is said to respond to stressors with denial and distortion. Overlooked in this stereotype is the role religion plays in the construction of some events and in the avoidance of others.

In the search for the spiritual, the world's religions have marked off the most critical junctions of the lifespan, setting them apart from ordinary times and wrapping them in religious garb. Oden (1983) captures the special sense of these "holy-days" from a Christian perspective:

> There are five incomparable days in the believer's life. The day one is born, when life is given. The day one is baptized, and enters anticipatively into the community of faith. The day one is confirmed, when one chooses to re-affirm one's baptism, and enter by choice deliberately into the community of faith and enjoy its holy communion. The day one may choose to enter into a lifelong covenant of fidelity in love. The day one dies, when life is received back into God's hands. (p. 85)

Through its association with religion, the event is fundamentally changed. The ritual circumcision of the infant within Judaism is something other than a medical procedure. A wedding within the Anglican church is not to be confused with a civil ceremony. Here, rituals and beliefs are more than window dressing; they add gravity and deeper meaning to the event, thereby altering the nature of the transition itself. This may help to explain the intriguing finding reported by Idler and Kasl (1992). Mortality rates among elderly Christians drop significantly in the 30 days prior to Christmas and Easter. A similar phenomenon occurs for elderly Jewish males in the 30 days before Passover and Yom Kippur. Apparently, the anticipation of these religious rituals and holidays has survival implications for the individual.

While religions remake the nature of the most inevitable and universal of life's events, they also create new demands and new presses of their own. Those involved in a religious world are likely to face some rather unique problems. One such problem arises when the truthfulness of religious claims is questioned. Kooistra (1990) studied the religious doubts of high school students in Roman Catholic and Dutch Reformed parochial schools. In this sample, 77% reported some doubts about their religion. These doubts were sources of distress in themselves. Active religious doubting (measured by the amount of time and energy spent in questioning basic religious tenets) was associated with higher levels of negative affect and anxiety.

Doubts are only one of the many unique problems and dilemmas that come with the religious territory. One person wonders how she can find a religious congregation where women are treated as equals to men. Another struggles with the fact that church leaders continually violate religious precepts. One person fights with his son who wants to marry someone outside of the faith. Another feels compelled by her congregation to remain in an abusive marital relationship. I could go on, but the central point here is that religions can create problems of their own, problems that may be especially painful, rooted as they are in a system that was expected to resolve existential crises, not engender them.

But if religions create some problems, they sidestep others. On the road map of religious paths and destinations, the routes to avoid can be drawn even more clearly than the roads to follow. They are marked by warning signs in capital letters: "profanity," "impurity," "sinful," "abomination," "taboo," and "defilement." The markers reveal that these paths and destinations have a sharply negative kind of religious significance of their own.

Murder, adultery, lying, stealing, cruelty, worshiping false gods—these are the ways people have traditionally strayed from the search for the sacred. The modern day continues to provide people with opportunities to take a wrong turn. Alcoholism and drug abuse, family violence, divorce, homelessness, and social and political oppression are, to many religious minds, some of the sins of our time.

Religions encourage people to avoid these paths. The encouragement comes, in part, from strong injunctions against the many forms of wickedness. One Biblical passage reads: "Ye shall not afflict any widow, or fatherless child. If thou afflict them in any wise, and they cry at all unto me, I will surely hear their cry; And my wrath shall wax hot, and I will kill you with the sword; and your wives shall be widows, and your children fatherless" (Exodus 22:21–23). The reader of the New Testament hears: "For the wrath of God is revealed from heaven against all ungodliness and unrighteousness of men who hold the truth in unrighteousness" (Romans 1:18). In a portion of the Koran we read: "And lo! the wicked verily will be in hell; They will burn therein on the Day of Judgment, And will not be absent thence" (Sarah, LXXXII, 14–16).

Religious encouragement to avoid the wrong turn is also expressed socially. Organized religions can, at times, reach out, grab people by the shoulders, and guide them away from these dead ends. Take the case of the meeting between Rev. Robert Smith of the New Bethel Baptist Church and Jerome, an unemployed 38-year-old crack addict, separated from his wife and living in abandoned buildings.

One morning in July, [Rev.] Smith reeled in Jerome. . . . Smith's bait
was simple. He invited Jerome to eat supper and attend a revival, and
Jerome agreed. . . .

But that was far from the end of Jerome's journey. His salvation
wasn't in the water that washed him; it was in the two religious
communities that adopted him afterward. . . .

"This church is a safe place. The people here have reached out to me,"
he says. "And I'm glad for that, because in the streets where I've been,
nobody does nothing for you—except abuse you and use you." . . .

It has been only four months since Jerome's baptism, but through New
Bethel and Narcotics Anonymous, he is back living with relatives. He
has stopped smoking crack. He is no longer committing crimes. And,
as the blue book preaches, he is taking his new life one day at a time.
(Crumm, 1991, pp. 8A–9A)

In addition to these informal encounters, many religious groups
offer more formal activities to help people steer clear of trouble and get
their lives back on track. Churches and synagogues support programs to
prevent many kinds of problems, such as drug and alcohol abuse, marital
distress, homelessness, and hypertension (see Pargament, Maton, &
Hess, 1992, for review). These programs should not be mistaken for
mental health programs. Unlike their mental health counterparts, they
have a specific religious intent. Their purpose is to protect people from
the sins of our times and to redirect them onto a spiritual path. But their
effect is to remake the character of situations people are likely to face
in living. By involving themselves in religious life, empirical studies
suggest, people are less likely to face the problems of substance abuse,
marital infidelity, suicidality (Payne, Bergin, Bielema, & Jenkins, 1992)
and high risk sexual behavior (Folkman, Chesney, Pollack, & Phillips,
1992).

It is important to remember, however, that in the effort to avoid
some problems, religions can create others. For example, while Mormons
have among the lowest rates of alcohol use of any religious groups, those
who do drink report a high rate of alcohol abuse (Strauss & Bacon,
1953). Those who break the strict religious code against drinking may
lack the knowledge of how to drink sensibly or may feel they have gone
too far to turn back. Thus, even though the religious injunction may
prevent alcoholism among most people, the same injunction may be the
source of problems for those who have transgressed. In this sense, Payne
et al. (1992) note, religion becomes "a two-edged sword, deterring

alcoholism and alcohol abuse, but resulting in greater abuse when the 'rules' have been broken" (p. 70).

Let me summarize. While religion is often described as a way of denying the painfulness of life, I have argued here that religion constructs situations in many ways. It is just as capable of increasing perceptions of threat and loss as decreasing these perceptions. It is also able to do more than react. It can remake the topography of life experience, dotting the landscape with some events and removing other features from the map. Once again, simple stereotypes cannot do justice to the roles of religion in the construction of the situation. The same point applies to the concrete methods of coping.

Merely Avoidance? The Many Methods of Religious Coping

People do many things with religion in stressful times. Consider, for example, the variety of ways one group of people reportedly coped religiously with the ordeal of waiting in the hospital for their loved ones who were about to undergo major cardiac surgery (VandeCreek et al., 1995). Their responses ranged from reading the Bible, watching religious television, and reciting sacred phrases to a period of quiet prayer, a conversation with clergy, and a religious ritual. Religion provides its adherents with a long list of coping options. While this list illustrates the varied sources of religious coping, it does not say much about the coping methods themselves. How, for instance, is the individual praying? What is he or she praying for? There are, after all, many forms of prayer (see Poloma & Gallup, 1991). Similarly, what kind of religious television is the individual watching? What portion of the Bible is being read? What is the individual searching for through a conversation with clergy or participation in ritual? Bare-bones descriptions of religious activities say little about the roles of these activities in the coping process. For that, we must go beyond description to a more functional analysis of religious coping.

Here we encounter another stereotype. In the attempt to reduce tension, this stereotype holds, religion resorts to inappropriate measures. As one reviewer of the field observed: "The psychological research reflects an overwhelming consensus that religion . . . is associated with [among other things] an array of what may be called desperate and generally unadaptive defensive maneuvers" (Dittes, 1969, p. 636). More specifically, religion has been accused of acquiescence and lethargy in response to stress. How accurate is this view? Is religion simply a passive, avoidant approach to solving problems?

Just as we can find examples of religiously based denial, we can find illustrations of religiously based passive and avoidant coping activities.

> I remember a young woman, Ellen, who came in for counseling after discovering that her husband had been having an affair with her best friend. The mother of four small children, unemployed, and distant from her family, Ellen was naturally enough uncertain about her marriage and her future. Adding to all of the confusion was the fact that her husband had asked her to return home; unfortunately, he refused to promise that he would stop seeing the other woman. After the initial session, Ellen agreed to return and try to sort through some of her questions and conflicts. Later the next week, though, she called me in a much cheerier voice saying a miracle had occurred to her over the weekend. God, she said, had come to her in a dream and told her to return to her husband. The following day Ellen went home to a joyous reunion with her spouse. Although her husband had made no commitment to end his affair, Ellen was confident that God would change him. In spite of my strong encouragement that she return to counseling, Ellen declined. Passivity and avoidance were central to the way she coped with her dilemma. These strategies were not without their advantages. By deferring to God, she was able to relieve herself of the responsibility for her very difficult decision. Not only that, by returning to her husband and trusting that God would show him the light, she neatly sidestepped both the threat of single parenthood and the threat posed by "the other woman." But the immediate gains associated with her passive–avoidant way of coping were purchased at great cost to her personal sense of competence and any chance of salvaging her marriage as well.

It is not hard to locate other clinical examples. In support of these clinical accounts, a few studies have tied various measures of religiousness to escapist forms of coping (Dunkel-Schetter, Feinstein, Taylor, & Falker, 1992; Rosenstiel & Keefe, 1983). Acceptance, resignation, deference, avoidance, forbearance, and submission can be important elements of religious coping. They are not the only elements, however.

There is more to religion than avoidance of pain. Rofe and Lewin (1980) surveyed the daydreams of Jewish high school students from two towns in Israel. One of the towns had been subject to a number of terrorist attacks; the other town had not. In both towns, the more religiously orthodox and traditional students had more Messianic daydreams than the secular students (e.g., I daydream of the rebuilding of the Holy Temple). However, they did not experience any fewer unpleasant daydreams. Religious students were as likely as secular students to visualize the people of Israel again being in exile, see themselves or their parents dead, or imagine themselves choking someone. These religious individuals did not appear to avoid the pain of their situations to a greater extent than their less religious counterparts. But they did seem to have another source of support and relief for themselves in their stressful circumstances.

There is also more to religion than submission; religion can express itself through active as well as passive coping approaches. For example, Horton, Wilkins, and Wright (1988) used questionnaires to compare the coping activities of abused wives who defined themselves as religious with victims of abuse who viewed themselves as nonreligious. While religious women remained in their marriages longer than nonreligious women, they were not acquiescent. In fact they appeared to work harder to save their relationship, using more resources (e.g., counselors, religious leaders) in their attempts to resolve their situation. Horton et al. conclude: "Religious women can no longer be considered as barefoot and pregnant, weak and unable to change. They have shown a very different character and a positive approach to violence in their lives and for their families. They are not disadvantaged, nor should they be 'treated' for religiosity instead of abuse" (p. 245).

This study is not unusual. In our review of this empirical literature, Park and I (Pargament & Park, 1995) reached several conclusions: (1) religion is not inconsistent with an internal locus of control; (2) religion is not commensurate with passivity in the face of social oppression; and (3) in many cases, perhaps more often than not, measures of religiousness are linked to active rather than avoidant forms of coping. These conclusions should not come as a complete surprise. Among the religious faiths we can find rationales for active approaches to coping. For instance, deism acknowledges the existence of a God, but a God who does not interfere with the natural laws of the universe. From this perspective, God has given humanity the ability to reason and resolve problems itself. Galileo (1614/1988) voiced this view in the 17th century:

> I do not feel obliged to believe that that same God who has endowed us with senses, reason, and intellect has intended to forgo their use and by some other means to give us a knowledge which we can attain by them. He would not require us to deny sense and reason in physical matters which are set before our eyes and minds by direct experience or necessary demonstrations. (p. 20)

The Protestant ethic has also encouraged vigorous activity and achievement in this world, not because God has set people free, but because worldly success is a sign of proof that one has been called by God.

Religious coping activities cover both ends of the spectrum of human initiative and divine power—from autonomy, industry, and diligence to deference, passivity, and resignation. Of course, these are the extremes. There are other possibilities. When people describe the role of religion in coping they often point to a third style, one in which they are neither passive nor autonomous but instead interactive with God. In this kind of religious coping activity, God and the individual are collaborators in problem solving. Responsibility for coping is shared, with both partners playing an active role in this process. Heschel (1986) puts it this way: "God is a partner and partisan in man's struggle for justice, peace, and holiness, and it is because of His being in need of man that He entered a covenant with him for all time, a mutual bond embracing God and man, a relationship to which God, not only man, is committed" (p. 172).

One of our interviewees from the Project on Religion and Coping (Pargament, Royster, et al., 1990) illustrated this collaborative approach. Joe was a 69-year-old man faced with a decision about whether to go through a risky heart operation or eventually become an invalid. When asked how religion was involved in his coping, Joe said he prayed to God for guidance, but not in a passive or deferring sense. In his prayers, God served as a supportive listening ear, a loving Being who helped him reflect on his situation and make the best possible choice. Together, Joe said, they decided that he would not make a very good invalid. So Joe went ahead with the surgery.

Self-Directing, Deferring, and Collaborative: Three Religious Approaches to Control in Coping

In the preceding discussion I have hinted at three distinctive approaches to responsibility and control in coping: (1) the self-directing approach, wherein people rely on themselves in coping rather than on God, (2) the deferring approach, in which the responsibility for coping is passively deferred to God; and (3) the collaborative approach, in which the individual and God are both active partners in coping. Several years ago, my students and I (Pargament et al., 1988) attempted to measure these three styles of religious coping. The short version of the three scales is presented in Table 7.2. We administered the scales to members of a Presbyterian and Missouri Synod Lutheran church and factor-analyzed the items. Three distinct factors emerged from the analyses, which paralleled exactly the three styles of religious coping. Furthermore, each of the three coping styles had different relationships with other measures of religiousness, and with measures of psychological and social competence.

TABLE 7.2. Three Styles of Religious Coping Scales

Self-directing
1. After I've gone through a rough time, I try to make sense of it without relying on God.
2. When I have difficulty, I decide what it means by myself without help from God.
3. When faced with trouble, I deal with my feelings without God's help.
4. When deciding on a solution, I make a choice independent of God's input.
5. When thinking about a difficulty, I try to come up with possible solutions without God's help.
6. I act to solve my problems without God's help.

Deferring
1. Rather than trying to come up with the right solution to a problem myself, I let God decide how to deal with it.
2. In carrying out solutions to my problems, I wait for God to take control and know somehow He'll work it out.
3. I do not think about different solutions to my problems because God provides them for me.
4. When a troublesome issue arises, I leave it up to God to decide what it means for me.
5. When a situation makes me anxious, I wait for God to take those feelings away.
6. I don't spend much time thinking about troubles I've had; God makes sense of them for me.

Collaborative
1. When it comes to deciding how to solve a problem, God and I work together as partners.
2. When considering a difficult situation, God and I work together to think of possible solutions.
3. Together, God and I put my plans into action.
4. When I feel nervous or anxious about a problem, I work together with God to find a way to relieve my worries.
5. After solving a problem, I work with God to make sense of it.
6. When I have a problem, I talk to God about it and together we decide what it means.

Note. The long form of the three styles of religious coping scales is available in Pargament et al. (1988). Copyright 1988 by The Society for the Scientific Study of Religion. Adapted by permission.

1. The self-directing style was negatively associated with most of the measures of religiousness. However, this was not a nonreligious approach. Even the more self-directing people in our study maintained an affiliation with their church. Moreover, self-directing scores were associated with higher scores on the measure of religious quest.

2. The deferring style was related to a greater sense of control by God, doctrinal orthodoxy, and extrinsic religiousness. The emphasis of this style was on dependence on external authority, rules, and beliefs as a way to meet particular needs.
3. In contrast, the collaborative style was associated with a greater frequency of prayer, higher religious salience, and intrinsic religiousness—indicators of a more committed, relational form of religion.

The three styles of coping were also connected to different levels of personal and social competence.

1. A more self-directing style was related to a greater sense of personal control in living and higher self-esteem. This finding is consistent with the general coping literature which emphasizes the value of proactivity and autonomy in problem solving.
2. A more deferring style was tied to a number of indicators of poorer competence: a lower sense of personal control, a greater sense of control by chance, lower self-esteem, less planful problem-solving skills, and greater intolerance for differences between people. These findings may not be too surprising; the deferring approach with its reliance on external authority seems to embody the passive, helpless kind of religiousness so heavily criticized by many psychologists.
3. Once again, in contrast to the deferring approach, the coping process involving an active give-and-take between the individual and God seemed to bode well for individual competence. A more collaborative style was associated with a greater sense of personal control, a lower sense of control by chance, and greater self-esteem.[1]

Other researchers using these measures of religious coping styles with other samples have also found them to be associated with different kinds of religious beliefs and practices, different levels of physical and mental health, and different approaches to health and pastoral care (Bransfield, Ivy, Rutledge, & Wallston, 1991; Casebolt, 1990; Hathaway & Pargament, 1990; Kaiser, 1991; McIntosh & Spilka, 1990; Pargament, Ensing, et al., 1990; Schaefer & Gorsuch, 1991; Sears & Greene, 1994; Winger & Hunsberger, 1988).[2]

These three religious coping styles may not be the only religious approaches to responsibility and control. Pleas and petitions to God for divine intervention represent another method deserving further study. Petitions for divine intervention are not uncommon. Forty-two percent of people in one national survey acknowledged that they prayed to God for material things (Poloma & Gallup, 1991). One pharmaceutical company recently established a prayer network that physicians can access to request intercessory prayers on behalf of the health of their patients (Wall, 1994). Requests for divine intervention have both active and passive elements. Ultimate control and responsibility for the outcome of the situation are seen as resting in God's hands. However, the individual who pleads for divine intercession is actively, albeit indirectly, attempting to shape the outcome of the situation. In self-directing coping, control is sought *by the self*. In deferring coping, control is sought *by God*. In collaborative coping, control is sought *with God*. And in petitionary coping, control is sought *through God*. In Chapter 10 we will review some evidence suggesting that petitionary coping has mixed implications for adjustment.

The point here is not that we have identified a few good ways of religious coping and a few bad ones. (Later I will consider how these styles of coping relate to other measures of personal and social well-being and how the helpfulness of these approaches may vary from situation to situation). Neither am I suggesting that these approaches to control are the only kinds of religious coping methods. What have been identified here are some of the distinctive ways people integrate their conceptions of divine power with human initiative. To define religious coping as passive is not incorrect. It is incomplete. Submission and deference to God are only two of the many faces of religion.

To the distant observer the involvement of religion in coping may appear to be uniform. But we have taken a closer look at religion and seen it to be many-sided, a force that can come to life in a variety of ways in every part of the coping process: in the ends we strive toward, in the construction of life events, and in the concrete steps we take in the midst of stress. I hope this discussion has left the reader with a healthy skepticism for stereotypes and simple descriptions of religious life.

Measuring the Many Faces of Religious Coping

A few researchers have developed measures of the degree to which people turn to religion for help in coping with negative events (e.g., Carver, Scheier, & Weintraub, 1989; Koenig, George, & Siegler, 1988). These scales are helpful in describing *how much* religion is involved in coping, but they do not specify *how* religion is involved. For this latter purpose, a more differentiated approach is needed.

In the Project on Religion and Coping, my colleagues and I (Pargament, Ensing, et al., 1990) assessed some of the many faces of religious coping in more detail. Unlike the measures of the three styles of religious coping that were developed around the theoretical construct of control, the approach we took to developing the religious coping activities scales was not explicitly theoretical. Questions were generated through interviews with church and synagogue members, personal accounts of religious coping, and a review of the literature. We tried to assess a wide array of religious coping methods, methods that embody thoughts, feelings, behaviors, and relationships. These questions were then given to a sample of church members who were asked to respond in terms of how they had coped with the most serious negative event they had experienced in the past year. Our questions focused on three dimensions: the purposes or ends of significance the members hoped to achieve through religious coping, the members' appraisals of the event, and their coping methods. To reduce the many questions about coping activities and purposes to a more manageable set of scales, we conducted factor

TABLE 7.3. The Religious Coping Items and Scales

Purposes of Religion in Coping[a]
  Spiritual
    Personal closeness with God
    A sense of meaning and purpose in life
    Feeling of hope about the future
  Self-Development
    Help in feeling good about myself
    Feeling more in control of my life
    Help in improving myself as a person
  Resolve
    Help in solving my problems
    A sense of peace and comfort
  Sharing
    Help in expressing my feelings
    A sense of closeness and belonging with other people
  Restraint
    Help in keeping my emotions or actions under control

Religious Appraisals of the Event[b]
  The event was God's will
  The event was a punishment from God
  My spiritual well-being was threatened

Religious Coping Activities[c]
  Spiritually Based
    God showed me how to deal with the situation
    Looked for the lesson from God in the event
    Took control over what I could, and gave the rest up to God
    Sought God's love and care
    Realized that God was trying to strengthen me

(continued)

Realized that I didn't have to suffer since Jesus suffered for me

In dealing with the problem I was guided by God

Trusted that God would not let anything terrible happen to me

Used Christ as an example of how I should live

My faith showed me different ways to handle the problem

Accepted that the situation was not in my hands but in the hands of
   God

Used my faith to help me decide how to cope with the situation

Good Deeds

Tried to be less sinful

Offered help to other church members

Confessed my sins

Tried to lead a more loving life

Attended religious services or participated in religious rituals

Participated in church groups (support groups, prayer groups, Bible-
   study groups)

Discontent

Expressed feelings of anger or distance from God

Expressed feelings of anger or distance from the members of the
   church

Questioned my religious beliefs and faith

Religious Support

Sought support from clergy

Sought support from other members of the church

Plead

Pleaded with God to make things turn out okay

Asked for a miracle

Bargained with God to make things better

Asked God why it happened

Begged for God's help

Religious Avoidance

Focused on the world-to-come rather than the problems of this world

Let God solve my problems for me

Prayed or read the Bible to keep my mind off of my problems

Let God worry about the problem for me

---

[a]Instructions: "In dealing with this event, what were you seeking or aiming for through your relationship with God, your church, and your religious beliefs and practices?"

[b]Instructions: "At the time the event occurred, to what degree did you have the following reaction to the event?"

[c]Instructions: "To what extent was each of the following involved in coping with the event?" Some items on the Religious Coping Activities scales were revised and added in Pargament et al. (1994)

analyses (Pargament, Ensing, et al., 1990). The Christian form of these scales and items are presented in Table 7.3, and briefly described here.

   1. The religious purpose items describe the ends the church member was seeking through religion in coping with their particular event. The Spiritual factor brings the desire for closeness with God together with the search for meaning and hope. Self-Development is made up of the

search for self-esteem, control, and self-actualization. The Resolve factor focuses on religion as an aid to the resolution of problems and emotional comfort. Sharing incorporates the search for intimacy and emotional expression with others through religion. Finally, Restraint reflects the members' desire for religious help in curbing emotions and behaviors.

2. The appraisal items include more benign assessments of the situation from a religious perspective (God's will) as well as more negative ones (God's punishment; spiritual threat).

3. The religious coping activities items reflect different uses of religion in coping. The Spiritually Based factor emphasizes the individual's relationship with God in coping. Through this relationship, problems are reframed positively, the limits of personal control are accepted, and guidance and reassurance are sought. The Good Deeds factor reflects a focus on action; in particular, on living a better, more religiously integrated life. In Discontent, we hear anger, distance, and questions about God and the church. Religious Support involves the attempt to obtain assistance from the clergy or fellow church members. Plead is made up of bargains with God and petitions for a miracle as well as questions about why the event happened. And the Religious Avoidance items involve activities that divert attention from the negative event through prayer, Bible reading, or beliefs in the afterlife.

The religious coping activities scales are not the last word in the conceptualization and measurement of religious coping. The scales are not explicitly theoretical and they do not measure some important coping approaches (e.g., religious forgiveness, conversion). In the next chapter I will take a closer look at religious coping methods from a more theoretical, purposive point of view. My colleagues and I are also in the process of developing a more comprehensive, functionally oriented set of religious coping scales as well as a brief measure of positive and negative patterns of religious coping (see Chapter 10; Pargament, Smith, & Koenig, 1996). Other measures of religious coping are also needed for groups outside of mainline Christian traditions. What these scales do capture are some of the many forms of religious coping among Christians (see Zerowin, 1996, for a Jewish form). As we will see, they have proven to be useful in understanding the factors that shape religious coping, in predicting how people adjust to crises, and in suggesting more helpful and more harmful methods of religious coping. Let us turn our attention to one of these issues now.

If it is true that religion has many faces in coping, then what determines its expression? Why, for instance, does one seriously ill person feel that God is punishing her while another faced with the same illness views her condition as an opportunity to grow spiritually? Why does a death trigger intense involvement in a synagogue for one man and solitary prayer for another? Why does one unemployed man plead with God for a miracle and another ask God for the strength to get through hard times?

SHAPING THE EXPRESSION
OF RELIGIOUS COPING

In the last chapter, I noted how individual, social, and contextual forces converge to affect whether people involve religion in their coping. However, these forces do more than influence *whether* people cope religiously. By making some religious options more available and more compelling than others, they shape *how* people choose to express religion in coping.

Situational Forces and the Shape of Religious Coping

Life events have pushes and pulls of their own. As noted in the last chapter, situations that highlight the frailty of the human condition and the power of forces far greater than ourselves often push for a religious response. But there are many kinds of boundary situations and, as we have seen, many kinds of religious coping; the particular expression of religion depends in part on the particular losses, threats, and challenges each situation poses to significance.

For example, wherever we find a major life transition, we are likely to see religious rituals and beliefs at play tailored to the distinctive tensions these situations raise. Circumcisions, baptisms, and naming ceremonies are some of the religious rituals that mark a birth; each facilitates the integration of the new member into community life. Communions, confirmations, B'nai Mitzvot, and initiation rites are some of the ceremonies that mark a child's coming of age; each calls for a change in the roles and responsibilities of the soon-to-be adult. Funerals, mourning practices, and commemoration ceremonies are some of the rituals that mark a death; each offers an outlet for the expression of loss, a forum for support to those in grief, and a mechanism for reuniting a disrupted community.

Other life crises also press for different religious responses, as religious leaders and clergy are well aware. Compare the religious advice offered by Christian chaplains to people dealing with three contrasting situations—imprisonment, divorce, and physical incapacitation. In the solace to the prisoner we hear an attempt to assuage guilt:

> You may feel guilty about the kind of life you have led, but that should not prevent you from experiencing joy. When the Israelites returned

> to Jerusalem after being in captivity for years, they felt guilty because
> they knew they had not been obeying the laws of Moses. But
> Nehemiah told them, "Do not be grieved, for the joy of the Lord is
> your strength." (Singer, 1983, p. 20)

In a prayer offered to the divorced, the spiritual response is tailored more
closely to the problems of isolation and loneliness:

> There is no one to reach out to me in my lonely bed. How I long to
> have someone to touch and hold, to laugh and talk with, to shout at
> and to hug. I reach for you and you are not there. Did you give me
> this seering loneliness so that it would be easier for me to give you
> everything? All of me? This I know, I need your love. Come, Jesus,
> come. Amen. (Payne, 1982, p. 13)

And the words to the physically incapacitated are particularly suited to
questions of the fairness and meaning of suffering:

> God does not make arbitrary choices about who shall suffer and who
> shall not, who shall live and who shall die. Nor does God desire to
> punish or humble us. . . . Knowing that difficulties are part of life and
> that God does not purposely send them our way enables us to move
> from the "Why me?" questions to the "How" questions—"How can I
> survive this trying time? How can I cope with my situation? How can
> I grow through what I am experiencing?" (Biegert, 1985, pp. 5–6)

As these vignettes show, the religious world can be "situationally
sensitive" (cf. Oden, 1983), molding its response to the problem at hand.
     Whether individuals show a similar sensitivity to the nature of the
situation in their own choices of religious coping is another question.
Religion is often thought of as a stable personality characteristic, an
orientation to life applied consistently and unvaryingly across time and
place. In the Project on Religion and Coping, we tested whether different
life events are linked to different religious and nonreligious coping
strategies (Pargament, Olsen, et al., 1992a). The religious coping methods were described earlier. The nonreligious coping questions focused on
(1) the degree the event was appraised as a threat, challenge/opportunity,
or harm/loss, and (2) the degree the person coped with the event by
focusing on the positive, problem solving, avoidance of the problem, or
interpersonal support (McCrae, 1984; Moos, Cronkite, Billings, &
Finney, 1984; Stone & Neale, 1984).
     We subdivided our sample into groups who had experienced one of
four negative events over the past year: (1) the death of a family member
or close friend; (2) a work-related problem such as unemployment, or

being fired or laid off; (3) an interpersonal conflict such as a divorce or separation; or (4) a health-related problem. We then compared the way the four groups coped. If religion were situationally insensitive, then we would expect to see few differences in the ways the groups coped with their respective problems. Religion would express itself similarly regardless of the negative event. If religion were situationally sensitive, then we would expect to find each group coping differently with their troubles. What did we find?

Our results lent some support to the situationally sensitive view (Pargament, Olsen, et al., 1992a). The four groups coped differently across the board: They appraised their situations differently, made use of different religious and nonreligious coping activities, and looked to religion for different purposes. Most distinctive of all was the religious response to death. More than those in other situations, people who had lost a loved one appraised their situation as the will of God. They took more religiously avoidant steps to help them shift their focus from their losses, and they looked more to their religion for sharing and closeness with others. Along with people facing health-related problems, they engaged more in spiritually based coping and received more support from their clergy and fellow congregation members. Interestingly, the group grappling with death was less likely than other groups to make use of nonreligious coping activities, such as problem solving or focusing on the positive. Clearly, death and religion were closely wrapped together. It is important to emphasize, however, that individuals who had suffered a death did not simply lay a "religious blanket" over their loss. Their approach to religious coping was selective. For example, they were as likely as anyone else to perform good deeds, plead with God, or voice their religious discontent in coping. In short, the religious response to death was not indiscriminate; it was molded to the needs among these people for emotional, social, and spiritual support.

The Project on Religion and Coping afforded us another opportunity to study the question of situational sensitivity. Because we followed up with these members 1 year later, readministering the same scales, we were able to measure how consistently the same person coped religiously over time and situation. Church members were placed into one of two groups: those facing similar situations and those facing different situations over the 1-year period. As expected, there was a strong degree of similarity in religious coping for people dealing with the same kind of situation 1 year later. Similar situations led to similar coping. But what about people confronting different situations? Would they apply the same religious solution to their new problems or a different one? Our results revealed a much smaller correlation in religious coping among people in this group. As the situation changed, people became less likely to use religion in the way they had before. In other words, different problems seemed to push for different religious solutions. Hathaway (1992) also reported day-to-day variations in several types of religious coping among people dealing with hassles over a 90-day period. These hassles included preparing meals, too many interruptions, not enough sleep, and difficulties at work.

To say that situations contribute to the shape of our lives seems obvious. But to say that situations also shape the nature of religion in our lives is less apparent. Because religion is so often seen as a stable part of personality, the power of the situation in religious experience and the capacity of a faith to adapt itself to a variety of circumstances may be underestimated. However, the evidence reviewed here, limited as it is, suggests that situations do affect the way religion expresses itself in coping. Of course, they are not the only determining force. As we have stressed, people do not cope alone nor do they come to coping empty-handed.

Cultural Forces and the Shape of Religious Coping

Culture makes some ways of thinking about and dealing with critical problems more accessible and more compelling to its members than others. This point holds true for religion. Culture selectively encourages some religious expressions in coping and selectively discourages others.

Stephenson (1983–1984) describes the case of a 48-year-old man suffering from lymphosarcoma who died 2 weeks after his initial collapse. Family members were particularly despondent. After the funeral, one brother of the deceased angrily said to another: "He died too quick, too quick. . . . he was so alive. Well I've seen worse cases . . . men who went out in the morning to work and who never came back! But, he just died too quick" (p. 131). This death caused a great deal of consternation and conflict in the community.

To members of Western culture, these reactions may seem a bit peculiar. A death of this kind would certainly lead to shock and sadness, but the grief might be cushioned by the recognition that the person went quickly and did not have to suffer. However, the death Stephenson described occurred within a Hutterian colony. In this culture, the ideal death is protracted. A prolonged death offers Hutterites the time to make amends for their sins, to forgive and be forgiven, and to prepare for eternal life. As one Hutterite put it: "We prefer slow deaths, not sudden deaths. We want to have plenty of time to consider eternity and to confess and make everything right. We don't like to see a grownup go suddenly" (Hostetler, 1974, cited in Stephenson, 1983–1984, p. 128). Here we have an illustration of culture shaping the religious interpretation of a situation. The quick and painless death is, to the Hutterite, a spiritual blow.

Cultures shape religious coping methods as well as religious appraisals. For several years ethnographer Unni Wikan (1988) lived and worked in two different cultures, Egypt and Bali, that share the religion of Islam. In spite of their common religion, Wikan found, the members of the two cultures cope very differently with death. In Egypt the death of a child precipitates intensive reactions of grief and suffering: "They will cry as if pouring their hearts out. Females will scream, yell, beat their breasts, collapse in each others' arms and be quite beyond themselves for days, even weeks on end" (p. 452).

Balinese respond quite differently to the death of a child: "They will strive to act with calm and composure, especially beyond the circle of closest family and closest friends. But even among intimates, their reactions will be moderate and laughter, joking and cheerfulness mingle with mutely expressed sadness" (p. 452).

Why such different responses to death from people of the same faith? Religion, Wikan maintains, is filtered through culture; Egyptians and Balinese alike draw on the elements of Islam most consistent with their ethos. In the world of the Egyptian, emotional expression is viewed as essential to health. "Unhappiness must find a way out of the body or it weighs upon the soul" (p. 458). Cultural norms encourage the open display of all feelings—sadness, anger, and conflict. And Islam, with its vision of a compassionate and merciful God, abets the emotional expression of the Egyptian.

Among the Balinese emotional expression has a different meaning. It represents a threat to oneself, others, and the soul of the dead. Bad feelings are said to interfere with good judgment. Not only that, they are contagious, putting others in the community at risk. As important is the danger emotional upset poses to the soul of the dead. According to Balinese Muslims, the fate of the soul is dependent on the actions of the living. One man said: "If we cry and are unhappy, the soul will be unhappy too, not free to go to the God. We must contain our sadness that the soul will be liberated to go to heaven" (p. 458). Like the Egyptians, the Balinese are supported in their approach to bereavement by aspects of Islam. But in the latter case the key Islamic tenet is the belief that death is foreordained by God and one must submit to God's will. "The Balinese often remind themselves that to give oneself over to grief is like opposing God's will" (p. 458).

Wikan concludes that culture plays the critical role in shaping the response of Balinese and Egyptians to loss. The religion of Islam is not unimportant here. But it is an Islam which takes different shapes across different cultures: " . . . despite its all-embracing and rigorous character

[Islam] is nevertheless always subjected to distinct and particularistic, locally produced interpretations, that lend a particular cast and character to its precepts, laws, and pervasive doctrines" (p. 451). Although Wikan focuses on Islam, her conclusions may apply equally well to other faiths.

Even in the so-called "melting pot" of the United States, the individuals' culture of origin continues to affect the response to questions of ultimate importance in living. McReady and Greeley (1976) asked a large sample of Americans how they would react to each of four hypothetical situations: one's own terminal illness, having a son drafted into combat, the slow and painful death of a parent, and the birth of a mentally retarded child. They categorized the responses into five groups: (1) Religious optimist ("God will take care of everything, so there is no need to worry"), (2) Hopeful ("There is no denying the evil of what is happening, but the last word has not been said yet"), (3) Secular optimist ("Everything will turn out for the best somehow"), (4) Pessimist ("There is nothing that can be done; what will be will be"), and (5) Diffuse ("Unsure, don't know") (p. 19).

Among their many comparisons, McCready and Greeley contrasted the ways people of different ethnic heritage responded to the painful scenarios. Even among members of the same religious group, differences in culture of origin were associated with varied approaches to coping. For instance, Catholics of Polish and Spanish background were more likely to be religious optimists or hopeful and less likely to be pessimists than Catholics of Irish, German, or Italian ancestry. Protestants of Scandinavian origin were more likely to respond with religious optimism and less likely to indicate secular optimism than British or German Protestants. The authors were not able to sort out the potential influence of other variables, such as socioeconomic status, on their findings. Nevertheless, their findings suggest that Americans continue to carry a legacy from the cultures of their ancestors that influences their responses, religious and nonreligious, to the most basic problems in living in the United States.

Individual Forces and the Shape of Religious Coping: The Orienting System

Important as the situation and culture are, neither can account for the diversity of religious coping. Cook and Wimberly (1983) underscore this point in their poignant study of religious coping among parents who had suffered the death of a child. Their sample of parents had many things in common: Most were white, married, employed, Protestant, had at least a high school education, and lived in the same geographical area. Most importantly, all had lost a child as a result of either cancer or blood disorders. However, in spite of similar situations and social backgrounds, their religious responses were far from identical. Many parents expressed the belief that they would one day be reunited with their child in heaven. The father of a 14-year-old boy who died of leukemia said: "I figure God gave me Gary for 14 years and it was super, he was a neat kid to have around, it was a wonderful experience for me. And if I play my cards right I'll see him again" (p. 229). Other parents viewed the death as a punishment for their own sins. One father who drank too much and had an extramarital affair during the illness of his son said: "[God] took him from me because of the rotten life that I lived. I think it was an awakening thing, that's the reason why [God] done it" (p. 228). Still another group of parents felt that the death of their child served a noble and divine purpose. As one parent said: "I believe that he was sent here for some reason and he had served his purpose and was taken back. He had faith in God, such faith . . . he touched so many lives" (p. 229).

If these parents were distinguished by neither culture nor circumstance, what accounts for their diverse responses? Cook and Wimberly do not focus on this issue, but one good hypothesis is that the parents were distinguished by the orientation they brought to the situation. Each came with a particular way of thinking about, acting, feeling, and relating to his or her world; each brought different resources and burdens to coping. Guided by their respective orienting systems, religious as well as nonreligious, these parents followed different paths in their struggle with loss. Those who generally look to religion as a source of comfort in living may have found the belief that they would join their child in the afterlife particularly compelling. Those who generally integrate their faith throughout their lives may have sought out ways to imbue their loss with religious purpose. Those who look to God for justice may have found it less frightening to view the death as a divine punishment than to consider the possibility that there is no God or that God is capricious.

As part of the orienting system, religion influences how situations are viewed and understood. In this vein, Kushner (1989) writes: "Religion is not primarily a set of beliefs, a collection of prayers, or a series of rituals. Religion is first and foremost a way of seeing. It can't change the facts about the world we live in, but it can change the way we see those facts, and that in itself can often make a difference" (p. 27). To use more psychological language, religion is, in part, a cognitive schema (McIntosh, 1995), a mental representation of the world that helps us filter and make sense of the massive amounts of stimulation we encounter.

But there are many ways of viewing the world religiously. Present the same information to people with different orientations and they will process it quite differently. Clergy are well aware of this point. Every week they present a sermon to their members and receive, in return, a bewildering array of reactions—from the yawn, polite nod, and "nice sermon, Reverend" to the frown, puzzled look, and desire to talk more after the service. Although the members belong to the same congregation and listen to the same sermon, they look at the world through different religious glasses; thus, the identical sermon takes on a very different appearance to the members (see Pargament & DeRosa, 1985, for an example).

The orienting system influences not only the way situations are viewed and understood, but the way they are handled. Depending on the nature of the orienting system, some religious options for coping become more accessible and more compelling than others. For example, Ebaugh, Richman, and Chafetz (1984) interviewed members of Catholic Charismatic, Christian Science, and Bahai faiths about their ways of coping. Although Ebaugh et al. had expected the groups to report different types and frequencies of life crises, these variations were relatively small and explained by demographic differences between the groups. What set the groups apart were their ways of coping. These differences could not be explained by demographic factors. Consistent with their theology, Christian Scientists engaged first and foremost in positive thinking. The other groups rarely used positive thinking to cope with their crises. Bahais and Catholic Charismatics were more likely to look for support than Christian Scientists. However, the two former groups seemed to want a different kind of support. The Charismatics sought out fellow members for emotional solace, while the Bahais looked to others for help in interpreting their sacred works. In contrast to the other two groups, Catholic Charismatics also engaged in more passive deferring religious responses, such as waiting for the Lord or putting the problem in God's hands. Ebaugh et al. tie these differences in religious coping to the distinctive theologies of the religious groups.

In the Project on Religion and Coping, my colleagues and I (Pargament, Olsen, et al., 1992b) took a closer look at the nature of the religious orienting system and its relationship to the concrete ways people cope with crises. Recall that a religious orientation was defined as a *general* disposition to use particular means in the search for particular ends. As a general disposition, a religious orientation is not involved with the details of any one situation. It comes to life only after it has been translated into a more concrete language that speaks to the problem at hand. We suspected that the three most commonly studied religious orientations—intrinsic, extrinsic, and quest—would translate into very different approaches to coping with critical life events. To test this hypothesis, scores on the measures of these three orientations were correlated with the coping responses of congregation members to the most serious life event they had experienced in the past year. Our hypothesis was confirmed. Each of the orientations was associated with a distinctive approach to coping, both religiously and nonreligiously.

1. The *intrinsic orientation* was closely bound to spiritual forms of coping. Those who were more intrinsic looked to their religion more for spiritual purposes and less for self-development in coping. They also were more likely to make use of spiritually based coping activities, such as seeking God's guidance in problem solving. Even though the more intrinsically oriented read the Bible more and thought about the hereafter more to take their minds off their problems, the orientation was not altogether avoidant or passive. In fact, intrinsicness was related to *lower* scores on the measure of nonreligious avoidance in coping and *higher* scores on the measure of problem solving. The appraisals associated with intrinsicness were also interesting: the more intrinsic congregation members viewed their events as a spiritual threat as well as an opportunity to grow. But they did not appraise their crises as any less harmful than other members. Apparently, intrinsic religiousness highlights only the spiritual risk of critical events, but the threat is counterbalanced by appraisals of promise and opportunity for growth in the situations.

2. People with a more *extrinsic orientation* looked to religion largely for their own personal development. There was a more defensive, even desperate tenor to coping here. In appraising the situations, extrinsicness was related to lower levels of self-blame, greater perceptions of personal threat to one's health, more of a sense that the situation cannot be personally handled, and less of a feeling that the event offers an opportunity for growth. Interestingly, the more extrinsically oriented more often reported that they could change the situation, but apparently not through their own actions. Extrinsicness was related to nonreligious avoidance and a focus on the positive. In the religious realm it was tied to pleading with God and performing good deeds; both of these religious coping efforts may reflect their efforts to sway God to intervene on their own behalf.

3. The quest orientation expressed itself in yet another way in coping. Like intrinsic religiousness, quest was associated with the search for spirituality through religion in coping. However, a finer analysis of the items on the spirituality scale indicated that quest was related only to the item dealing with the search for meaning. Consistent with Batson et al.'s (1993) description of this construct, the quest orientation was marked by signs of active struggle. Quest, like intrinsic religiousness, was tied to appraisals of the event as both a spiritual threat and an opportunity to grow. The religious coping methods related to quest were

action oriented, focusing on efforts at personal improvement through good deeds and expressions of discontent to God and the church.

It seems clear that the individual's orienting system has important implications for the way religion is expressed in specific situations. But, as yet, only a few facets of the orienting system have been studied. In all likelihood, religious coping is shaped by other orienting variables as well, such as gender, race, socioeconomic status, development over the lifespan, personality, mental health, and still other religious orientations.

CONCLUSIONS

"When my son was killed in 1975, that was the first time my faith was really tested. Before that everything was just theory" (Cobble, 1985, p. 140). It is one thing to think about religion apart from immediate problems and concerns. It is another to apply it to real tragedies and losses. Much of the psychology of religion has focused on the former approach—the religion of general beliefs, practices, and orientations that may have little to do with the down-to-earth predicaments of living. The psychology of religion and coping, however, shifts our attention from heaven to earth, to the specifics of religious expression in troubled times.

In this chapter we have seen that religion is not "one thing" in coping. It takes on different forms at different times and in different places. It appears in the ends sought, the construction of events, and the coping methods themselves. Religion is a force that helps shape the coping process and is, itself, shaped in turn. Stereotypical views of religion as a form of tension reduction, denial, or passive–avoidant coping do not do justice to the varied manifestations of religion in critical times.

But in moving away from simple description and stereotypes, in shifting from the macroanalytic to the microanalytic, from the distal to the proximal, the task of studying religion has become more complex. Some readers may wonder whether all of this is really necessary. After all, what difference does it make how religion expresses itself in the concrete? Isn't it enough to know about the individual's general religious approach to life? Or do we even need to know about the religious dimension of coping? Isn't it enough to know about how the person copes more generally? These questions cut to the very heart of the psychology of religion and coping. They challenge the assumption that how religion comes to life in critical situations is indeed important. In Chapter 10, I will present evidence that these concrete manifestations of religion are significant predictors of how particular situations will unfold. In fact, we will see that measures of religious coping predict the outcomes of negative events more strongly than standard measures of general religious orientation (e.g., frequency of prayer, frequency of church attendance, intrinsic religiousness). We will also see that the measures of religious coping add something beyond what we already know about crises from the secular study of coping. When religion is entered into the coping equation, it increases our ability to predict outcomes beyond the effects of secular coping methods. The main conclusion is this: Any understanding of religion and any understanding of coping remains incomplete when we overlook the transition from heaven to earth and the roles of religion "in the dust of our trials."

In this chapter I have described many of the faces and expressions of religion in coping and the forces that shape them. To stop here, however, would leave the mistaken impression that religious coping is totally determined by the larger context, the event, or what the person brings to the event. While these forces encourage some ways of coping and discourage others, they do not dictate the response to crisis. There is a pull as well as a push to coping. And the pull comes from the character of significance. People generally choose ways to cope from their available options in an effort to maximize significance. But when viable options are not available, they can create new ones or change the nature of significance. In the next two chapters I consider the religious search for significance in coping from this more purposive, volitional point of view. I will focus on the involvement of religion in the two central mechanisms of coping—conservation and transformation.

Chapter Eight

RELIGION AND
THE MECHANISMS
OF COPING
The Conservation
of Significance

In 1942 a Jewish couple in the Kovno ghetto defies the German ban against having children. As the ritual circumcision for their newborn boy is about to be performed, Gestapo agents come to the door. The mother shouts: "Hurry up! Circumcise the child. Don't you see? They have come to kill us. At least let my child die as a Jew."
—BERKOVITS (1979, p. 45)

Every religious coping effort represents a response to values under fire, values that are tested, endangered, or lost through life's events, and every religious coping effort has a common end, the enhancement of significance. Of course, there are many ways to enhance significance, but from a functional perspective, it comes down to one of two strategies in coping: to try to hold on to what matters most or to try to let go and change. To put it another way, the choice in coping is to conserve or to transform. In conservation, the emphasis is on attempts to protect or maintain what is of significance. This is usually the first and preferred strategy in coping. Yet there are times when old values can no longer be sustained, when old hopes and dreams must be abandoned if life is to go on, and when the search must begin for new things that matter. In

198

transformation, significance is maximized by attempts to change the nature of significance itself.

While both conservation and transformation are key mechanisms in the search for significance, they are very different choices in coping. The religious lexicon provides an unmistakably clear and distinctive set of labels to describe those committed to the tried-and-true (fundamentalists, traditionalists, conservatives, orthodox) and those convinced there is a better way (reformationists, modernists, revivalists). And there is no shortage of labels each group can use to derogate the other (heretics, infidels, heathens, disbelievers, pagans). The history of the world's religions has been sharply punctuated by periods of conflict between the standard bearers of the status quo and the advocates of profound change. Out of the collisions between Hindus, Buddhists, Jews, Christians, and Muslims, civilizations have been torn apart and reformed. *Within* major religious groups, the clashes between the old and the new have had similar effects. The social, political, and economic history of the United States has been shaped by every great religious awakening, from the Puritan departure from Anglicanism to the New Age response to conservative Christianity (McLoughlin, 1978).

The tension between conservation and transformation is not limited to organized religious groups; it occurs within the individual's religious world as well. Faced with life-shaking events, the individual must also choose between profound change and the status quo. In this chapter and the one that follows we will see how religion is engraved on both sides of this coping coin—in attempts to perpetuate the world, and in attempts to destroy old worlds and re-create new ones. We will examine religious coping methods that appear to have "built-in" conservational or transformational designs. But a word of forewarning. The focus on these mechanisms of coping will take us beyond the description of coping activities to a functional analysis of the purposes they serve. Thus, we will not be talking about prayer, beliefs, or congregational involvement in general; rather, we will consider particular religious expressions that serve particular purposes. In this functional shift from the "whats" to the "whys" of coping, we will have to rely less on empirical study and more on "softer" data—the kinds of inferences and interpretations many social scientists dislike because they can be disputed so easily. Yet if we are to understand this process, we have to dive into murkier waters, and feel for some of the underlying currents that direct the flow of coping.

From the outset I should also make my own views clear on the merits of conservation and transformation. Neither mechanism is necessarily good or bad in and of itself. Attempts to conserve or transform significance may or may not meet with success. (We will examine the relationship of religious coping methods to outcomes in Chapter 10).

Furthermore, conservation should not be equated with pathological defensiveness, and transformation with growth. In Chapter 11, I will make the case that the value of both mechanisms depends on *what* is being conserved or transformed and *how* this conservation or transformation takes place.

RELIGION AND THE CONSERVATION OF SIGNIFICANCE

Change can be a scary thing. "By nature we like the familiar and dislike the strange," Maimonides once said (Minkin, 1987). That is one reason why the new is not always welcomed. But it is not the only reason; after all, the familiar can become tiresome and the strange can be curious and exciting. Change may be less scary than it is costly. With change may come depleted resources, added burdens and diminished significance. Certainly, change can also lead to new resources and new value, but oftentimes the costs of change seem to outweigh the benefits. Thus, people generally prefer to protect and cling to their values. Under stress this tendency may become still stronger. Earlier we noted how people struggle tenaciously to maintain themselves and their way of life, even in the worst of situations. Here we turn our attention to the involvement of religion in these efforts to conserve significance.

In the minds of many, religion is first and foremost an instrument of conservation. "The core of religion," philosopher Harald Höffding (1914) wrote, "consists in the conviction that no value perishes out of the world" (p. 6) and later, "the innermost tendency of all religions, is the axiom of the conservation of value" (p. 209). Sociologists have made similar points (Berger, 1961; Yinger, 1970). For example, Berger (1961) sees religion as a defender of the social and psychological status quo, an author of integrative symbols, practices, and theologies rather than revolutionary ones: "When crises threaten the everyday taken-for-granted routine of the individual and there looms the ecstatic possibility of confronting directly his own existence, society provides the rituals by which he is gently led back into the 'okay world' " (pp. 121–122). Many psychologists have echoed this sentiment—that religion is a method of maintaining personal stability in the face of deprivation, undesirable impulses, death-related fears, and guilt (Argyle & Beit-Hallahmi, 1975).

Below we examine the involvement of religion in the two general mechanisms of conservation: preservation and reconstruction (see Table 5.1). Recall that both approaches attempt to protect the ends of greatest significance to the individual. In preservation, the person tries to hold on not only to the ends of significance, but to the means to attain it.

The effort here is to preserve an entire way of life. In reconstructive coping, the individual tries to conserve the ends of significance through a change of the means to achieve it rather than a change of significance itself. Here a different path is taken to an old familiar destination. It is not hard to find religion at work in both the preservation of significance and the reconstruction of the path to significance.

HOLDING FAST: RELIGION AND THE PRESERVATION OF SIGNIFICANCE

There are a number of mechanisms people draw on to sustain the means and ends of significance. In this section we will consider three of these methods: marking boundaries, religious perseverance, and religious support.

Marking Boundaries

One way to try to preserve a lifestyle that has come under threat is to draw an unmistakably clear line between one's own world and the forces outside of it. A bulwark is established on this line that safeguards against intrusion by foreign elements, draws people together, and discourages them from venturing outside the protective shield. Go beyond that wall and face danger, stand behind it and remain secure.

In some respects religious institutions operate as "boundary markers" that encourage their members to maintain a distinctive set of values and lifestyle, particularly in times of trouble. The immigrant church is a case in point. Traditionally, this institution has been an anchor in the community for members caught up in the wrenching transition from familiar to unfamiliar culture. The church responds to this disruption with a set of boundary mechanisms that reminds its members of who they are and, as importantly, who they are not. Palinkas (1982) describes some of the mechanisms immigrant Christian Chinese churches use to sustain the identity and cohesiveness of their members in the chaotic environment. In the religious services, Chinese proverbs are selected to illustrate Christian principles. Members address each other as "brothers," "sisters," "aunt," and "uncle" to underscore their special closeness. Sermons in the church have a dual function. They emphasize the dissimilarities of their members from the larger culture: In contrast to *non-Christian Chinese*, church members are less sinful and self-indulgent. In contrast to *non-Christians*, church members are more concerned with family values and less concerned with social gain. And in contrast to *non-Chinese*, church members are not prejudiced toward others. The sermons also emphasize the common values and practices among the members of the audience: the love of God, the respect for traditional values and customs, a shared language, the sense of filial piety, and the fact that every Chinese Christian is ultimately "saved" from the struggles of this life. Through boundary mechanisms such as these, the Chinese Christian is set apart from the larger culture, the bonds among church members are strengthened, and something of the old world is preserved in the new.

Sometimes it is not the individual's personal and social world that is challenged, but the religious world itself. These threats are, according to Paden (1988), the most dangerous and subversive of all: "If the sacred is the foundation of a world, then whatever denies that sacredness will be intolerable" (p. 61). With its own well-being at stake, the religious world may respond by marking its boundaries. Chidester (1988) illustrates this point in his description of the American response to the tragedy of Jonestown. It was hard enough for many people to fathom why the leader of the People's Temple and his followers would leave the United States and establish an alternate religious community in the jungles of Guyana. But the mass murder/suicide of 913 men, women, and children from cyanide was virtually incomprehensible. It struck at the core of the religious values most Americans hold: the sacredness of life, the belief that there is hope in the most desperate conditions, the commitment to personal freedom.

Most Americans, Chidester believes, viewed the Jonestown experience as demonic or insane; it was an aberration falling outside the boundaries of reason and decency. Many barriers were established to seal the experience off from national consciousness. Particularly telling were the efforts to keep the remains of the Jonestown dead from returning to the United States. In spite of the fact that morticians had taken extreme steps to sanitize the bodies (applying 10 times the usual amount of disinfectant and embalming fluid), concerns were raised that the poison from the corpses would pollute the earth. Others voiced fears that the mass grave would become a ritual site for unstable religious cult members. As the mayor of Dover said: "I don't need a bunch of weirdoes here in Dover" (Chidester, 1988, p. 17). Many others wrote letters to the state and federal government expressing their spiritual alarm that the bodies of the Jonestown dead would defile sacred American soil and come back to haunt the community. Ultimately, the remains were interred without religious ceremony in unmarked graves near San Francisco, with one exception. The body of Jim Jones was cremated (again without ceremony) and the ashes were thrown into the Atlantic Ocean.

The boundaries could not have been drawn any more sharply. In an effort to preserve the religious and social order, a physical wall was constructed that separated the community from the most visible symbol of a deeply disturbing event. In this case, the order was preserved. Chidester (1990) writes: "Clearly, faith in the American way was not shaken by the Jonestown deaths. Rather, an American faith was reinforced by the ritual exclusion of the Jonestown dead" (pp. 286–287).

It is not always so easy to draw such a clear line around religion. In our pluralistic society, most religions exist side by side with other faiths that have very different perspectives and practices. It can be an uneasy coexistence, for the presence of so many religious alternatives may threaten the most basic assumption of the faith—that it has a special grasp on the truth. Like the neighbors in a small town, religions often respond by putting up fences to mark off where their land begins and ends and to protect their property. Rules are defined for what makes someone a Protestant, Catholic, Muslim, Hindu, or Jew. Contact with other religions or the secular culture may be discouraged. The line between the sacred and the profane, the pure and the impure is clearly demarcated, and sanctions are established for those who might think about crossing the line—from raised eyebrows and criticism to shunning and excommunication. Even these rules and prohibitions, though, may not be enough to sustain a religious system in a multifaith, highly interconnected world where it is almost impossible to avoid others who say, in effect: "The way you see the world is not the way I see it."

There are, however, individual boundary mechanisms that buttress and reinforce the dividing lines marked by religious social systems. Some religiously committed people move away from the contaminating influences of society, literally or figuratively. The religious saint "may well find the outer world too full of shocks to dwell in, and can unify his life and keep his soul unspotted only by withdrawing" (James, 1902, p. 290).

Boundaries can be marked psychologically as well as physically. People are quite capable of selectively filtering or blocking information that threatens or challenges religious beliefs, practices, and values. In this vein, Brock and Balloun (1967) asked groups of more religious and less religious people to listen to a message attacking hypocrisy within organized Christianity. The message was intentionally filled with a great deal of static in the background that made listening very difficult. Compared to the less religiously involved, those who attended church and prayed more frequently were less likely to make the "Christianity is Evil" message easier to hear by pressing a "static-eliminating button." These findings were replicated over four separate experiments. Confronted with danger, these studies suggest, people make use of a protective screen that filters out threatening information (see also Pargament & DeRosa, 1985).

A related psychological boundary-marking response is to intensify the commitment to the religious world, a psychological "circling of the wagons" against threat. Batson (1975) examined this process of intensification in a laboratory study of female high school students. The students were asked to make a public commitment to their faith by sitting with one of two groups in the room: those who felt they could affirm that Jesus Christ is the Son of God or those who could not. The students were then presented with an article containing "conclusive proof" that the writings of the New Testament are false and the body of Jesus was, in reality, stolen by his followers to justify the claim that he was resurrected. Batson predicted that the students who made a public commitment to their religion and accepted the truth of this dissonant information would be more likely to intensify their beliefs as "their only recourse . . . to defend their present cognitive integration against the attack" (p. 182). In fact, the students in this group did increase the intensity of their beliefs following disconfirmation. Batson explains his results in the language of boundaries: "Defensively, it [cognitive mobilization] would provide a tightening of the ranks . . . offensively, it would imply threats of retaliation, both against the information and against the source (e.g., 'I *still* believe in Jesus'; 'I think whoever wrote that article should be locked up, and then throw away the key')" (p. 183).

It seems almost instinctive; many of us are quick to put up a barrier to protect ourselves from the perilous forces swirling around outside. Paden (1988) sums it up this way: "The subject matter here: worlds shut out, profanity shunned, bulwarks erected, lines not crossed, refusals to follow 'man's law, instead of God's law.' The results: existence unified, the sacred kept intact, integrity maintained" (p. 154). Paden may have overstated his case here. The motivation for marking boundaries seems to be conservational—to protect and preserve a world of values, beliefs, and practices—but the result is not always successful. In spite of the best efforts of individual and groups, threats cannot always be warded off. Yet even when these threats are realized and the boundaries of the world are violated, religions have at their disposal other ways to respond.

Religious Perseverance

Tenacity is one such way to deal with adversity. History is filled with accounts of determined, unyielding people who, under terrible pressures, refused to recant their religious beliefs and practices. We do not have to look too far back in time to find striking examples of religious perseverance. Take the case of the Amish. Descendants of the Swiss Anabaptists who fought against pressures to join the state churches of Europe in the 16th century, the Amish came to the United States over 250 years ago. Since that time they have been able to preserve a unique way of family and community life. Physical separation from the larger society, home-made clothing of plain colors, rejection of modern devices, a religiously based agrarian lifestyle, and a distinctive language are some of the markers that set the Amish apart from others and bond them more closely to each other. However, the task of perpetuating this time-honored mode of living has become increasingly difficult in today's world. Compulsory public school education laws in some states, technological developments in agriculture, tourism, the increasing scarcity of farmland, and governmental incursions have all posed serious problems for the Amish community.

Thompson (1981) describes how one small Old Order Amish community in Oklahoma has dealt with these encroachments of modern society. Although the young Amish must attend public schools until the age of 16, their clothing remains distinctive; German continues to be the primary language at home, and the English spoken by Amish students at school is often broken. While tourists bring traffic problems, litter, rudeness, and increased crime, the Amish typically respond by ignoring the outsiders and going on about their regular activities. Two proposed construction projects, a nuclear power plant adjacent to their land and a four-lane highway that would bisect their community, posed serious threats to Amish life. Nevertheless, they refused to take part in social protests or legal action that would call into question their patriotism or draw attention to their community. In each of these responses the attempt was to minimize the harm of external intrusions by clinging steadfastly to traditional values, beliefs, and practices.

It would not be accurate to say that the Amish resist all change. Despite the injunction against modern devices, Amish farmers do make use of tractors and modern electric milking machines. Prior to the introduction of any modern device into the community, church elders consider whether the instrument is needed to perpetuate the "living off the land." Tractors and milking machines are two of the modern devices seen as essential to maintaining the community. Thus, Amish society is not static, but the changes that do take place are slow in coming and methodically evaluated according to their impact on the traditional life style. What remains the most prominent approach to coping with threat and harm is a dogged determination to preserve a way of life.

This kind of persistence could be viewed as simply a reaction to external pressures, a form of psychological reactance in which threats to religious freedom are met with even greater commitment to the religious world (Brehm, 1966). However, there is an important distinction to be made between an intensification of religious commitment (the psychological "circling of the wagons") and religious perseverance. The former is a *re*action to threat, the latter a *pro*action—an effort to perpetuate a way of life *despite* the obstacles that block the path.

This is the point Berkovits (1979) makes in his powerful accounting of Jewish survival in the ghettos and concentration camps of Nazi Europe. "Forever preoccupied with the problem of faith after the Holocaust," he writes, "many of us often overlook the fact that in the ghettos and concentration camps there were untold numbers of Jews who to the very end lived and died as Jews" (p. ix). Berkovits supports his thesis with a number of poignant illustrations of those who were unswerving in their practice of the faith in the most desperate conditions. For instance, one Jew went to great lengths to find a place of prayer in the concentration camps. "In one of the various camps in which he stayed there was a vast open pit in which they used to bury the people who were killed. In that pit he found a quiet corner where he could pray regularly. From then on, his comrades would call that death pit *Das Beit-medreshei,* the little *Bet haMidrash* [house of study]" (p. 5).

For the "authentic Jew," Berkovits maintains, spirituality was not a reaction to the horrors of the camps. Neither was it a form of escape. "What was right before remained right and what was wrong remained wrong even after the dark age of the ghettos and the camps descended on him. . . . He had no need to find a 'new inward center of gravity' " (p. 54). Those who persevered in their religion, then, were not passive "sheep led to slaughter." Their relentless practice of the faith gave forceful expression to their most fundamental values. Berkovits captures the power that lies behind this spirit of perseverance:

> Had I wanted it, I could always have escaped the suffering of exile—as indeed many have—by surrendering to the dominant majority, to its culture, its religion. The arms of the churches were stretched out toward me, inviting me into their bosom. But I made a stand. I remained true to myself and refused. I remained captain of my soul. True, I have paid a terrible price for this stand. But no one forced me to do it. I chose it myself again and again. Is this passivity, inaction? Nonsense! It is the most intense form of activity. With a gun in your hand, with a country of your own, with a government behind you, it is comparatively easy. But without all that and defying all that, to choose your own way requires strength and dedication. (p. 148)

To persist in a religious expression is a choice. As Berkovits notes, other choices were available to the Jews. Similarly, at any time, the Amish could have decided to assimilate into mainstream culture. Why did people choose to persist in a faith when it became so very costly? The answer from our coping perspective would be that the costs of change were greater than the price of religious perseverance. Even if the price to be paid was one's own survival, continuity in the faith remained more compelling than the alternative. Here is what Berkovits says: "The authentic Jew wanted to survive like anyone else, but not at any cost; not at the cost of betraying the meaning of his own life. We have seen how devastating were the consequences of attempting to survive at any cost. It meant the betrayal of all human values and ultimately . . . it brought about the adoption of the SS values by the prisoners themselves" (p. 96).

Evidence from empirical studies suggests that many people do persevere in their religious beliefs and practices in times of stress. Over the course of a crisis, the majority of people report that their religious faith has been strengthened or remains unchanged. This finding holds true for many groups: widows of miners killed in a fire (Bahr & Harvey, 1979b), war veterans (Allport, Gillespie, & Young, 1948), and adolescents and adults following the deaths of loved ones (Balk, 1983; Loveland, 1968). For example, working with heart attack patients, Croog and Levine (1972) examined changes in ratings of the importance of religion over a 1-year period following the episode. Almost two-thirds of the group did not change their assessments. Attendance at religious services also remained unchanged for 73% of the sample over the same time period. Even an event as cataclysmic as the Holocaust did not lead to wholesale changes in religious faith and practice, according to most of those who lived through the upheaval. Brenner (1980) surveyed 708 Jewish survivors and found that 61% indicated no change in religious behavior before the Holocaust, after the Holocaust, and today. Only 29% reported that their belief in God had changed during or immediately after the Holocaust. While most of those who did describe a change reported a weakening rather than a strengthening of religious observance and faith, stability of religion seemed to characterize the majority of survivors.

Those who are more religious to begin with appear to be particularly likely to persevere. McIntosh, Silver, and Wortman (1989) illustrate this point in their study of mothers who had recently lost an infant to Sudden Infant Death Syndrome (SIDS). Mothers who defined religion as extremely important to them 3 weeks after the fatality (Wave I) were less likely than other mothers to change the importance they attached to religion 3 months later (Wave II). Similarly, mothers who made more use of religious coping at Wave I were less likely than other mothers to change their ratings of religious importance and religious coping at Wave II.

The weight of empirical evidence suggests that most people, particularly the highly religious, "keep the faith," sustaining their religious orientations throughout their ordeals. How is it that people stand firm in the face of hardship? Is it purely a matter of personal will or is there more to it than that?

Religious Support

Sheer force of will may help to explain the unflagging devotion to a faith; however, will power is only part of the story. Those who persist in their religion are not totally self-contained individuals; they are involved in a greater field of forces. When events threaten to upset their equilibrium, they often reach out beyond themselves for balance, or they may find that a helping hand is extended to them without asking for it. In either case, the function of the support is the same: to uphold and sustain the person through hard times—to preserve. Religious support comes from many sources.

Spiritual Support

Some people seek support from the divine directly. Listen to one of our interviewees from the Project on Religion and Coping. Sue Ellen, a 40-year-old Roman Catholic, had rushed to the hospital to be with her teenage son, who had collapsed on the court at basketball practice.

> Arriving at the emergency room, Sue Ellen was greeted by the sight of many of Jim's friends and teammates weeping in the hall, and in the room, Jim, unconscious on the bed, with tubes stuck in him everywhere. Sue Ellen recalls thinking, "This isn't happening. I'm dreaming this." The doctors approached her and told her they believed Jim had experienced a stroke.
>
> She recalls asking God for help and quickly receiving it: "If you expect this of me, help me. I can't do this alone. . . . Immediately it felt like someone came and held me up." Later that night with Jim now in a coma, Sue Ellen stood quietly over his bed, alone with her son for the first time all day. She described another mysterious physical sensation which overcame her then: "It was almost like someone had thrown a soft blanket over me. . . . I felt a tremendous sense of peace. . . . I tell people I have felt the peace of Christ."
>
> The next day her son died. Immediately after, Sue Ellen felt and saw a presence over the right side of his bed. I don't know if it was the angels or Jim himself, but the presence told me, "It's O.K." Driving home from the hospital that night, Sue Ellen had a feeling much like the warm blanket in the emergency room. "It was a washing of warm, like love . . . it's too hard to describe."

Calamity, in this instance, was counteracted by a "divine visit" (cf. Pruyser, 1968); the sense of a spiritual presence offered this mother emotional comfort and reassurance in the most wrenching moments of her tragedy. Not only that, it gave her the strength to make it through. In this sense, the spiritual support she sought not only comforted, but empowered as well.

Kushner (1989) speaks to this latter function: "We turn to God and He renews our strength so that we can run and not grow weary, so that we can walk and not feel faint. . . . the man or woman who turns to God is like a tree planted by a stream. What they share with the world is replenished by a source beyond themselves so that they never run dry" (pp. 137, 139). For those who feel they have this sense of God's presence and power, life crises of even the worst sort are met with unlimited resources. Empowered by God, virtually any situation can be viewed through the secondary appraisal process as manageable. For example, one father who had lost members of his family to a natural disaster was still able to say shortly afterward, "I lost two of my three children, and I lost my first wife, and we almost got ourselves killed that night, fo'sure. But the Lord say He won't put more on us than we can stand. If we can't take it, He'll be right beside us giving stren'th we didn't know we had" (Yancey, 1977, p. 127).

It is this sense of spiritual support, both comforting and strengthening, that many people seem to look for in times of stress. An empirical study by Shrimali and Broota (1987) is illustrative here. These researchers examined changes in beliefs in God and anxiety among surgical patients from a nursing home in New Delhi. Thirty patients who were about to undergo major surgery were compared to an equivalent group of patients who were to have minor surgery and to a matched control group. Before their operation the major surgery patients reported greater levels of anxiety and belief in God than the other two groups. After surgery the degree of anxiety and belief in God for the major surgery patients decreased to the same level as those of the minor surgery and control groups. What was a "dull habit," Shrimali and Broota conclude, became an "acute fever" in a stressful moment, and when the moment passed so did the need for spiritual support. Belief in God, they feel, helped the major surgery patients manage their fears and "bear their burden." They add that the patients may have also hoped to effect a direct intervention in the event from forces outside themselves; superstitious beliefs in luck and astrology rose and fell following major surgery just as belief in God did. The support these patients sought, then, may have been instrumental as well as emotional and empowering.

Religious faith and the perception of direct experiences with the divine are only one source of support. In hard times, some look to religious literature for help. Images of a loving, supportive God, always there to comfort and sustain, fill the hymnals, devotional literature, and scripture. In fact, the Bible has been described as a "Book of Comfort"

(Oates, 1953). Perhaps no portion is better suited to this end than the Book of Psalms. The psalms, particularly those of the lamenting type, have a structure designed to help the sufferer endure (Capps, 1981). Consider the following example:

> Unto thee will I cry, O Lord my rock; be not silent
>   to me: lest, *if* thou be silent to me, I become
>   like them that go down into the pit.
> Hear the voice of my supplications, when I cry unto
>   thee, when I lift up my hands toward thy
>   holy sanctuary. . . .
> Blessed *be* the Lord, because he hath heard the
>   voice of my supplications.
>   The Lord *is* my strength and my shield; my
>   heart trusted in him, and I am helped:
>   therefore my heart greatly rejoiceth; and with
>   my song will I praise him. (Psalm 28:2–3, 6–7)

In this psalm, we first hear the speaker's cries of distress and pleas for help from God. This is followed by a change in tone from supplication to resolution, one in which the individual is supported, the deity praised, and the covenant between lamenter and God reaffirmed. The predicament may be an illness, an injustice, a personal sin, the threat of enemies or of death. But neither the specific problem nor the specific resolution is spelled out. Because of that, the psalm can be extended to changing times and circumstances. Readers struggling with diverse problems of their own can identify with the psalmist's pain and petition for help; comfort and hope can be drawn from the account of fellow sufferers who, in spite of their afflictions, have been touched by God's presence.

Interpersonal Religious Support

There is a horizontal as well as a vertical dimension to religious support. The followers of most traditions are asked to express their faith not only in relationship to the divine, but in relationship to others. Interpersonal support works in two directions: It is sought and it is offered. Many people turn to their religious communities for help in sustaining themselves through stressful times. It may come as a surprise to mental health professionals, but the average citizen is more likely to seek out the clergy for help than any other professional (e.g., Chalfant et al., 1990; Veroff, Kulka, & Douvan, 1981). For example, 41% of one random sample of community members reported that they have used or would use their clergy for help with personal problems. In contrast, 29% said they would use their medical doctor, 29% a psychiatrist or psychologist, 18% a social service agency, 13% an attorney, and 12% a marriage counselor (Chalfant et al., 1990). Informal support from fellow congregation members is also commonly sought by at least some groups. In a national sample of black Americans, Taylor and Chatters (1988) found that only 18% reported that they never needed help from their church members.

The offering of support is as relevant as the seeking of support. There are those who respond to stress by devoting themselves to others. The motivations for these altruistic acts may be at least partly religious. Listen to the reasons one seriously ill man offered for agreeing to undergo painful tests and procedures even though they would be of little medical value to him personally: "I hope that my submission to these experiments will restore men and women to normal living in years to come. . . . If they do, I will have aided the scientific advances and repaid those who helped me, in the manner which I think God would expect" (Fichter, 1981, p. 61). Preservation appeared to be the goal here; not self-preservation but the preservation of the well-being of others. This is not to say that the individual in this case did not gain from the process. The attempt to sustain other people may have helped him sustain himself emotionally and spiritually. This case does not appear to be unique. In one study of oncology nurses, 40% reported that their patients offered *them* spiritual support (Taylor & Amanta, 1994a).

Religious support can be offered by groups as well as individuals. Indeed, congregations come together in part to minister to the needs of fellow members. The term "minister" is important here, for service to others is not understood as a secular task, but as a form of spiritual service—a way of sharing God's presence with those in distress. In this sense, efforts to sustain people physically, materially, and psychologically are completely compatible with the larger spiritual mission of the congregation, to know and serve God. In fact, religious institutions provide a wide array of supportive activities to their members and, in some instances, the larger community (Pargament, 1982). The support may be formal in nature; most congregations offer their members pastoral counseling by the clergy or lay ministers, and many churches and synagogues sponsor support programs for members struggling with particular problems: marital enrichment, parental effectiveness, divorce recovery, or visitation for shut-ins. The support may also come from participation in regular worship services or from the more informal day-to-day exchanges among members.

Clergy and congregation members are in a unique position to support people through difficult times (Taylor & Chatters, 1988). Next to the family, no other institution offers the possibility of such sustained contact throughout the lifespan. From birth, through the major transitions of life, to death, the congregation member can be accompanied by a "convoy" (cf. Kahn & Antonucci, 1980) of friends and acquaintances who share a history of experience and concern for one another. Though the members of the convoy may change over time, the convoy itself stays intact and the expectation remains that members will be there for each other in times of need.

Both the seeking and the offering of religious support play important roles in the preservation of significance. In fact, some evidence points to psychological advantages for people who are involved in both sides of this helping coin. Maton (1987) asked a group of members of a nondenominational Christian fellowship to complete daily logs of the degree to which they provided or received material assistance from their fellow members over a 9-month period. He divided his sample into several groups: those who were both providers and receivers of assistance (bidirectional supporters), those who were primarily providers or receivers (unidirectional supporters), and those who neither provided nor received support (nonsupporters). The bidirectional supporters reported greater life satisfaction and more positive attitudes than the unidirectional supporters or the nonsupporters. Unidirectional support, Maton concludes, has its costs. The unidirectional receiver may feel a sense of indebtedness and inferiority. The unidirectional giver may develop feelings of resentment, burnout, and struggle with unmet personal needs. Bidirectional supporters, however, are able to achieve a sense of balance between giving and receiving and, perhaps as a result, experience greater satisfaction with relationships and life more generally.

To conclude, we have considered many sources of religious comfort and strength in coping. Spiritual experiences, religious beliefs, religious scriptures, and congregations come together to form a system of religious support that individuals can draw on in their efforts to sustain themselves and each other in the midst of turmoil and change. In the following chapter, we will see that people can turn to these same religious sources for more transformational purposes as well.

In this section, we have reviewed the involvement of religion in three mechanisms of preservation—marking boundaries, religious perseverance, and religious support. These are some of the religious coping efforts designed to hold on to both the means and the ends of significance in stressful times. Often they may be the strategies of first choice in coping, for the desire to preserve may be the most basic instinct when people are under stress.

However, preservation is not always possible. Neither is it always prudent. Well-trodden paths of coping may be blocked, or crises may reveal weaknesses in old familiar ways of looking at and dealing with the world. The religious system itself may be found wanting. Many people report religious doubts and dissatisfaction after they have suffered a tragedy. In one study, 33% of parents who had experienced the death of a child reported doubts about God in the first year of their bereavement (Cook & Wimberly, 1983). In another study, 90% of mothers who had given birth to a profoundly retarded child voiced doubts about the existence of God (Childs, 1985). Painful disorientation, religious and nonreligious, can result when old systems are no longer capable of handling new demands. Preservation, in this case, can provide no relief, for the old solutions no longer work or, even worse, they have become a part of the problem. The times call for a change of paths, not to transform significance but to conserve it.

ANOTHER WAY TO AN OLD DESTINATION: RELIGION AND THE RECONSTRUCTION OF THE PATH TO SIGNIFICANCE

Most people do not associate religion with the idea of change. Instead, we tend to think of religion as a constant, a force that encourages stability and continuity. On closer inspection, however, we find that reorientation and change are integral parts of religious experience. To renew and sustain the individual's relationship with God, the world's religions make every effort to shift the physical, temporal, and psychological landscape from the profane to the sacred. From the moment of physical entry into a religious setting, Paden (1988) notes, the individual is encouraged to reconstruct the place of the human in the spiritual universe: "A cathedral," for instance, "declares the smallness of human stature within the divine majesty of the house of God" (p. 99).

Time as well as place undergoes a metamorphosis within the religious world. Certain periods are set apart from the ordinary flow of time. These are holy days when "the sacred gets restored" (p. 101). Heschel (1986) speaks to this point within Judaism

> The Sabbaths are our great cathedrals. . . . Six days a week we live under the tyranny of things of space; on the Sabbath we try to become attuned to *holiness in time*. It is a day on which we are called upon to share in what is eternal in time, to turn from the results of creation to the mystery of creation; from the world of creation to the creation of the world. (pp. 302–303)

In these special times and places rituals are performed that reenact and regenerate the community's vision of the world. "Every time the Catholic Mass is performed," Paden (1988) says, "Christ's sacrifice for humanity reoccurs. . . . Every Christmas Day Christ is born again. Every Passover, the Exodus is recalled" (p. 101). These observances are extraordinary. Set apart by time, place, and the practices themselves, they are radically different from anything we experience in day-to-day life. Yet they are not so radical in purpose; they are designed to revitalize and sustain the relationship with the significant.

Change, then, is not at all foreign to the religious world. It is in fact regularly encouraged and practiced. In stressful times, however, the individual may look beyond the regular rituals of religion to one of several reconstructive coping mechanisms. Change is sought here—change in religious thoughts, actions, relationships, or feelings. However, it is important to stress that the ultimate goal of the change in reconstructive coping is to conserve significance. (In the following chapter, conservational forms of coping will be contrasted with transformational religious coping methods designed to change the character of significance itself.) We will now consider three reconstructive coping mechanisms: religious switching, religious reframing, and religious purification.

Religious Switching

Switching Gods

One of the interviewees from the Project on Religion and Coping described a crisis period in her life and the changes that followed in her concept of father and God.

> Laura, a 22-year-old graduate student, was raised as a Roman Catholic. As a child, her relationship with her father was ambivalent. Although she knew he cared about her, she felt that rules, order, and the Catholic church were more important to him than her mother or herself. She saw God very much like her father. He "loves you, but you'd better stay on the straight and narrow or he's going to zap ya!" In adolescence, Laura began to experience problems: Her parents' marriage was failing, she was overweight, and the other kids picked on her at school. Laura felt she had strayed off the "straight and narrow," and had no place to go for help. Religion was no solace. "Go to God?" she asked, "RIGHT! God gave me ALL THIS!" After an aborted suicide attempt, Laura asked her father for help, but none was received. "Dad told me, in a not-so-nice tone of voice, that he didn't ever want to hear anything like that again and that I should just forget about it."
>
> In the next few years Laura began to change. She grew attracted to her mother's Methodist church, which portrayed the deity in more personal, less fearful terms. Over time, God took on the characteristics of the father she wanted but never had, someone who

would love her unconditionally. In fact, she now refers to God as her "papa." Her new "father," she says, "never falls short of expectations. He fills a gap in my life that my family and friends can't. . . . It's O.K. to screw up, God will still love you anyway." Laura's spiritual relationship is now the constant in her life. While her religious beliefs have changed many times, she no longer questions God's love for her.

In her search for nurturance and reassurance, Laura made a religious switch. The switch is not to be confused with a religious conversion (which as we will see later also involves a change in the ends of significance). Laura's goal, her desire for love and nurturance, remained constant; what changed was the path she took to attain her goal. In her adolescent struggle, Laura's father, her church, and her own conception of God proved to be insufficient. Her response was to modify her religious orientation—to switch, in essence, from one "papa" to another better suited to her ends.

Laura's case is not unique. The religious switch can offer a substitute for many strained, inadequate, or lost relationships.

> . . . the thought of our Maker becoming our perfect parent . . . is a thought which can have meaning for everybody, whether we come to it by saying, "I had a wonderful father and I see that God is like that, only more so," or by saying, "My father disappointed me here, and here, and here, but God, praise His name, will be very different," or even by saying, "I have never known what it is to have a father on earth, but thank God I now have one in Heaven." (Packer, cited in Carlson, 1988, p. 194)

Kirkpatrick and Shaver (1990) provide empirical illustration of this coping process. Drawing on attachment theory, they suggest that children with insecure attachment relationships to their parents may compensate later by turning to "a loving, personal, available God" as a substitute (p. 320). To test this "compensation hypothesis," they administered a survey to 200 adults. The results were consistent with the hypothesis. Participants in the study who described their mothers as nonreligious and cold, distant, and unresponsive to them prior to adolescence were more likely than others to believe in a personal God and feel they had a personal relationship with God. Children of these avoidant mothers were also more likely than others to report that they had had a sudden religious conversion in adolescence or adulthood. The large majority of those who indicated a sudden religious change made mention of a precipitating crisis, one which often involved the disruption or loss of an important relationship such as a divorce, or marital or family problem. To many people with a history of poor relationships, Kirkpatrick and Shaver conclude, God may become an ideal substitute attachment figure, a haven of safety in turbulent times and a secure base for exploring the world.

Switching Religious Groups

Religious switches are not limited to new or different gods. People switch religious groups as well. Not all of these changes from denomination to denomination or congregation to congregation are ways of coping. Many follow a move to another community, a step up the socioeconomic ladder, or a marriage to a spouse who belongs to another church (see Newport, 1979). But there are times when the switch to another religious group becomes a solution to problems. Empirical studies indicate that changes to different denominations are often preceded by stressful episodes and periods of brief or extended unhappiness (e.g., Sales, 1972; Tamburrino et al., 1990; Ullman, 1982). For example, Ullman (1982) compared people who had switched to Jewish Orthodox, Roman Catholic, Hare Krishna, or Bahai groups to a control sample of people who had remained Jewish or Catholic. (A control sample of Hare Krishna and Bahai groups could not be found.) Switchers reported more problematic relationships with their fathers and mothers than controls. In addition, the former group described greater turbulence, trauma, and unhappiness in childhood and adolescence than controls. Perhaps most strikingly, 80% of the switchers reported some kind of emotional trauma immediately prior to their shift. A similar percentage indicated that they felt relief from their distress following their change ("I did not feel so desperate anymore"; "I knew He [Christ] will take care of me") (Ullman, 1982, p. 190).[1]

From the perspective of coping theory, religious switches become more likely when life stresses call into question the adequacy of the religious group in problem solving and when alternative religious groups are available and offer more compelling solutions. Gartrell and Shannon (1985) provide some data that supports this point of view. They listened to the stories of how 25 people became deeply involved in the Divine Light Mission (DLM). Involvement in the DLM was preceded by a clear rejection of the mainstream religious institution. One hundred percent of the group reported that the mainline church was hypocritical, and 80% indicated that the mainline church was unable to help them solve their personal or social problems. Conventional nonreligious alternatives to the religious institution were also rejected as sources of help. One hundred percent of the converts felt that colleges and universities, political and reform groups, and therapy were unable to solve personal or social problems. Most of these individuals, however, had an alternative available to them; 73% had experimented with Eastern religious beliefs and practices before they joined the DLM. All of the participants reportedly felt that the DLM offered viable solutions to their personal and social concerns.

Old religious structures may fail, but that does not mean religion will be rejected in its entirety. There are many spiritual homes. When gods or religious groups are no longer adequate to the tasks of coping or when they become stressful in themselves, the individual can make a move. Be it a new god or a new group, the religious switch represents a changing of the way, a new path to an old destination of significance. Switching is, however, only one method of reconstructive coping. Religion is also involved in reconstructive methods that call for more of an internal change.

Religious Purification

Virtually every faith recognizes that people occasionally stray from the religious path. But they do not treat the matter lightly. To turn away or against the religious design is not to be confused with a simple mistake or error; to many religious minds it becomes a sin. What makes an act of transgression so significant is that it undermines the relationship of the individual to the sacred (Tillich, 1951). The three Hebrew words that come closest to the terms "evil" and "sin"—*ht* (missing a mark), *psh'* (breaking of a relationship), and *'awon* (crooked, twisted, or wrong)—refer to a breach of the covenant between God and the Jewish people (Taylor, 1985). Satan himself, the religious personification of evil, was originally portrayed by the Hebrews as an obstructor or a tester of the relationship between humankind and God, and later as a disrupter of this relationship. Still later within Christianity, Satan became the embodiment of all forces opposed to God. There is a parallel within Buddhism in its description of Mara (the Evil One) who presents Siddhartha Gautama with a variety of temptations to lure him away from his search for enlightenment. Here again it is the violation of the relationship between the individual and the sacred that is most reviled.

What qualifies as a breach of the relationship varies from tradition to tradition and person to person. The form of sin takes as many forms as definitions of the sacred. "To those for whom authority is the supremely sacred thing, disloyalty and apostasy are the ultimate threats. To those for whom enlightenment is the supreme goal, ignorance is [the greatest impurity]. To those living a monastic life for whom chastity is the supreme gift to God, concupiscence is the direst seduction and sin" (Paden, 1988, p. 143).

But religions do more than define transgressions; they provide coping mechanisms for reorientation, a return to the right way. Through rituals of purification, the sin, evil, or uncleanliness associated with religious violations are removed, and the individual is reconciled to God. The actual methods of purification vary quite a bit. They include sacrifice, isolation, exorcism, repentance, punishment, and apology. Physical elements also play a prominent role in these rituals—water, fire, rain, ashes, sun, oil, and blood, to name a few (Paden, 1988).

Rituals of purification can be found in every faith and in every phase of life. For example, among Roman Catholics, the baptism ritual is said to wash away the original sin all people bring into the world. At the other end of the life cycle, those who have died with sins that have gone unconfessed are offered a final cleansing in purgatory before they are admitted to heaven. Among Muslims, purification has been described as half the faith. Prior to handling the Koran, entering a mosque, or prayer, the Muslim is required to remove physical and spiritual pollution through explicit rituals such as ablution: "O ye who believe! When ye rise up for prayer, wash your faces, and your hands up to the elbows, and lightly rub your hands and (wash) your feet up to the ankles. And if ye are unclean, purify yourselves" (Sarah V:6). Once a year on Yom Kippur, Jews are asked to confess their sins against God and repent by abstaining from eating, drinking, washing, and sexual intercourse. Sins committed knowingly and unknowingly, by the community as well as the individual, are all confessed in the liturgy of atonement. Although God is always receptive to repentance, Yom Kippur is an especially important time of confession, for on that day one's fate is said to be sealed for the following year.

Purification rituals may vary in form, but they share a common function, to reorient the individual to the sacred. Consider, for example, some excerpts from the confession of one Roman Catholic to his priest.

> PENITENT: . . . it seems the past month has been all work with very little time for my family. . . . In this past month, I have been too tired to give [my children] any attention or time. I really regret how cold I have been to them and how I yelled at them this week. I feel terrible about slapping Joey. He really was being a good boy, but he just happened to be the nearest one around when I finally lost my cool. I regret the hurt I have caused my children, especially Joey. . . . They seem to have a sense that I don't love them. I guess they aren't experiencing me the way I experienced God in that reading we just heard. . . .
>
> PRIEST: I hear your regret, Joe. And I hear you wanting to be more like the loving Father you know God to be with you. You seem

to be telling me that love has grown cold in your life because you have become so caught up in your own achievements.

PENITENT: Yes, my preoccupation with my work is taking its toll on the life and love in our family. How can I make things different?
. . .

PRIEST: If healing and reconciliation are going to take place in your family, then, it sounds as though you will need to examine your priorities and create some space in your life. What can you do to show your children you love them and that your work doesn't have to come first all the time?

PENITENT: (*Pausing to think*) I need to give them some time and attention for one thing. And it is time we did something playful together. . . .

PRIEST: Sounds like a good idea to me. . . . Let's take a moment to pray together, Joe. You pray your prayer of contrition in the way you would be most comfortable, and then I will pray for you in my own name, and then in the name of the Church by praying the prayer of absolution while imposing my hands on you. (Gula, 1984, pp. 276–277)

The emphasis here is not on a wholesale change of values. Penitent and priest recognize that this father loves his children. The problem is defined as a failure to live by these priorities. In his confession, the father admits his sins and the priest encourages him to realign his practices to fit with his religious values—to be more like "the loving Father you know God to be with you."

This is not an isolated example. Empirical studies in this area are scarce; however, there is some evidence that others look to religion for this kind of reconciliation. Lilliston and Klein (1989) compared the religious coping practices of college students who reported a discrepancy between their *actual* selves and the selves they feel they *ought* to be with those of students who did not have this discrepancy. Although Lilliston and Klein did not focus specifically on rituals of purification, they did find that students with an "actual–ought" discrepancy were more likely to report that they would use religion in coping. "For these people," Lilliston and Klein conclude, the response to crisis is "to live more fully in accord with the religion they have chosen" (pp. 8–9).

Religious rituals of purification seem designed to conserve not only spiritual ends but psychological ends as well. By encouraging admissions of personal failure, these rituals increase the tension of the moment. This exacerbation of stress sets the stage for the resolution to come; confessions of shortcomings are met with acceptance and forgiveness rather than condemnation, and relief and comfort seem likely to follow. A study by Pennebaker and Beall (1986) is relevant here, although it did not focus on religious confession per se. Over four consecutive days, a group of healthy undergraduates were asked to write about either the most traumatic event they had ever experienced or a set of unimportant assigned topics. Students assigned to write about the traumatic event were placed into three subgroups: (1) those who were told to describe only the facts about the trauma, not their feelings (trauma–factual), (2) those who were asked to write only about their emotions about the trauma, not the facts (trauma–emotion), and (3) those who were told to write about both the facts and their feelings surrounding the incident (trauma–combination). Participants in the trauma–emotion and trauma–combination groups reported themselves to be the most upset after writing about the trauma. However, follow-up data over the next 6 months showed that people in the trauma–combination group visited the student health center for illness less often than others. Furthermore, in comparison to the other groups, students in both the trauma–combination and trauma–emotion groups reported fewer illnesses and less restricted activity as a result of illness. "Confession," it appears, increased tension and discomfort in the short-term, but enhanced physical health in the long run.

Of course we do not know how well these findings apply to *religious* confession. The presence of a religious authority who offers absolution to the individual could add to the relief the individual ultimately experiences from disclosure. On the other hand, this same presence could inhibit the person from making a more emotional and complete confession. In fact, Pennebaker, Hughes and O'Heeron (1987) found that people revealed less about personally traumatic events in which they felt some guilt when asked to do so in front of a confessor (a faculty member unknown to the students). Moreover, they were less physiologically aroused when speaking with a confessor present than when speaking alone. Still, confession to a stranger in a psychology department may be quite different from confession to a better known and trusted religious leader. Further study will be needed to sort out the psychological motivations and impact of various religious rituals of purification.

It is important to point out that when purification is sought only to alleviate guilt or distress, that is, when it is unaccompanied by a desire for change, the ritual no longer qualifies as a mechanism of reconstruction. Instead, it becomes a method of preservation, a bromide allowing the individual to continue comfortably on the same path rather than a stimulus encouraging the individual to take a new path or return to an old one. Clearly, this is not the religious intent behind rituals of purification. As a case in point, the Roman Catholic priest may refuse to give absolution to the penitent who shows no sorrow for the sins that have been committed, no plans to make reparations for these transgressions, or no intention to avoid the same sins in the future. But, to the sincerely repentant, the sacrament of penance is said to promise a fresh start on life and the path to significance:

Religious Reframing

In his studies of Javanese culture, Geertz (1966) witnessed an unusual event. A large, oddly shaped toadstool was spotted in front of the home of a carpenter and, although the mushroom had no particular social value to the community, it caused quite a stir. Villagers from near and far came to see and wonder about the toadstool. Why the fuss? "It was just that this [toadstool] was 'odd,' 'strange,' 'uncanny,' " Geertz explained, "and the odd, strange, and uncanny simply must be accounted for. . . . One does not shrug off a toadstool which grows five times as fast as a toadstool has any right to grow" (p. 16). In this sense the mushroom was not trivial at all; because it was so unusual and could not be easily explained, the toadstool threatened their understanding of the world.

This example may seem outlandish, but Western culture has toadstools of its own. We, too, make some basic assumptions about the world that help to orient and guide us in our encounters with the usual and not-so-usual. Many situations can be easily assimilated into our worldviews, but others, like the mushroom, disturb and disorient. They reach out to shake our "assumptive worlds" (cf. Janoff-Bulman, 1989). Events like these call for a reconstruction of beliefs to conserve what we find significant (see Park & Folkman, in press).

Religion is often involved in the reconstruction of traumatic events. In fact, Geertz (1966) argues, an essential task of religion is to cope with "crises of interpretability":

> Bafflement, suffering, and a sense of intractable ethical paradox are all, if they become intense enough or are sustained long enough, radical challenges to the proposition that life is comprehensible and that we can, by taking thought, orient ourselves effectively within it—challenges with which any religion, however "primitive," which hopes to persist must attempt somehow to cope. (p. 14)

To what may seem the most senseless accident, the most unbearable pain, or the most unjust outcome, religions have their responses. Most suggest a different way of thinking about hardship, about people, or about the sacred. Beliefs about events, oneself, and the world are realigned with each other and placed in a new perspective. In this process of reframing, suffering may become something explainable, bearable, and even valuable. Reframing is designed to conserve significance: to soften the blows of crisis, to reaffirm that life has meaning in spite of its pain, to protect the sacred, however it may be defined.

Let us take a closer look at three of the more common types of religious reframing: those that involve, respectively, the event, the individual, and the sacred. These three factors form the tripod of a belief system that many people hold. Central to this belief system is the idea that *a benevolent God participates in our lives to ensure that bad things will not happen to good people* (Kushner, 1981). The world is just, many say, and God is one of the reasons why. But when traumatic events strike, this belief may be threatened. Serious questions may arise and shake the delicate balance among the three factors in this conceptualization, that is, the event, the person, and the sacred: How could a bad thing happen if I am a good person and God truly watches over me? How can I be a good person if such a bad thing happened and God allowed it to happen? How can God really be watching over me if I am a good person and such a bad thing happened?

Questions raised by the catastrophic experience may lead to a rejection of the belief system in its entirety. More often than not, however, one or more of the elements is reframed in an effort to establish a new balance within the belief system, a balance that conserves the sense that the world is ultimately just, that the individual is worthwhile and safe, and that there is a loving God.

Religious Reframing of the Event

A Spiritual Opportunity

One way to reconstruct a shaken belief system is to redefine the traumatic experience so that it is not so pointless. Attributions to the divine can play a part of this process. Consider the response of one victim, paralyzed by an accident to the spinal cord, to the question "Why me?": "I say, 'Well, I'm put in this situation to learn certain things, 'cause nobody else is in this situation.' It's a learning experience; I see God's trying to put me in situations, help me learn about Him and myself and also how I can help other people." (Bulman & Wortman, 1977, p. 358). Or listen to one parent who found this way to make sense of the death of a firstborn infant: "They say there's reasons for God to do everything you know. I think that's very true because I think I love him (second child, born after the death of first child) a lot more now than I would of had our first son been here" (Gilbert, 1989, p. 10).

These kinds of religious attributions are not at all unusual. In Bulman and Wortman's (1977) study of paraplegics, the most popular response to the open-ended question "Why me?" was that God had a reason. Similarly, in the Project on Religion and Coping (Pargament, Ensing, et al., 1990), church members confronting a serious negative event were more likely to attribute it to God's will than to themselves or chance. In another study, students from a state college were presented a set of hypothetical life events and asked what would cause these events. On several of the health-related items (e.g., I develop a brain tumor; I live a long life), students on average attributed greater responsibility to God than any other locus of control, including natural forces, significant others, chance, or themselves (Pargament & Sullivan, 1981).

Perhaps it should be no surprise that people commonly attribute certain life events to the divine. A God with a plan for the individual may offer an explanation far more benign than the external alternatives—the belief that life is determined by chance, powerful others, or nature (Pargament & Hahn, 1986). Viewed as the will of a benevolent God, events are cast in a new, softer light. Pain is not a divine punishment; it is God's way of hitting my "reset button for change," says one person (Siegel, 1986). I know God will not give me more than I can handle, says another. Death is not a final exit, says yet another, it is just God's way of opening the door to a greater realm. When the sacred is seen working its will in life's events, what first seems random, nonsensical and tragic is changed into something else—an opportunity to appreciate life more fully, a chance to be with God, a challenge to help others grow, or a loving act meant to prevent something worse from taking place. In any case, the incomprehensible turns into the interpretable, the unbearable becomes "sufferable" (Geertz, 1966).

This is not to say that everyone attributes negative events to the will of God. To do so may come too close to blaming the sacred for the misfortune, something, we will see shortly, most people are quite reluctant to do. However, negative events can continue to be reframed in positive spiritual terms, even when the notion of divine providence is rejected. God may not be the author of pain, to this way of thinking, but suffering still offers the opportunity to attain something of spiritual significance.

A religious reframing of the event says that what seems to be so terrible is not in fact so terrible. Though the event may hurt or threaten, there is another and more important dimension to it. Beneath the surface of the situation, we can find God working his will; we can find a spiritual companion who makes the trauma more manageable; and we can find opportunities and challenges for spiritual growth. This is a powerful coping strategy. By redefining the negative situation more positively, the relationship between God, oneself, and the world remains in balance; the benevolence of the divine, the fairness of the world, and the basic worth and security of the individual can be conserved.

Powerful as this way of coping may be, not everyone can view traumatic situations in a positive light. Kushner (1981), for one, drew little solace or meaning from efforts to reframe his situation, the death of his 14-year-old handicapped son. To the notion that God planned for good to come out of the loss, Kushner retorts: "If a human artist or employer made children suffer so that something immensely impressive or valuable could come to pass, we would put him in prison. Why then should we excuse God for causing such undeserved pain, no matter how wonderful the ultimate result may be?" (p. 19). To the idea that God is testing us and never gives us more than we can handle, Kushner responds: "If God is testing us He must know by now that many of us fail the test. If He is only giving us burdens we can bear, I have seen Him miscalculate far too often" (p. 36). To the idea that his son's death was really a blessing, Kushner has this to say: "We try to persuade ourselves that what we call evil is not real, does not really exist, but is only a condition of not enough goodness, even as 'cold' means 'not enough heat,' or darkness is a name we give to the absence of light . . . but people do stumble and hurt themselves because of the dark, and people do die of exposure to cold" (pp. 27–28).

Like Kushner, many people may find religious attempts to reframe negative situations in a more positive light far from compelling. There are, however, other ways to shift perspectives on the world and our place in it.

Religious Reframing of the Person

Human Sinfulness

Confronted with a catastrophe, it may be more plausible to change the way we think about *people* in the situation than about God or the situation itself. Mahedy (1986), a chaplain in Vietnam, came to terms with the war in this way. Earlier in the book, we noted how many soldiers felt betrayed by a God they had assumed would be on their side. Mahedy, however, reached a different conclusion. The problem was not that God had betrayed the soldier. No, the soldiers had turned their backs on God through their involvement in a sinful war. To expect the support of the sacred while evil acts were being perpetrated would have been ludicrous: "One cannot be immersed in sin and at the same time expect to feel the loving presence of God" (p. 131). Mahedy is very clear on where the responsibility rested for the war and the spiritual desolation that came with it: "God indeed checked out of our lives in Vietnam because we 'checked out' on Him" (p. 131). Much as God would have liked people to follow a different path, He was not willing to interfere with their freedom to choose. People then, not God, bore the responsibility for the tragedy of Vietnam. In this way, Mahedy attempted to conserve the benevolence of God.

This type of personal attribution for negative situations is not uncommon among the religiously involved. For example, McGuire (1988) studied middle-class suburbanites who were involved in alternative healing groups. When failures in healing occurred, human limitations were often perceived as the culprit. One woman explained that she had not been healed because she had to "become more worthy of a healing" (p. 72). Another said: "Some people don't know how to accept the healing. They go all out and do completely wrong things. People, most of the time, make their own mistakes by not thanking the Lord every day" (p. 75). Among Hindus, the belief in Karma is another commonly held way to hold people accountable for their fate. According to this doctrine, what happens in this life is determined not by God, but by one's past deeds, including actions that occurred in earlier incarnations. Furthermore, the doctrine states, one's actions in this life will eventually receive their just reward or punishment. By extending the temporal line of personal responsibility, even the most unfair experience can be explained in a way that absolves God of blame and offers the reassurance of ultimate justice in the world. Narayanan, Mohan, and Radhakrishnan (1986) suggest that the doctrine of Karma may help to explain the relative lack of bitterness among common people in India when they encounter pain and sorrow. "When any misfortune befalls them, they blame neither God nor their neighbour, but only themselves for it" (p. 63).

The price of this kind of reframing may seem high. A benevolent God and a just world may appear to be purchased at the expense of the third element of the triad, the sense of personal worth. But to say that someone has erred or sinned is not to say that he or she is worthless or irredeemable. Many theologies offer the possibility of redemption through atonement, forgiveness, grace, or good deeds. As we have seen, religions also provide rituals of purification to return the person to a better path. In this vein, Mahedy concludes his book on Vietnam with a liturgy of reconciliation in which the participant confesses his sins. Thus, even when problems are reframed as the result of human failure, the worth of the person can be conserved, along with the benevolence of the sacred and the sense that the world is just.

The Limited Ability to Understand

Another type of person-centered reframing focuses less on human responsibility for suffering than the limited human ability to understand it. This type of reframing has a paradoxical quality. Here we make sense of a life crisis by concluding that we cannot make sense of it; some things, we decide, are just beyond our comprehension. Take an example from Corrie Ten Boom's (1971) account of her experiences in a concentration camp during World War II. After her father died in a German prison, she was asked by an officer: "What kind of God would let that old man die here in Scheveningen?" She answered with a phrase her father had repeated to her: "Some knowledge is too heavy . . . you cannot bear it . . . your Father will carry it until you are able" (p. 163). Admitting that she was unable to understand the death of her father did not reflect poorly on God or the situation; Ten Boom's belief in a sacred design in all things, even the most terrible, remained unchanged. What changed was her assessment of her own ability to see into this design.

From this perspective, some problems must remain mysteries never to be fathomed, puzzles too complicated ever to solve. That does not mean there is no ultimate answer. (As one bereaved parent put it: "There is a God. And it's an explanation that there's no explanation" [Gilbert, 1989, p. 9]). But it does mean that as human beings we will never be able to see clearly into the divine plan. Efforts to understand why we must suffer will prove futile. Indeed, when the problem is reframed in this way, the question "Why me?" becomes the wrong question; it is better to focus on the response to bad times and good times as well. Krauss (Krauss & Goldfischer, 1988) illustrates this point. After his wife's funeral he was asked by a young, distraught member of his congregation why God had taken her away. Krauss responded this way: "You know, I never asked that question. That's a question a shattered heart asks. . . . These are the questions to ask: Was her life rich? How many lives did she touch? . . . Did she take her joys humbly and gratefully? Did she meet her sorrows courageously? Was God present? Who can doubt it!" (pp. 52–53).

Religious Reframing of the Sacred

A Punishing God

One final form of reframing focuses on the deity itself. Typically this is a *last* resort. People are for the most part quite reluctant to change their conception of the sacred. They are particularly wary of blaming the sacred for the bad things they encounter. When, on occasion, negative events are attributed to a punishing God, the punishment is usually seen as deserved, not random, and not malicious. In this sense, the penalty, while delivered by the deity, is ultimately brought on by the person. God may be stern but He is not unjust. His punishments are reserved for those who have sinned and tailored to fit the crime, as we hear in this description of the supreme criminal court in Bali:

> Presided over by high priests, the ceiling is decorated with vivid paintings of the punishments in Hell for wrongdoing in life. Apart from the more obvious crimes, the scenes depict aborted fetuses pushing their mothers off wobbly bridges into well-stoked fires; butchers' heads being sawn open by the animals they killed; the indolent inverted in mortars to have the behinds on which they sat while others worked, pummeled by giant pestles; and fornicators having their genitals scorched by flaming brands. (Hobart, 1985, p. 182)

These are vivid portrayals of divine vengeance in action. But attributions to a punishing God may be preferable to the belief in an unjust world, even if it means that the deity can be so fearsome and that the fault for pain and suffering lies with oneself or others. Illustrating this latter point, we found that several of our college student participants refused to accept the possibility that an unjust event could happen to them (Pargament & Hahn, 1986). When presented with a situation that described responsible behavior on the part of the individual followed by a negative outcome (e.g., walking carefully to class on an icy day and falling and breaking an arm nevertheless), one student said she would tell God: "I'm sorry if I did anything to offend you. Please forgive me and I'll try and do better." Another said "God never punishes when there is no reason. Did I act wrong?" (p. 202). Along similar lines, one woman gave this advice to her friend with cancer: "Surely, there's something in your life which is displeasing to God. . . . You must have stepped out of His will somewhere. These things don't just happen" (Yancey, 1977, p. 13). These people were holding tightly to their belief in a just world, in spite of the emotional cost it carried for themselves or their friends. God, they insisted, would not cause pain unless it was in some sense deserved.

Attributions to a vengeful God may do more than redress the imbalance in the scales of justice. A certain sense of security and control may accompany the belief in a God who punishes fairly, for as long as transgressions can be avoided, retribution can be avoided as well. Only when the moral order is violated does the individual risk spiritual penalty. Those who live within this order have nothing to fear, but those who live outside it run a greater risk. This is what one person seemed to intimate in a comment made following an earthquake in South America: "Did you know that a much lower percentage of Christians died in the earthquake than non-Christians?" (Yancey, 1977, p. 63).

Extrapolating from this remark, we might expect notions of a wrathful God to be applied more often to members of other religious groups than to members of one's own group (provided they are in good religious standing).

Reframing negative events as well-deserved divine punishments may offer the individual some sense of security, control, and justice. However, as we have noted, the cost is pretty steep, for this kind of reframing can be accomplished only by derogating oneself or others and only by placing some limits on the benevolence of God. Perhaps that is why it is not often we find God reframed in punitive terms. In fact, the proportion of people who attribute negative events in their lives to a punishing God is small (Bearon & Koenig, 1990; Croog & Levine, 1972; Pargament & Hahn, 1986; Pargament & Sullivan, 1981; Pargament, Ensing, et al., 1990). For example, Croog and Levine (1972) asked victims of heart attacks to explain what caused their illness. The idea that the illness was a religious punishment was ranked the lowest of 16 possible etiological factors. Only 13% felt their illness was a "payment for sins" or a "punishment for doing wrong in life." Interestingly, 40% of the group felt that the heart attack was the "will of God." In the Project on Religion and Coping (Pargament, Ensing, et al., 1990), church members were more likely to attribute a serious negative event in their lives to God's will, themselves, or chance than to God's punishment. Finally, only 25% of a sample of elderly community residents agreed with the statement that "Physical illness comes from God and is a punishment for sin" (Bearon & Koenig, 1990).

Those feelings of spiritual punishment that do occur are often most pronounced immediately after the tragedy (see Cook & Wimberly, 1983; Gilbert, 1989). Even C. S. Lewis (1961), the well-known Christian apologist, was unable to avoid some feelings of religious victimization of his own soon after the death of his wife: "What chokes every prayer and every hope is the memory of all the prayers H. and I offered and all the false hopes we had. . . . Step by step we were 'led up the garden path.' Time after time, when He seemed most gracious He was really preparing the next torture" (p. 27). But this type of feeling is usually short-lived. The next day C. S. Lewis begins to recant: "I wrote that last night. It was a yell rather than a thought. Let me try it over again" (p. 27). Similarly, in the Croog and Levine (1972) study, only one-third of those who felt their illness was a punishment from God continued to feel the same way 1 year after their heart attack. In contrast, more than two-thirds of those who felt their illness was the will of God continued to make the more benevolent religious attribution 1 year later.

In short, people are very hesitant to see God as the punitive being responsible for their pain. Rather than attribute their woes to the sacred, they are more likely to redefine the situation in positive religious terms, or blame themselves or others alone. Even no religious belief may be preferable to the belief in a hostile deity, as we hear in the words of one Holocaust survivor who explained his loss of religious faith this way: "Maybe man's existence without God is meaningless, but I'd rather have a meaningless life than a God who allows pogroms and the slaughter of the innocent. And I refuse to believe God is a horrible sadist" (Brenner, 1980, p. 111).

The Devil's Doing

Reframing the sacred then does not usually involve a shift to an angry, vindictive, or malevolent God.[2] However, the sacred can be reframed in other ways. One approach is to split the sacred into two competing forces—those of good, and those of evil. Belief in the "forces of darkness" is not at all rare. Gallup and Castelli (1989) find that 37% of Americans reportedly believe in the devil. Through the years, the figure of Satan and his followers has been invoked to explain many a puzzling or tragic situation. Listen to the words of one grandfather on the anniversary of the death of his two grandsons, killed in the Oklahoma City bombing: "A year ago this week, Satan drove up 5th Street in a Ryder truck. He blew my babies up. He may have looked like a normal man, but he was Satan" ("Anniversary . . . ," 1996, p. 19). Rumors and panics about cults of Satanic worshipers provide another case in point. These rumor-panics are often triggered by unusual or disconcerting events, such as a violent local crime, cemetery vandalism, or "satanic" graffiti (Victor, 1991).

Balch and Gilliam (1991) describe one rumor of devil worship that swept a western Montana town in 1974. What started the rumor was the brutal murder of a 39-year-old woman. The woman had been sexually assaulted, bound, gagged, and shot five times in the head. Adding a bizarre quality to this murder, small ropes were found in the house attached to bedposts and bathroom fixtures. A few days later, a rumor began circulating that this woman had been sacrificed by devil worshippers. As the rumor spread, new details were elaborated. Signs of the devil reportedly had been cut into the woman's body and painted on the wall of her home. The ropes were supposedly symbolic of the ropes that hung witches in Salem. These same Satanic forces were then used to account for another unexplained crime that had taken place 2 months earlier involving a 5-year-old girl who had been kidnapped and stabbed to death. Finally, a future death was predicted. The devil-worshipers, it was said, required three victims: "a Christian woman, a virgin, and a betrayer" (p. 249). These were powerful rumors. Even the first author of this paper admits to becoming so fearful, he slept with a loaded gun next to his bed. The rumors turned out to be false. No Satanic markings had been found on the body of the woman or in her home. Furthermore, her killer was eventually arrested and there was no evidence that he had been involved in a Satanic cult. Nevertheless, to this day many people continue to hold Satan responsible for these deaths.

Why were so many people so willing to accept these seemingly outlandish stories? Among other factors, the rumors offered a neat and simple explanation for some very troublesome and threatening circumstances (Balch & Gilliam, 1991). The terrible events that had befallen the town were the result of the devil at play. But this Satan was not a completely mysterious force. The townspeople were well acquainted with the devil from movies, television, books, stories, family, and church. Not only was he a familiar force, he was a force that could be reckoned with. Speaking out against cults, eliminating courses on the occult from the high school curriculum, protesting against satanic lyrics in rock music, returning to church—these were things people could *do* to reduce the chances of any more tragedies. In fighting the devil, the people of this town could find a measure of comfort and control in their lives. Moreover, by reframing the events as the work of Satan, God remained a benevolent being, and there remained the hope of ultimate justice in the world. True, bad things happened to good people, but they were the work of the devil, not the deity, and ultimately God could be expected to triumph over the forces of darkness.

A Limited God

There is another way to reframe the sacred, one that explains pain and suffering not by carving out the evil, menacing figure of Satan from the sacred, but by absolving the sacred of any responsibility for life's events. Here, the power of the deity to intervene directly in the sufferings of the world is delimited, but it is God's omnipotence that is questioned, not God's love and compassion—his goodness and caring remain a constant. God may be unable to prevent our pain or erase it, but he is there by our side with us and his presence may make our suffering more bearable.

Earlier I noted how Kushner (1981) refused to reframe the death of his young son in spiritual terms. He could see no religious opportunity or purpose in his loss. Neither could he hold himself or his son responsible for his death. Like the biblical Job, Kushner refused to believe he had been guilty of sins that in any way justified his suffering. But relinquishing his faith in a loving God was as untenable as either of the other alternatives. The resolution for Kushner involved a reframing of God's powers:

I believe in God. But I do not believe the same things about Him that I did years ago, when I was growing up or when I was a theological student. I recognize his limitations. He is limited in what He can do by laws of nature and by the evolution of human nature and human moral freedom. I no longer hold God responsible for illnesses, accidents, and natural disasters, because I realize that I gain little and I lose so much when I blame God for those things. I can worship a God who hates suffering but cannot eliminate it, more easily than I can worship a God who chooses to make children suffer and die, for whatever exalted reason. . . . Because the tragedy is not God's will, we need not feel hurt or betrayed by God when tragedy strikes. We can turn to Him for help in overcoming it, precisely because we can tell ourselves that God is as outraged by it as we are. (p. 134)

Within the Judeo-Christian tradition, images of omnipotence are an important part of most people's conceptions of God (Foster & Keating, 1992). Thus, it is unclear how often people engage in the type of coping illustrated by Kushner, which sets limits on God's authority. The advantage of this approach to reframing is that, when tragedy does occur, comfort can be gained from the belief that the misfortune is not a punishment from God, and strength and courage can grow from the belief that God is, in fact, sharing the person's ordeal. However, by stripping God of his power to prevent calamities, the individual is forced to look elsewhere for the roots of injustice and its cure; ultimate justice will not be meted out by the deity. A less ascendant God may feel compassion for human suffering, but He can no longer intervene to ensure that good things will happen to good people.

I have reviewed several of the ways religion can be involved in the reframing of negative events. The focus may be the event, the person, the sacred, or some combination of the three, but each form of reframing calls for a reconstruction in beliefs about the world and the place of the person and God within it. In its own way, each form is designed to conserve some semblance of justice, comfort and control, and sacred benevolence in the world.

It is important to note that once a reconstruction occurs, the new orienting system becomes the filter for viewing and dealing with life events. The reframed event, person, or God becomes a part of the individual's new worldview; experiences that come after are now *framed* rather than *reframed* through this changed perspective. Similarly, those who make a religious switch now handle their hardships through an orienting system of new gods and new congregations. After reconstruction, pressures also mount to conserve the now-changed perspective. Renewed through religious purification, the individual faces the fresh challenge of staying on the religious path. Similarly, the person who has found a new god tries as hard to protect his or her new deity as he or she once did the old. Thus, once a reconstruction takes place, the focus shifts from rebuilding the orienting system to sustaining it. It is a shift from reconstruction to preservation. In this sense, we find that the two mechanisms of conservation grow out of each other. Just as the failed effort to preserve significance is often followed by reconstruction, the reconstructive effort is often followed by the attempt to preserve the new path.

CONCLUSIONS

To say that someone prays or goes to church to cope with crisis says little about the role of religion in that individual's search for significance. People pray and attend congregations for many reasons and in many ways. In this chapter, I have considered religious coping from a functional point of view, one that takes us beyond general descriptions of religious beliefs and practices to an analysis of their underlying design. My focus has been on methods of religious coping that appear to have a "built-in" design, methods that are particularly suited to the conservation of significance. Unfortunately, I could not cover every method of religious conservation here. Involvement in religious healing, for instance, deserves more attention as a method of conservation that appears to include elements of religious reframing, purification, and support (see McGuire, 1988). The religious coping methods of children; of nontraditional, emerging religious groups; and of other cultures also merit further study (see Grzymala-Moszczynska & Beit-Hallahmi, 1996). Here I have simply sampled some of the more common ways religion is involved in efforts to protect the ends of greatest significance in coping.

Admittedly, reading into the underlying design of religious coping is a pretty subjective business. Others might see preservation where I have seen reconstruction, or vice versa. And not everyone will necessarily use these methods of religious coping for the purposes I have described here. (Recall that an iron can do many things besides remove wrinkles.) To decipher the functions of religion in coping for any individual, we have to have to take a close look at that person's history of experience, motivations, and life situations as well as his or her methods of religious coping.

Finally, it is important to remember that methods of religious coping are not simply "psychological"; they are designed to conserve spiritual as well as psychological, social, and physical ends. They help to explain the resilience of religion to withstand, assimilate, and adapt to a variety of negative experiences (Calhoun & Tedeschi, 1992). Thus, religions are not only conservational mechanisms, they are part of the world that is conserved.

Some psychologists might say that the story of religion and coping ends here, that religion is a method of conservation plain and simple. I disagree. Conservation may be part, even a big part of the story, but it is not the whole story. There are occasions when we can find religion deeply involved in upheaval and change of the things we care most about. It is time to consider some of the transformational roles of religion in the coping process.

Chapter Nine

RELIGION AND THE
MECHANISMS
OF COPING
The Transformation
Of Significance

An elderly Mormon describes the car accident which took the life of his wife: I knew that she was killed. There was a big gash on her wrist, and it wasn't bleeding, and I couldn't get any pulse. And I felt that I could lay my hands on her head and bring her back [a healing practice in the Church of Jesus Christ of Latter-Day Saints]. And a voice spoke to me and said: "Do you want her back a vegetable? She's fine. She's all right. . . . Let her go."
—Pargament, Royster, et al. (1990, p. 9)

Conservation may be the first reaction in coping, but conservation is not always possible. There are times when dreams must be deferred or when dreams must come to an end. Some events throw up barriers that make it impossible to realize a dream. Others point to the foolishness of the ends we have sought. Some experiences open up the possibility of new values that make others pale by comparison. Still others shatter the things we cherish most. These are the times when the purpose of life is called into question. These are the times that insist on a change in values, a transformation of significance.

Transformation is difficult. It requires a shift in direction from old destinations that no longer seem viable to new, more compelling ones. Giving up deeply held values and discovering replacements can be a wrenching experience. Perhaps that is why transformation may be attempted only when every other conceivable way of conserving the ends of significance has been exhausted. Yet, painful as it may be, transformation remains a necessary part of coping, for at times the only way to maximize significance may be to transform it.

In the midst of transformation, we often find religion. Every religious tradition has its exemplars of people who find themselves tested or lost in a real or symbolic wilderness (e.g., Ratliff, 1989). For 40 years, the Israelites wandered the desert of Sinai uncertain at times whether to return to Egypt, take up idol worship, or pursue the Promised Land. For forty days Jesus Christ lived in the wilderness and faced temptations by the devil. In moments of desolation, something of the sacred is encountered, a new sense of direction and purpose emerges from the trials.

The stories of religious transformation are not a thing of the past. Unfortunately, only a few systematic studies have focused on the nature of religious transformation, perhaps because the study of change is so difficult or perhaps because social scientists have viewed religion more as a conservative force in coping. Whatever the reason, we must rely more on case studies, anecdotal accounts, and interpretations than "solid data" here. But "soft" as these data may be, I think they illustrate some of the important ways religion is involved in attempts to give up old dreams and create new ones.

In this chapter we will examine religious transformation in coping, focusing specifically on the roles of religion in the two types of transformation described in Table 5.1: (1) re-valuation—the effort to change the destination of significance while leaving the pathways to significance intact, and (2) re-creation—the effort to change both the destination of significance and the pathways to reach it.

CHANGE OF HEART: RELIGION AND THE RE-VALUATION OF SIGNIFICANCE

Re-valuation has a paradoxical quality. On one level, *change* is the focus; old objects of significance must be relinquished and replacements must be found. On another level, *continuity* is the central issue; in the midst of loss and change, a way of life must be sustained.

Managing the conflicting demands for change and continuity is not an easy task. For thousands of years, people have looked to religion for help in navigating their way through situations that call for a change in significance. In this section, we will take a closer look at two of the ways religion is involved in re-valuative coping: seeking religious purpose and rites of passage.

Seeking Religious Purpose

There are some life events that are so disruptive, they throw an entire set of values into disarray. Preservation or reconstruction is no longer feasible because the old destinations of significance are no longer viable. The task for coping is to find a new set of priorities or goals to pursue. The focus is not on a total life change (though it may come to that eventually), but on a change in values. This type of coping process is re-valuative—means are conserved, at least for the moment, while ends undergo a transformation. The search is on for a new sense of purpose.

Some people look to religion for help in this process.

The story of Kathy Hughes (1990) is a nice example. Recently graduated from college and involved in a relationship with a boyfriend, she was sure of herself and her direction in life. Marriage, children, and a career in social work were all a part of her future. All of her plans, however, were shaken when she suffered a life-threatening injury in a car accident. A trauma to her head was accompanied by expressive aphasia, making it unlikely that she would be able to find employment as a social worker. Other physical injuries made it impossible for her to have children. And when she discovered her boyfriend with another woman, she wondered whether she would ever be a wife. Throughout the account of her ordeal, Kathy comes back to the question, what should she do with her life? Having lost her objects of greatest significance, she struggles to find a new purpose in living.

In this process, she prays to God for a fresh sense of purpose. After she learned that her boyfriend was involved with someone else, she asks of God: "I see I'm not to be a mother. I'm not even to be a wife, it seems, at least for now. Well what, what in heaven's name do you want me to do?" (p. 83). The initial response she felt from God was a re-valuative one: "She felt a welcoming warmth spread through her, illuminating her mind. A tiny voice seemed to whisper, 'Just get better and the rest will follow' " (p. 83). In this account, God seemed to be encouraging Kathy to conserve herself, while offering her the promise that she would find a new sense of direction in life. Further along in her physical recovery, she receives her answer from God: "Then, deep inside her mind, Kathy felt a stirring, an opening. A familiar voice rang out. 'Kathy, start a support group. Finish your book. And I will take care of the rest'" (p. 113). Her search for a religious direction, she concludes, had ended: "A sense of purpose pervaded everything she did. She finally knew why her life had been spared. She was part of a plan, and she intended to fulfill her role to the best of her abilities" (p. 114).

Underlying the search for religious purpose is the belief that life has an ultimate goal. What gives the search its *religious* quality is the belief that purpose is transcendental in nature, going beyond whatever the individual may make of it on his or her own. According to most religious perspectives, each of us has a reason for being; no matter how terrible our situation may be, every person is said to have a special mission or calling in life. The mission is not constructed *by* the person; it is constructed *for* the individual. When old purposes are no longer viable, the individual does not have to create a new reason for living—the work in coping is to discern the transcendental design.

This is the way Frankl (1984, 1988) speaks of meaning in life. There is, he says, a "right" and "true" meaning for every individual and every situation, one which exists apart from the individual's own "closed system." In the midst of turmoil and despair, the individual must find this meaning. The appropriate question, he believes, is not what do we expect from life, but what does life expect from us. "Someone looks down on each of us in difficult hours," Frankl told his fellow prisoners in a concentration camp, "a friend, a wife, somebody alive or dead, or a God—and he would not expect us to disappoint him. He would hope to find us suffering proudly—not miserably—knowing how to die" (Frankl, 1984, p. 104). Meaning for Frankl is clearly a transcendental phenomenon. It is "something to be found rather than to be given, discovered rather than invented" (Frankl, 1988, p. 62). In this respect, Frankl's theory is fundamentally religious.

When successful, the search for a religious purpose places the individual's life into a different context. The focus shifts from immediate, personal goals to longer-term, loftier ends. Purposes become destinations (Johnson, 1959). In the case of Kathy Hughes, we hear how a concern with personal suffering is replaced by a sacred vocation—to help others who have suffered a similar disability.

Whether God has, in fact, revealed to the person a glimmer of his or her destiny is another question, one the scientist cannot answer. Certainly, the perception that the person has received spiritual direction may be a way to satisfy one's own desires while avoiding the responsibility for them at the same time. Projected on to God, human aspirations of all kinds may receive the spiritual stamp of approval. Many in the religious world, however, caution against this type of projection and encourage their members to distinguish a true religious calling from a false one (Ratliff, 1989).

While the reality of religious inspiration cannot be determined through scientific methods, other questions about the search for a religious objective are testable. For one, we might ask how often people look beyond themselves to religion for purpose in coping. How typical is the kind of experience described by Kathy Hughes? We can find anecdotal accounts similar to hers, but empirical research in this area is scanty. One study by Cobble (1985), however, suggests that it may not be all that unusual. He interviewed and surveyed a sample of adult Christians from ages 18 to 81 about the ways they express their faith in God. "Seeking direction from God" emerged as one of the most prominent themes. The search for religious direction was most common in periods of transitions. A majority of both men and women looked for religious direction in the shift from adolescence to adulthood (ages 18–23). Men also frequently sought direction from God in the transition to age 30 and in their 40s. Women were more likely to seek religious guidance in their mid-20s and from their mid-30s to mid-40s, a reflection, Cobble suggests, of greater turmoil for women in the child rearing and career-oriented phases of life.

Even more interesting are questions about why people seek out spiritual guidance. From a secular perspective the idea of turning to God for purpose in times of crisis may seem a bit peculiar. If significance is lost, why doesn't someone like Kathy Hughes simply develop a new set of goals for herself? Why instead does she look beyond herself for spiritual guidance? Without much empirical research on this question, we can only speculate, using our framework of coping as a guide. First, the individual must find herself inadequate as the sole arbiter of significance. In appraising her ability to find her own direction in life, she concludes that she is in some way insufficient. Perhaps she questions her own authority to define the values of greatest significance in life. Perhaps to this point she has not been successful in finding a fulfilling direction for herself. Perhaps she has entered a dramatically different phase of life, pushing her beyond her own resources to generate new directions. Or perhaps she has a new and troubling sense of the fragility of what she has come to value, a sense of how precarious many objects of significance, including life itself, can be.

In response to this sense of insufficiency, religious sources of guidance must be accessible to the person and must offer a compelling alternative. Certainly, religious institutions try to be both available and compelling. To those who have become disenchanted with their dreams, the church suggests a different vision. The sign in front of one suburban church reads: "Tired of money, sex, and power? Check in with God." Another sign calls out to the unfulfilled: "If you're heading in the wrong direction, God allows U-turns." To those who may feel confused and lost at a critical juncture, clergy offer pastoral direction. Finally, to those who may question the legitimacy of their own values or find them too fragile, religion offers a source of authority and permanence. Secularly based values may come and go, but the significance rooted in religion has the potential for great staying power (see Klinger, 1977). Kathy Hughes's desire to help others faced with similar disabilities, once transformed into a holy quest, may be more resilient to future crises and disappointments.

In short, we would expect people to seek out a religious purpose in coping when religious objectives are available and offer a more compelling sense of direction than the alternatives. Unfortunately, researchers have not examined how religion shapes values in times of stress. Systematic study is needed (see Schoenrade & Leavitt, 1989, for a promising start).

The search for religious purpose involves continuity and change. The individual attempts to maintain a way of life as he or she seeks out religious direction. But this method of coping is time-limited. Ultimately, the search for religious purpose may lead to a reaffirmation of the individual's way of life. But not always. The search for a religious direction may be simply the first step in a process of change. Having discovered a new purpose in living, life must be reshaped to fit with the new mission. In the language of coping, re-valuation (the transformation of ends and conservation of means) will be followed by reconstruction (the transformation of means and conservation of ends) to bring pathways and destinations into closer alignment with each other.

Rites of Passage

Over the course of the lifespan, we experience moments that have a special "once and for all" character (Smith, 1968). These moments coincide with life's most important transitions—birth, coming of age, marriage, and death. Oftentimes they elicit feelings of mystery, awe, and trepidation. Powerful forces seem to be at play, unseen but sensed, just beneath the surface of everyday life. These are also unsettling moments, periods of sharp discontinuity, when people leap (or are pushed) from one status to another.

Every religion provides its members with rituals to accompany life's transitions. Pierced flesh, enforced separations, fasting, exchanges of gifts, immersion in water or milk, ceremonial meals, special language, song, and dance are just a few of the distinctive rituals that mark the specialness of these occasions (see van Gennep, 1960). Although these rituals take many different forms, they share a common function and a common structure; their purpose is to mark and facilitate the transition through what Friedman (1985) has called "hinges of time" (p. 164). In this sense, they are rites of passage.

It is important to note that, unlike many of the other religious coping methods considered to this point, rites of passage are, in some sense, externally imposed. Their function and structure are largely a social construction. The individual may choose whether to engage in a rite of passage and, if so, how seriously to take it. There also may be some room for "tinkering" with the passage to accommodate individual needs and preferences. Even so, the rite of passage has a design of its own that imposes clear demands and expectations on the individual in transition.

Rites of passage have the dual nature so characteristic of re-valuative coping. They encourage change and continuity. At the same time, they signify transformation while lending stability to the individual and community in crisis. In these passages, we find people asked to give up old values and take on new ones, just as they are encouraged to keep themselves together emotionally and remain a part of a historical, social, and spiritual community. Sacred power is called on to assist in both functions—to facilitate the shift from one value to another and to provide reassurance that in the midst of all this upheaval there is an underlying continuity. Life may ebb and flow, but God remains eternal.

Rites of passage also have a common structure, one that involves more than just a religious ceremony. Certainly, the ceremony is the most visible sign that an important change has occurred, but the transition itself does not begin and end there. As Edwin Friedman (1985), rabbi and family therapist, notes: "Some people were married (emotionally) long before the ceremony, and some never emotionally leave home after it; some were 'buried' before they died, while deceased others remain around to haunt for years" (p. 167). Anthropologist Arnold van Gennep (1960) studied the rituals of primitive and modern cultures in the early 20th century and concluded that rites of passage have three phases, each distinguished by its own rituals: separation, transition, and incorporation. Others have reached similar conclusions (e.g., Roberts, 1988). I will illustrate these points by focusing on the final rite of passage.

From Life to Death

A death creates holes in the structure of significance and some new imperatives: An individual has died and roles have been lost, relationships ended, old plans abandoned, and terrible challenges raised. How can these losses be acknowledged and accepted? How do the survivors manage to keep themselves and their way of life intact while grieving their losses? How are lost roles, statuses, and commitments replaced with new sources of significance? Death elicits the need for both continuity and change. Oftentimes death is enveloped in religious rites of passage designed to respond to just these needs.

If we focus on death-related beliefs and practices in the United

States, we might conclude that religious rituals deny this rite of passage rather than foster it. In this country (and other Western nations as well), the firsthand encounter with death has become an unusual event. What used to occur at home among close family now unfolds in a hospital room among medical professionals. From there the body is whisked to a funeral parlor where specialists embalm the corpse, restore it to a more life-like appearance with the help of make-up products such as "Nature-Glo" and the artful rearrangement of facial features (e.g., parting the lips to leave the impression that the deceased is still breathing), and place it in an impermeable casket (Chidester, 1990). The funeral itself is a briefer affair. The long stately funeral procession to the graveyard that used to stop pedestrians and traffic in a final tribute to the deceased has given way to a fast-moving line of cars difficult to distinguish from the rest of the traffic (Griffin & Tobin, 1982). Children who used to witness death close up are now sheltered from the experience. The mourners themselves are expected to accept death stoically and return to work within a week.

It would appear that death has become sealed off from American consciousness. But the problem may be rooted less in religion than in the secularization of what was once a profoundly religious event. If we turn our attention to religious rites of passage in the United States and throughout the world, we find that, far from denying the event, they mark the fact that a terribly important change has occurred. Moreover, they encourage adherents to accept and interpret this new reality, protect them from the threats it brings, and, with time, guide them back into the community. It is important to add that, from the religious perspective, the rite of passage addresses the deceased as well as their survivors. While the survivors are introduced to the role of mourners, assisted through their grief and reintegrated into the community, the deceased is shepherded through the transition from life to death to incorporation into a transcendental realm. In the following sections, I examine the phases of this rite of passage with illustrations from many different religious perspectives.

Preparation and Separation

Even before a death has occurred, we can find religious rituals that attempt to prepare the individual, family, and friends for the event and to ease the transition. Popular Buddhist belief, for instance, holds that the individual's frame of mind at the moment of death determines his or her status afterward. The dying person whose soul is still trapped by earthly desires risks drowning in a treacherous river made up of three dangerous currents (fearsome human beings, vicious animals, and hungry ghosts) (Long, 1975). By freeing the self from worldly attachments, however, the individual can achieve a successful passage. Meditation, the technique for raising consciousness, plays a particularly important role in the preparation for death. This is the focus of *The Tibetan Book of the Dead,* one of the most widely sold books in the world. In the face of death, the person is instructed to focus consciousness on the "luminous splendor of the colorless light of Emptiness" (cited in Long, 1975, p. 69). In fact, the supreme mantra the Tibetan Buddhist is taught to meditate on is the last sound the dying person will hear.

Anglicans also call on religious rituals to assist the dying in the transition from life to afterlife before the death has occurred, as we hear in the final prayer of the Anglican litany for the dying: "Depart, O Christian soul, out of this world, in the name of God the Father Almighty who created you, in the name of Jesus Christ who redeemed you, in the name of the Holy Ghost who sanctifies you. May your rest be this day in peace, and your dwelling place in the Paradise of God" (*Book of Common Prayer,* cited in Oden, 1983, p. 306).

The moment of death itself is quickly followed by many religious rituals to mark the sacredness of the event and announce new separations in the community. One separation involves the departure of the dead from the living: Across many cultures, the bodies of the dead are hastily removed from the home according to religious rituals designed to speed the departure of the dead and prevent their return to haunt the living or tempt their loved ones into joining them (Bendann, 1930). Windows may be thrown open, allowing the souls of the dead to escape, or the body may be carried out feet first through a special exit in the house so the spirit cannot make its way back home. Rituals underscore another separation—the living from the dead: In some cultures the grieving family changes residence; physical reminders of the deceased are destroyed, given away, or placed in the coffin with the corpse; and the mention of the name of the dead is taboo (Rosenblatt, Walsh, & Jackson, 1976). Rituals also mark the separation of the bereaved from the rest of the community: special dress, cutting the hair, uncleanliness, seclusion, or other methods signify the unique social status of the survivors.

Transition

All of these important changes are formally acknowledged in the funeral ceremony. Among those groups that believe in a period of transition between death and an afterlife, the funeral incorporates prayer and rituals to ease the entry of the dead into the next world. For instance, in their prayers for the dead, Roman Catholics ask God to be merciful and release the departed from the burdens of their sins so they may enjoy a better place in the hereafter. Muslims whisper into the ear of the deceased answers to questions the angels may ask them about their deeds in life; according to tradition, this "trial of the grave" determines whether the dead will go to the garden of paradise or the torments of hell (Chidester, 1990). And according to traditional Hindu custom, the dead could be spiritually reborn into the world of ancestors through the assistance of an elaborate and lengthy funeral ritual. Lest we dismiss the focus on heaven as unusual, it is important to point out that 71% of people in the United States reportedly believe in a life after death of one sort or another (Gallup & Castelli, 1989). These beliefs are common even for the least religiously active. Fifty eight percent of those who do not belong to a church believe in an afterlife.[1]

The funeral serves the living as well as the dead. It confronts the bereaved with the fact that a loss has occurred, and encourages them to accept this fundamental change. Rosenblatt et al. (1976) elaborate on this point. The passage from old commitments to new ones is exceptionally difficult, they say, and the natural tendency of the bereaved is conservational—to reject change and hold on to the familiar. The funeral ceremony, however, forces them to face the reality of the event. Here, in front of a group of caring witnesses, the bereaved view the body in the casket, carry the coffin to the grave, or shovel dirt onto the coffin in the grave site. These are public, voluntary, and effortful behaviors on the part of the mourners (cf. Bem, 1972) that run counter to any tendency to act as if the event had not happened. After all, how can the participant in this most basic rite of mourning deny that something momentous has occurred?

The funeral is designed to protect the bereaved while encouraging their acceptance of the death. Expressions of grief are supported and even prescribed, but some limits are set. The widow who throws herself on her spouse's coffin is led gently away. The despondent parent is accompanied by others to prevent self-harm. Friends and family try to calm and soothe the agitated widower. Clergy help mourners keep their emotions in check, particularly those of anger, guilt, and frustration.

The protection offered by the funeral extends beyond the bereaved to the larger community. As many sociologists have pointed out, deaths are social losses, not just personal ones (Riley, 1968). With every death comes the loss of an actor playing important social roles in the community. Mortality, in this sense, weakens the social structure. The funeral ritual offers a social response. Here, in the face of this threat, the group comes together to reassert its solidarity and renew itself through ceremonies of mourning. Durkheim (1915) wrote, "Since they weep together, they hold to one another, and the group is not weakened, in spite of the blow which has fallen upon it . . . The group feels its strength gradually returning; it begins to hope and to live again" (pp. 447–448).

Incorporation

In Western culture, the funeral service often marks the end of this final rite of passage. Though the funeral helps the mourners manage their first shock and initial grief, they may be left with little support as they go through the even more trying time of bereavement ahead (Gorer, 1965). Many religious groups, however, offer their members final ceremonies of bereavement. They take the form of prayers for the dead, the lighting of a memorial candle, graveside rituals, or special Masses on the anniversary of the death. These ceremonies are integrative in several respects. For one, they symbolize the incorporation of the deceased into the afterlife (van Gennep, 1960) and permit the bereaved to imagine their loved ones secure and cared for, as we hear in one father's description of his daughter in heaven:

> My picture of God is that F. is up there running through a field picking flowers and bringing them. And Jesus is sitting there on a rock. She is gathering flowers for Him. I feel that she is right there in his lap. I feel that even though I still grieve and still have the pain and the tears, I have this picture of Jesus on a rock with a little girl in his lap. And all these other little kids there, and Him telling them stories. (Klass, 1988, p. 143)

In addition, final ceremonies help reintegrate the mourner into the group by imposing a time limit on the period of grieving that, once past, signifies the mourner is now ready to take on new roles in the community. For example, before the first year of mourning has ended, Jews are expected to participate in a special "unveiling" ceremony in which the grave is visited and the tombstone consecrated through appropriate prayer. The mourner's clothes, rended as a sign of grief before the funeral, can now be sewn and reworn as a sign that the wounds are healing and life, even with its scars, must go on.

In their empirical analysis of ethnographic descriptions of 78 cultures, Rosenblatt et al. (1976) found that members of cultures with final ceremonies experienced far fewer signs of prolonged grief, such as suicidal behavior, work-related difficulties, troubled dreams, and mental and physical illness. Like the funeral service itself, they explain, final ceremonies encourage the bereaved to drop the symbols of mourning and commit themselves publicly to new status and full participation in the community.

Final ceremonies also symbolize the integration of the living with the dead. Though they remind the survivors of their loss, the very act of remembering binds the mourner with the deceased. Consider the Reform Jewish prayer recited in memorial services:

> In the rising of the sun and in its going down,
> we remember them . . .
> When we are lost and sick at heart,
> we remember them.
> When we have joys we yearn to share,
> we remember them.
> So long as we live, they too shall live,
> for they are now a part of us, as
> we remember them.
> (*Gates of Prayer: The New Union Prayerbook*, 1975, p. 552)

In acts of prayer and ritual such as this one, the dead are addressed, not so much as entities with physical presences of their own, but as departed ones who have left the living with a legacy of memories, images, and emotions. In this sense, these final ceremonies help the living take on a new representation of the dead. To put it another way, final ceremonies symbolize a transformation of the dead, from physical beings to spiritual beings whose essence has been incorporated into the inner experience of the survivors.

This functional analysis has jumped from religion to religion, cutting across many important differences in belief and tradition. Religious groups vary widely in the relative emphasis they place on the different phases of the passage from life to death (i.e., preparation, separation, transition, incorporation). They also vary in the degree to which they respond to the needs of the deceased, those of the bereaved, or those of the larger community. In spite of these differences, there is a common underlying purpose to this last rite of passage. It is a rite that encourages continuity and change at the same time. In the midst of their greatest losses, the individual and the community are sustained. Meaningful connections are formed between what has occurred in this world and what will come after, between the living and the dead, and between those in mourning and the rest of the community. Death becomes integrated into personal and social life, ensuring the continuity of all experience. However, this is not a stability purchased through denial. The rite of passage confronts the participant with the fact that something momentous has indeed occurred. It pushes the mourner out of grief and confusion into new identities and new roles. The bereaved may reenter the world, not as they once were, but fundamentally changed through the transformation of significance.

The transformations involved in re-valuative coping are not total. Attempts to find new significance in living are likely to be followed by other changes as well. New pathways will be needed to reach new destinations. Thus, re-valuative coping may be followed by a period of reconstructive coping. Not all coping, however, follows this rule. In some cases, the transformation of means and ends occurs not sequentially, but simultaneously. These are times of most radical change. Here, too, we find religion at work. We now turn our attention to this fourth and final type of coping.

RADICAL CHANGE: RELIGION AND THE RE-CREATION OF SIGNIFICANCE

Twenty-nine years old, Brenda was at the end of her rope (Project on Religion and Coping). The daughter of an abusive father, Brenda had married as soon as she could to get out of the house. When her husband left her, she began to drink heavily to cover up her feelings: "I was trying to let other people know that it didn't matter to me," she said, "I was happy this way, better off." Brenda met her second husband in a bar, and although she quit drinking during her pregnancy, she started up again when her son was very young. After her second husband left her, she stopped eating, lost a great deal of weight, and drank heavily every night: "I'd put my son to bed and I'd sit out on the steps and wonder why I had no friends, no life, no money, didn't know what I was going to do, and why me?" Over the next few years she drifted from relationship to relationship and her drinking continued. Her third marriage was abusive from the start: "The first week I started going out with him, he (physically) pushed me around a little. Every weekend, we would do the same thing, we would get drunk together, and he would get mad at me, and then something would happen, and then the next day, always a Sunday, he would say he was sorry, and that it would never happen again." But the cycle of violence continued, reaching its peak a few years later: "We got in the biggest fight we ever had, and I ended up in the hospital. I'm sitting there on the table, and they were taking pictures of all the marks and bruises, and I was waiting to hear whether or not my skull was fractured. They had just told me that my eardrum was broken. I was sitting there thinking it hurt a lot. I felt like I was going to faint, and I knew, sitting there on that table, that there had to be something different, there had to be a better way, there had to be more than this."

Brenda was at a turning point. The despair she felt with her life had set the stage for a radical change. She was not looking for partial adjustments in her situation. She was not seeking a transformation of means alone (i.e., reconstruction) nor ends alone (i.e., re-valuation). Brenda was looking for a very different life. To effect this total transformation, she was about to experience a radical religious change. In this section, we will consider religious conversion and religious forgiveness, two powerful coping mechanisms designed to re-create both the means and ends of significance.

Religious Conversion: From Self to Sacred Concern

Probably no subject in the scientific study of religion has generated as much attention and debate over the last 100 years as the topic of conversion. Psychologists, theologians, mental health professionals, and sociologists have all taken their turns at describing and explaining this uniquely human phenomenon. In the late 19th century, religious revivals, baptisms, and dramatic accounts of conversion experiences were commonplace in the United States, particularly among the more evangelical Protestant groups (Spilka et al., 1985). For the founding figures in psychology, these experiences represented important psychological processes that deserved serious attention. Drawing from rich personal accounts, interviews, surveys, and in some instances, quasiexperimental studies, psychologists such as William James, Edwin Starbuck, James Pratt, George Coe, and Elmer Clark explored conversion as a normal human experience. They were most interested in describing the experience, understanding its causes, and distinguishing the sudden, dramatic religious change from the gradual, less intense transformation.

With the advent of behaviorism, psychologists shifted their attention away from processes as subjective and phenomenological as conversion. Mental health professionals, however, began to write about conversion from a clinical evaluative point of view. Freud (1928/1961) viewed this process unfavorably. From his perspective, conversion represented a regressive attempt to resolve early oedipal hatred of the father by complete submission to a higher power. Others, however, evaluated conversion more positively: For Jung, conversion was a method of balancing personality; for Adler, it aided in the transition from inferiority to superiority. Some argued that it was important to distinguish the regressive, dysfunctional type of conversion described by Freud from the progressive conversion designed to achieve new, more mature values (Salzman, 1953). In more recent years, some mental health professionals have raised concerns that religious conversion may be a form of "brainwashing" or "thought reform" used by cults and new religious movements to coerce the unsuspecting individual into membership (e.g., Sargant, 1957; Singer, 1979). Some clinicians, however, have argued that this is an oversimplistic and stereotyped view of the conversion process (e.g., Galanter, 1989).

Over the last 25 years, the lion's share of research on conversion has come from sociologists (e.g., Richardson, 1978; Robbins & Anthony, 1979; Snow & Machalek, 1984). Not coincidentally, their interest in this topic has paralleled the sharp increase in new religious movements and cults in the West. How and why people come to experience such dramatic change in their group identity is a central concern in this body of work. From the sociological perspective, conversion is as much as a social transformation as it is a psychological one.

Given the many attitudes and interests people have brought to the study of conversion, it should not be surprising to find that the term has taken on very different meanings and uses. We cannot settle these differences here or provide a comprehensive model of religious conversion. Most social scientists would agree that there is no such thing as "the" conversion. The goal here is more modest: to consider conversion as a radical way of coping toward significance.

We start with a working definition. *In an effort to re-create life, the individual experiences a dramatic change of the self, a change in which the self becomes identified with the sacred.* This is the essence of religious conversion as the term will be used here. There are two key features of this perspective.

Life Transformation as the Goal of Conversion

While scholars debate the exact meaning of conversion, most agree that it is radical in purpose: "the notion of radical change remains at the core of all conceptions of conversion, whether theological or social scientific" (Snow & Machalek, 1984, p. 169). Life is out of kilter and small changes will not do. To say that there is a specific problem in need of solving misses the point. Existence itself has become the problem and a fundamental change is called for. The objective of conversion is to create a substantive change in both destinations and pathways of living.

In this sense, conversion is unlike conservational approaches to coping. We would not apply the term to someone who switches religious groups simply to find a greater sense of belonging, nor to someone whose idea of God changes from a punitive power to a loving being in an effort to find greater comfort in life. These are reconstructive approaches; new steps may be taken here but the goals are old and familiar. In a similar vein, we would not label a change in one particular attitude, feeling, or behavior as a conversion. Toch (1955) describes what seemed to be a last minute "change of heart" by anti-Semite Julius Streicher at the close of the Nuremberg Trials, but his purported conversion was only a "switch of valences" within the same framework:

> ... now I see that the Jews have determination and spunk—They will still dominate the world, mark my word!—And I would be glad to lead them to victory because they are strong and tenacious, and I know Jewry.... If the Jews would be willing to accept me as one of them, I would fight for them ...! (from Gilbert, cited in Toch, 1955, p. 64)

The function of conversion is more far-reaching. Consciously or unconsciously, the potential convert is hoping to relinquish an old life and replace it with something new. Improvement, growth, and development are terms that do not capture the fundamental change the individual seeks. Transformation comes closer. Images of this kind of radical change can be found in many religions. They are particularly abundant in Christianity: "Death to sin in order to live in God; conversion from the status of slave to that of son and heir; transformation from darkness to light and from the way of the flesh to the way of the spirit" (Whitehead & Whitehead, 1979, p. 34).

It is important to note that the immediate impulse leading to conversion may be an emotional, moral, social, or intellectual problem, but only by grasping that there is something fundamentally wrong with one's life can conversion occur. One recovering alcoholic put it more plainly: "I came here [Alcoholics Anonymous] to save my ass. And then I found out it was attached to my soul" (Robertson, 1988, p. 122). The convert attempts to give up not just old "love objects" (e.g., alcohol, sex, unfulfilling relationships, anger, guilt, or helplessness), but the life built around them. In their place, the convert looks for another organizing force, a new "center of loyalty" (Pratt, 1946). With destiny hanging in the balance, the individual attempts to change the whole course of life (Johnson, 1959).

Self-Transformation as the Method of Conversion

Although theorists think of conversion in different ways, most believe that a change of self lies at the heart of the experience. In conversion, James (1902) said, a "self hitherto divided" becomes unified. Conversion for Coe (1916) was an intense and abrupt self-realization. Recent writers have placed a similar emphasis on self-transformation in their descriptions of conversion. They speak of change in the "core identity construct" (Thumma, 1991), a transcending self (Nino, 1990), and identity consolidation (Gordon, 1974).

How does this transformation take place? If we take a closer look at this experience, we can discern two separated but related processes: (1) an admission that the self is limited, and (2) an incorporation of the sacred into the self.

Admitting the Limitations of the Self

Radical change does not come easy. Some type of stressor, tension, conflict, or uneasiness seems to be a prerequisite. The trigger may be an important transition or major negative events, such as the death of a loved one, a health threat, a divorce, or a critical loss. Former President Jimmy Carter, for example, experienced a religious conversion after a devastating loss in his election for governor of Georgia (Norton & Slosser, 1976).

Empirical studies also point to a connection between stressors and conversion. In one retrospective study, Kox, Meeus, and Hart (1991) compared a group of young converts to a charismatic Christian denomination to a group of matched controls. Sixty-seven percent of the converts reported personal problems within 3–5 years before their conversion, as opposed to 20% of the controls. Converts were also more likely than the nonconverts to report a major life event (e.g., a move, the death of a parent, or parents' divorce) prior to their conversion. This study was limited by its retrospective design. To testify to the power and value of their transformation, these converts may have overstated the stressfulness of their preconversion lives. Some doubts on this interpretation are shed by Galanter (1980), however. In one of the few prospective studies in this area, he examined potential converts to the Unification Church *before* they made the decision to join. Compared to those who chose not to join and a comparison group of nonmembers, the converts showed higher levels of emotional distress 1 month before becoming a member of the church. These results offer stronger evidence of the role immediate tensions can play in the conversion process.

The stress and trauma leading to conversion do not have to be sudden or acute. A significant percentage of converts do not report crises just prior to their conversion (Heirich, 1977; Kox et al., 1991; Seggar & Kunz, 1972). In many instances, conversion appears to grow out of a longer history of tension and conflict. Chronic feelings of depression, loneliness, and unsatisfactory parental relationships have been noted by investigators (Deutsch, 1975; Schwartz & Kaslow, 1979). Similarly, researchers have found higher than usual rates of major psychopathology and hospitalization among converts to some religious groups (e.g., Galanter, Rabkin, Rabkin, & Deutsch, 1979; Witztum, Greenberg, & Dasberg, 1990). Some of these findings may be biased by raters well aware that the participants in their studies are members of religious groups or, in some instances, cults. Nevertheless, the weight of the evidence indicates that, for many, it is the accumulation of distress over time rather than one particularly powerful stressor that sets the stage for conversion.

Whether it is an acute crisis or a longstanding sense of unease, tension of some kind is an important precursor of conversion. Of course, not everyone under tension experiences a conversion. For example, 46% of the *nonconverts* in the Kox et al. (1991) study reported major life events in recent years. More than life stress is needed to precipitate this experience. For a conversion to occur, the usual forms of coping with stress must also be found wanting. Typically, the individual has engaged in many coping strategies before he or she is willing to even entertain the thought of a drastic departure in living. Only after these efforts have failed, and failed repeatedly and convincingly, does radical change become a serious possibility.

These failures in coping demonstrate the limited power of the self to reach its goals. By the time a conversion occurs, what were once seen as unsuccessful attempts to cope have become demonstrations of personal futility. As a self-contained being, the individual is simply unable to effect change. This was the situation confronting Brenda, the alcoholic abused woman previously described. She was faced with the fact that all of her attempts to end her drinking and find meaningful relationships had failed. She had reached the limits of her control (Soper, 1951).

Failures in coping underscore not only the limits of a person's power, but the inadequacy of what the person has been striving for. Significance has been shaken to the core. The individual may feel a loss of ultimate grounding and meaning (Heirich, 1977; Proudfoot & Shaver, 1975), a sense of worthlessness and incompleteness, or a conflict between base desires and more elevated ends (Starbuck, 1899). Typically, however, self-centeredness is defined as a key part of the problem by the religious convert.

Take, for example, the story of Asa Candler Jr. (1951), second son of the founder of the Coca-Cola Company. Unable to resolve his depression and unable to quit drinking, Candler (with some assistance from a divine voice) identifies his own pride and vanity as the cause of the problem:

> I was unusually troubled in my soul. Suddenly I heard a voice, just as clearly as I have ever heard anyone. . . . The voice said to me, "You must get rid of your *self*; you must renounce your *self*; you must reject your *self*." These were surprising words. I should not have been surprised if the voice had commanded me to stop drinking. But this was not the message at all. It was my *self* that I was commanded to

give up. My *self* was my trouble—my love of myself, my fear of anything that might frustrate my wishes. My will had always been the central interest in my life. False pride had erected a barrier between my soul and God. (pp. 55–56)

Admissions of the limits of personal power and the limits of the self as the object of greatest significance pave the way for another critical, yet paradoxical part of the process. Starbuck (1899), in what remains one of the richest accounts of religious conversion, described this process as self-surrender, "the giving up of personal will" (p. 98). The person who has been struggling to reject the old life and find a new one, he writes, "is striving at a wrong angle" (p. 115). The act of resistance only gives more power to what is being resisted. The solution cannot be found in further expressions of the will. Instead, the person "must cease trying; he must relax, and . . . fall back on the larger 'Power that makes for righteousness,' " (p. 115). Starbuck (1899) provides a number of examples of self-surrender from his interviewees who had experienced conversion:

> [Male, 15:] "All at once it occurred to me that I might be saved, too, if I would stop trying to do it all myself, and follow Jesus. . . ." [Male, 15:] "I finally ceased to resist, and gave myself up though it was a hard struggle. Gradually the feeling came over me that I had done my part, and God was willing to do His." (p. 114)

The language of Starbuck and his converts, "ceasing to resist," "giving up," and "self-surrender," may be red flags to many people, including mental health professionals, who look critically on terms that fairly shout "loss of personal control." Giving up seems to contradict everything we have been told about how to solve problems. Yet there are times and situations when surrender may be the most appropriate form of coping.

This is the point Brenner (1985) makes in her book *Winning by Letting Go*. She presents this illustration:

> Barry had been skin-diving near a sewage plant at the local beach. Venturing too close to the intake pipe, he'd been sucked in a flood of seawater into the pipe. He struggled against the violent pull of the water until he died, not from being mangled, but from exhaustion. "There's a flotation tank in all those plants," sighed [his friend] Steven. "If he hadn't struggled, he would have floated unharmed to the top." (p. 36)

Brenner admits that surrender can turn into fatalism—an excuse for passivity when action is called for. However, she goes on to note that surrender has its more constructive side. In contrast to the experience of losing control, surrender has a voluntary dimension to it. The individual can choose to give up; this willingness to give up allows the individual to explore very different, potentially more adaptive modes of experience. In fact, she argues (not unlike the Zen devotee), surrender is a necessary part of living: "Every muscular movement is based on one muscle group's 'letting go' while its complement tenses up. We cannot live unless we are willing to let go of each breath to make room for a fresh one" (p. 113).

How is it then that the concept of surrender or giving up elicits such different reactions? Why, Brenner asks, do mystics, prophets and politicians seek surrender, while politicians and generals do everything they can to avoid it? The answer may be that it makes a great deal of difference what the person is surrendering *to*. In the case of religious conversion, admissions of personal limitations are followed by surrender to a particular kind of object—the sacred.

Incorporating the Sacred into the Self

In a religious conversion, the sacred is incorporated into the identity of the individual. A force perceived to be far greater than the self is experienced as a new and central part of the self. One convert says, "God entered my life and I became a new person." A second says, "I felt filled by the Holy Spirit and nothing else mattered." Still another proclaims, "I no longer lived, but Christ lived in me."

As we hear in the last words, some have described the process of religious conversion as a loss of self, a "dying unto oneself." However, to be more precise, what is lost in this process is not the self, but self-absorption. One of Starbuck's (1899) interviewees talked about his conversion this way: "The chief change was in my inmost purpose. I was no longer self-centered. The change was not complete but there was a deep undercurrent of unselfishness" (p. 127).

In a religious conversion the sense of self is not erased, it is expanded. Leuba described it this way: "When the sense of estrangement fencing man about in a narrowly limited ego breaks down, the individual finds himself 'at one with all creation.' He lives in the universal life; he and man, he and nature, he and God, are one" (Leuba, 1896, cited in James, 1902, p. 241). Starbuck (1899) used similar language. Through the act of yielding, he wrote, the self becomes a part of a new world and "the 'ego' is lifted up into new significance . . . into the life of God" (p. 119). Through the conversion experience, the individual has gone beyond exclusive self-preoccupation to an identification with something larger than the self, something sacred.

There are important differences in what this "something" is. The religious world offers many objects of sacred devotion. They run the gamut from the benevolent God to the despotic religious leader. Because the sacred force varies so greatly from person to person and culture to culture, we cannot form a single conclusion about the value of conversions. How the conversion unfolds will depend a great deal on the nature of the sacred the individual comes to adore. Typically, a religious conversion involves an identification of the self with one of three classes of sacred objects: a spiritual force (spiritual conversion), a religious group (religious group conversion), or the whole of humanity (universal conversion). Though none of the types of conversion is necessarily exclusive of the other two, each represents a distinctive organizing force for the transformed self. As James (1902) noted, it makes a great deal of difference whether one object or another becomes the center of a person's energies.

Spiritual Conversion. The prototypical religious conversion centers around a spiritual force. In the conversion process, the individual experiences a feeling of connectedness with a power that goes beyond his or her own self-contained world. But the power is not simply transcendent; it is immanent as well, very much concerned with the individual's immediate experience. Oftentimes the spiritual convert reports feeling loved, understood, forgiven, and at one with God (Starbuck, 1899). In some cases, it is as if the person has been "swept up" by this power, as we hear in the following account:

> . . . the Holy Spirit descended upon me in a manner that seemed to go through me, body and soul. I could feel the impression, like a wave of electricity, going through and through me. Indeed, it seemed to come in waves and waves of liquid love; for I could not express it in any other way. It seemed like the very breath of God. I can recollect distinctly that it seemed to fan me, like immense wings. (James, 1902, p. 250)

Feelings of love from God do not go unreciprocated. The spiritual convert responds with feelings of gratitude, attachment, and devotion of his or her own. "I determined to yield my heart and life to God's service," as one of Starbuck's (1899, p. 91) converts put it. The spiritual convert finds a new organizing force for the self in the spiritual. To live in harmony with the divine will becomes the overriding goal (Starbuck, 1899).

Religious Group Conversion. Although psychologists have tended to focus their studies on spiritual conversion, higher powers are not the only objects of sacred devotion. In some instances, the religious leader or religious group represents the focal point of conversion. Take the case of Ed, a member of the Unification Church, who spent 2 full days in isolation praying for a revelation. When Ed receives an answer to his prayers, it comes from a sacred encounter not with the divine but with Reverend Sun Myung Moon. Psychiatrist Marc Galanter (1989) describes the experience:

> On the second night, he finished his prayers and read from the Divine Principle [the Church's major religious document based on the revelations of Reverend Moon] while alone in his apartment. Suddenly he felt he was in the presence of Reverend Moon, and heard the minister speaking to him directly "as real as we're talking now. I didn't turn around but I knew that Reverend Moon was there. His presence was as real as any person I've sat with. He told me that I was doing the right thing and should continue on my course, that I would find spiritual enlightenment." (p. 75)

The similarities between Ed's experience and an encounter with the divine are striking. In fact, replace Reverend Moon with "God" or the "Holy Spirit" in this account and it would be impossible to distinguish his experience from the spiritual conversions I have already described.

In the religious group conversion, the group, its leader, and/or its mission are defined as sacred. By converting to the group, the individual is able to appropriate its special force into his or her own sense of self. Listen to the way one woman, addicted to drugs, draws on the sacred power of the members and leader of the Divine Light Mission.

> Once I got to know them, I realized they loved me. They took me up, and it was as if they were holding me in their arms. I was like a baby whose mother guides its moves and cares for it. When I wanted to take heroin, or even to smoke [marijuana], I knew they were with me to help me stay away from it, even if I was alone. And their strength was there for me, even before I could hardly meditate at all, I could rely on their invisible hand, moved by Maharaj Ji's wisdom, to help me gain control. (Galanter, 1989, p. 30)

Examples of people who convert to religious cults provide vivid illustrations of the group conversion process: Attributions of divine power to the leader, the group, and its mission are commonplace, and dramatically different lifestyles replace old routines, commitments, and relationships. But religious group conversion is not limited to cults. Sacred power can be attached to the local mainstream congregation and clergy as well as the nontraditional group. The loyalty and devotion the individual feels for the neighborhood church and its leader can also become a new organizing force for the self. Every clergy person knows (and appreciates) the converts to the church who fill their calendars with congregational involvements. Life, for these converts, revolves around the congregational hub, and personal identity is best defined by their newfound devotion to the church.

Universal Conversion. In some cases, the conversion process takes the individual beyond an identification with a spiritual presence or a religious group to a sense of connectedness with the larger natural and social world. The world's great religions present models of this process. The spiritual encounters of great figures from Moses and Muhammad to the Buddha and Joseph Smith were followed not by lives of religious retreat and isolation, but by a return to the world to serve others and share their messages of revelation. This kind of experience is not limited to major religious figures. Approximately one-third of Starbuck's (1899) religious converts spontaneously stated that they had experienced a stronger love for others and desire to help others as an immediate result of their conversion. One said: "I had more tender feeling toward my family and friends" (p. 127). Another said: "I felt in harmony with everybody, and all creation and its Creator" (p. 128). Spiritual conversion in these instances was followed by a universal conversion, an identification of the self with the whole of humanity. As Starbuck concluded, these people were called out from themselves "into active sympathy with the world outside" (p. 128).

Universal converts hope to re-create not only the self in the image of God but the larger social whole. Social change, for them, becomes a form of religious expression and a mark of personal identity. Thus, we can find religious prophets speaking out against injustice, Mahatma Gandhi and Martin Luther King Jr. promoting nonviolent resistance to social and political oppression, established churches challenging banks to treat Third World countries more equitably (Kowalewski & Leonard, 1985), Quakers protesting apartheid in South Africa, and religious coalitions developing housing for the homeless (Cohen, Mowbray, Gillette, & Thompson, 1992). The list goes on.

Suffice it to say here that for the universal convert, the identification with humanity and the desire to make the world a better place become hallmarks of the transformed self; they are orienting points for a radically different approach toward significance in stressful times. This type of conversion should not be mistaken for a secular coping mechanism. Through their association with the transcendent, universal concerns take on a religious aura. Because the world contains a spark of the divine, it is believed, the world deserves our attention, care, and even devotion.

In this sense, the search for a more just, loving society becomes a sacred task—a way to experience the holy, a way to move the world closer to an ideal transcendent vision, or a way to bring disparate people together beneath the umbrella of a loving God (Wells & Maton, 1992).

Whether the object of devotion is a spiritual power, a religious group, or humankind, religious conversions offer the same hope to the potential convert: the chance to resolve the tensions brought on by the encounter with personal limitations. Dissatisfactions with self-centeredness may be eased by the incorporation of broader concerns into the self. A greater purpose in living has been found and a new hub for the individual's energy and affection has been discovered. Similarly, frustrations with the limits of personal power may be countered by perceptions of a self newly empowered through its association with the sacred. By surrendering to "unlimitedness," the self can take part in unlimited possibilities (Brenner, 1985). In this sense, the religious conversion is a well-designed response to the confrontation with human limitations in the search for significance. Armed with a new object of significance and a new sense of power to reach out and sustain it, the individual has found a powerful mechanism for radical change.

The Question of Choice

Conversion, for many, raises concerns about coercion. Has the person been forced or tricked into radical change? Has the convert been engulfed and overpowered by negative circumstances, unconscious conflicts, or social pressures? In short, is the convert a victim?

Again, as with most stereotypes, there is a grain of truth to this one. Conversion typically occurs under pressure. As we noted earlier, chronic or acute tensions often precede radical religious change. The failure of existing resources and old coping efforts is another source of tension. In some instances, religious groups add pressure of their own: The individual may be confronted with his or her spiritual shortcomings, or dire predictions of what lies in store for the unconverted may be made to heighten tensions and make current conditions even more untenable. Religious groups offer a solution to the dilemma they have helped create that, by way of contrast, looks all the more attractive. To anyone who is willing to make the leap into a new identity, the groups pledge, will come the support and affirmation of the network itself. In this sense, Galanter (1989) writes: "The [religious] group acts like a psychological pincer, promoting distress while at the same time providing relief" (p. 93).

In some instances, religious groups have gone beyond social pressure and influence to acts of deception and coercion. For instance, in the 1970s numerous complaints were lodged against one Family of the

Unification Church for its deceptive recruiting practices. Potential members were approached by attractive, friendly men and women their own age (who did not identify themselves as Moonies) with invitations to participate in ostensibly nonreligious programs such as "Creative Community Workshop" and "New Educational Development System." Once there, participants were gradually introduced to the principles of the church in a group context, unaware that several group members were established church members who had been taught to ward off doubts or reservations with love and affection. Only weeks later, when the members' attachment to the group had become more secure, did they become aware that they had joined the Unification Church (Galanter, 1989).

Clearly, conversion does not occur in a vacuum. Like other psychological processes, it unfolds within a field of forces that puts the person under considerable pressure. In some instances these forces may become coercive. Does that make the convert a victim? Probably not, in most cases. The problem with the perception of the convert as a victim is that it focuses on only one side of the equation. It neglects the fact that there is a pull as well as a push to conversion, an active dimension as well as a reactive one. In the midst of personal and social pressures, the individual is still attempting to maximize significance and, in the process, still making decisions and choices.

Of course, to the outsider, new cult members, engaged in radically different practices and beliefs, may appear to be anything but rational. Yet many of those who have studied cults closely describe prospective members as "seekers," people interested in discovering a more satisfying religious lifestyle (Richardson, 1985; Straus, 1979). What may look like an impetuous irrational act to the outsider is often the result of a conscious decision to step into a new role and try out new behaviors, even though it may be impossible for the potential convert to fully imagine where this new life will lead. In this vein, Melton, author of the *Encyclopedic Handbook of Cults in America* (1986), notes that before joining the Hare Krishna movement, the large majority of converts had read about Eastern religion and experimented with vegetarianism. Many had tried and rejected a variety of groups before they settled on the group most comfortable for them. In fact, he points out, of those who attend the recruitment programs sponsored by various religious cults, less than 10% join. Add to that the fact that the great majority of the people who do join will leave the cult within 2 years, with most of these people returning to the religion they grew up in, and these statistics begin to challenge the stereotyped view that cults are luring large numbers of unsuspecting, gullible people away from mainstream religious traditions. Further challenge to this stereotype comes from the stand many nonconventional religions have taken toward new converts. Some will not recruit new members. Other groups put prospective members through a series of tests before they can become a part of the group. Still others, such as the Church of Scientology, ask potential members to sign a form indicating that they are aware they are participating in a church program. Because many cults adopt unusual dress and practices, Melton adds, it is virtually impossible for them to hide who they are.

From the outside, new cult members may look as if they have taken leave of their senses, their judgment, and their will. A closer examination, however, suggests that many are actively experimenting with new lifestyles. Though they have taken on radically different roles, they have not necessarily been coerced, nor, for that matter, have they necessarily made wholesale changes. The act of joining a new religious group may simply be a first and tentative step in the process of transformation. Sociologist Roger Straus (1979) writes: "It is not so much the initial action that enables the convert to experience a transformed life but the day to day actions of living it" (p. 163). Balch (1980) makes a similar point when he cautions against drawing too many inferences from the sharp changes in behavior of the new cult member. The public facade of conviction and commitment may cover significant uncertainty and doubts. "Many cult members never become true believers," Balch writes, "but their questioning may be effectively hidden from everyone but their closest associates" (p. 142).

This review suggests that fears of brainwashing, coercion, and deception by cults may be blown out of proportion. True, some groups have put prospective members under intense pressure and, in some cases, misled or coerced them into joining. And, true, some people are vulnerable to false promises and outlandish messages of hope. But this does not make the convert a victim. Decision making and choice are as much a part of the conversion process as social influence and pressure. Even in coercive conditions, people have their ways of maintaining some level of autonomy and choice. The bottom line is this: the process of group conversion involves a blend of action and reaction on the part of the convert. While the group is looking for new members, the potential member is on a search of his or her own for a new center of identity. As Straus (1979) notes, "The two approaches are complementary, not antagonistic" (p. 160). In the religious conversion, as in every other mechanism of coping, we find an individual searching for a way to maximize significance in the midst of a larger constellation of social, situational, and personal forces.

In some ways, this seems like the logical place to conclude this chapter on religion and transformation in coping. Conversion is, after all, a culminating experience within certain religious traditions. It is not, however, the *only* way to achieve radical change. This point was underscored in a retrospective study directed by Zinnbauer who put to test several of the assumptions about religious conversion noted earlier here (Zinnbauer & Pargament, 1995). Three groups of college students were compared: those who reported a spiritual conversion within the last 2 years, those who had reportedly become more religious in the last 2 years without experiencing a religious conversion, and those who had not changed in their religiousness during this time period. Consistent with our predictions, the spiritual converts reported greater stress in their lives prior to their conversion than the "no change" group at a similar point in time. In comparison to the "no change" group, the converts also described greater identification with the sacred and greater change on several dimensions of self-functioning (e.g., esteem, confidence, identity) before and after the conversion.

Interestingly, however, the group of spiritual converts did not differ substantially from the group that had become more religious over the same time period without a conversion. Like the converts, the "more religious" group perceived greater stress prior to their religious change than the "no change" group. And like the converts, the "more religious" participants also reported significant increases in self-functioning and greater identification with the sacred over time. We should be careful interpreting these results. Perhaps the "more religious" had indeed experienced a religious conversion but failed to label it as such. Nor can we rule out the possibility that, in looking back over their experiences, both convert and more religious groups were simply exaggerating the degree to which their lives had been transformed. But if we take these results at face value, they suggest that conversion is not the only method of transformation. Other methods of religious thought and practice can also lead toward profound change. I conclude with a discussion of one other coping method whose design is re-creative in nature—religious forgiving.

Religious Forgiving: From Anger to Peace

It may be surprising to see forgiveness in this section on radical change. In many of the ways the term is used, forgiveness does not appear to be particularly transformational. Forgiveness has been described as a form of denial, a way to overlook an offense or pretend as if it never happened. "Forgive and forget," the old saying goes. Forgiveness has also been viewed as condonation, a form of excuse or pardon for misdeeds, illustrated by Gerald Ford's controversial pardon of Richard Nixon for his role in the Watergate scandal. Forgiveness has been equated with reconciliation, a way to restore a relationship, even if that relationship places the victim at further risk of abuse. Forgiveness also has been described as self-serving, a way to "get even" by asserting one's moral superiority over a perpetrator. There is nothing particularly "radical" about forgiveness from any of these perspectives, in which it is portrayed as a protective method, one designed to limit the pain and hurt of injustice.

However, not everyone shares this view. Many philosophers, theologians, and a growing number of psychologists see forgiveness as a more profound process. Anger, resentment, and hatred, they note, are natural consequences of mistreatment. In forgiving, however, the individual is essentially "giving up the right to hurt back" (Pingleton, 1989, p. 27). This act seems counterintuitive. How could anyone truly let go of an anger that is so well deserved? Not easily. Forgiving has been described as one of the hardest things in the world to do and one of the greatest of human achievements (Augsberger, 1981). It calls for change at many levels: cognitive, affective, relational, behavioral, volitional, and spiritual. From a coping perspective, I believe forgiving represents an act of re-creation.

Forgiving as Re-Creation

Mistreatment comes in many guises: abandonment by a parent, humiliation at the hands of a teacher, betrayal by a confidante, victimization by a stranger, deception by a boss, or abuse by a spouse. Few of us offer immediate forgiveness when we have been treated so poorly. Something of significance has been taken away unfairly, and the response may be one of anger, fear, hurt, or resentment. These are more than just feelings. They represent coping devices aimed at conserving what is left of significance (see Simon & Simon, 1990). With anger and fantasies of revenge come energy and power to counteract the feelings of paralysis and loss of control so often a consequence of personal assault. With fear and wariness come efforts to avoid a repeat of past mistreatment. With hurt comes the belief that one is a decent person who deserves better treatment. With resentment and hatred comes a clear explanation for why life is not any better. As importantly, the expression of these feelings communicates the person's plight to others and gives them a chance to respond.

These coping methods are only partially effective, however. Anger also brings with it a reminder of the individual's powerlessness to change the past. Embedded in fear is the realization that violations can indeed occur again. Implicit in hurt are nagging questions about one's own worth. Beneath the surface of resentment and hatred are reminders of the individual's great shame. In each of these feelings the pains of the past continue to intrude into the present.

Negativity in response to injustice has costs that go beyond the individual's relationship with the perpetrator. Memories of the violation can interfere with the capacity to develop new ties. Assuming that old patterns are likely to be repeated, the individual may opt for safe yet ultimately unfulfilling relationships. Communicating the sense that he or she is somehow owed something by other people, the victim of injustice may end up alienating those who could be potential sources of support. When people fail to respond to this sense of entitlement, the individual may react with anger, bitterness, and violations of his or her own, thereby perpetuating the cycle of abuse. Feelings of hostility can also pose physical health threats. Research has tied these feelings to heightened risks for serious medical illness, such as coronary heart disease (e.g., Diamond, 1982). In short, there is a heavy price to be paid for the limited protection afforded by feelings of anger, fear, hurt, and resentment.

Forgiveness is designed to produce a radical change from a life centered around pain and injustice. It is a method of coping that involves a shift of both destinations and pathways. Implicit in the act of forgiving is the effort to transform significance—to depart from protection as the best that can be hoped for to what has been described as "a boldly, venturesomely, aspiring, and active pursuit of Value" (Kolnai,1968, cited in Rowe et al., 1989, p. 236). In forgiveness, the individual pursues the dream of a newfound peace, both personal and social. Forgiveness offers the possibility of peace of mind, that is, the hope that painful memories can be healed, that the individual will no longer be held emotionally hostage to acts of the past. Forgiveness also offers the possibility of peace with others. Coming to terms with the hurt and injury inflicted by another person opens the door to a future of more fulfilling relationships.

A new path is required in the search for the new destination of peace. Grudges and grievances can no longer be nursed and nourished. Old enmities must be relinquished. But the answer is not as simple as saying "I forgive you." To facilitate a metamorphosis in affect, attitude, and action, a radically different path is needed. Theorists, practitioners, and a few researchers have begun to identify a number of "active ingredients of forgiveness" that prompt this fundamental shift in orientation.

First, forgiveness cannot occur without the experience of anger, hurt, fear, or resentment. To put it another way, without injury there is nothing to forgive. It follows that denial, minimization, or condonation of an offense are at odds with an essential part of forgiving. Trainer (1981) found some empirical support for this notion in a retrospective study of divorcées. Those who reported more genuine forgiveness of their ex-spouses indicated higher levels of anger and hostility than others at the worst moments of their experience. Later in the process they reported more resolution of their anger than others. Clinical interventions designed to promote forgiveness also generally start with this ingredient, encouraging people to face, explore, and express the hurt and pain associated with an injustice (e.g., Hebl & Enright, 1993; McCullough & Worthington, 1995; Rosenak & Hamden, 1992).

Second, forgiveness involves a tertiary appraisal: The costs of negativity in the service of self-protection are judged to be greater than the risks of letting go of negativity in the search for peace. This decision-making process does not have to be particularly deliberate or conscious, but at some level the person comes to a realization that negativity in response to injustice only increases the torment for oneself and others. Releasing animosities, it is hoped, will lead to peace rather than further abuse.

Third, forgiveness grows out of a humanization of the offender. Labels such as "evil" and "bad" that permanently set the wrongdoer apart from the rest of society give way to more compassionate terms, such as "wounded" and "unhealthy," more suggestive of possibilities for change and healing (McCullough, 1995). The gap between victim and offender is further bridged by the victim's openness to examining the hurts he or she has caused others and his or her own needs for forgiveness (Patton, 1985). Ultimately, it is the victim's willingness to empathize with the pain of the offender that reconnects the offender and the victim to each other and to the larger human community. Empathy, McCullough (1995) has argued persuasively, is what makes forgiveness possible.

Finally, forgiveness involves action; attempts are made to change ways of thinking, feeling, and relating (Rye, 1996). The past cannot be undone, but the response to the past can be changed. Rumination is not inevitable; new ways can be found to remember (Smedes, 1996). Neither is bitterness nor social isolation a foregone conclusion. Even if the individual does not feel especially forgiving, it is still possible to act that way. With changes in behavior, changes in feelings may follow.

To extend good will to the offender may be the most challenging act of all. Good will should not be equated with complete reconciliation. Many writers in this area note that reconciliation can be foolish if one-sided (e.g., Enright, Eastin, Golden, Serinopoulus, & Freedman, 1992; Simon & Simon, 1990). Unless the perpetrator expresses remorse and takes responsibility for his or her actions, reconciliation can have dangerous consequences. But, writers also assert that it is possible to find peace within oneself and with others without reconciliation.

Hope (1987), for instance, presents the case of Tom whose hypersensitivity to criticism and hostility to any perceived slight led to difficulties holding a job and problems with his wife and children. Tom's problems were traced to his ambivalent relationship with his alcoholic father, a man who had been verbally abusive and critical to Tom throughout his childhood. At the prompting of his church, Tom decided to offer forgiveness to his father. Although Tom's father responded with tears and a hug, Hope found little evidence of change in their relationship or in the father's abuse of alcohol. Reconciliation did not happen here, but Tom was still able to set his animosity aside and wish his father well. This was a gift, an act of altruism all the more remarkable by the fact that it was unearned.

Forgiveness has been defined here as a re-creative form of coping, a method of radical change. It is an effort to find peace by letting go of the deep anger, hurt, fear, and resentment associated with an offense, even though these feelings are deserved. There is, however, one element missing from this discussion—the religious dimension.

What Makes Forgiving Religious?

"To err is human, to forgive, divine." Religion and forgiveness are intimately tied, as we hear in this famous quotation by Alexander Pope. Virtually every major religious tradition speaks to the values of mercy and compassion and the dangers of vengefulness and hatred. The value of forgiveness is perhaps most deeply and explicitly rooted within Judaism and Christianity. In both of these traditions, we find exemplary figures who return hatred with love and good for evil. Each tradition strongly encourages its adherents to follow these models and practice forgiveness in their lives. Maimonides, for example, states that the failure to forgive someone who sincerely requests it is as great an offense as the initial wrongful act (Minkin, 1987). The New Testament is replete with encouragement to forgive: "Be tolerant with one another and forgiving, if any of you has cause for complaint: you must forgive as the Lord forgave you" (Colossians, 3:13, *Revised English Bible*). Perhaps then it should not be surprising to learn from research studies that people who are more religiously involved also place more value on forgiveness (Gorsuch & Hao, 1993; Rokeach, 1973).

Religion can contribute to forgiveness in two ways. It can lend significance to the act of forgiving. It can also provide a set of models and methods to facilitate this process.

The Spiritual Significance of Forgiving

Human relationships are, from many religious perspectives, working models of an ideal, namely, the relationship between the individual and the divine. From this point of view, a breach between two people that goes unrepaired involves more than the two parties and even more than the larger community; it is an offense against the sacred. Forgiveness takes on a larger significance in the religious context. It offers the possibilities not only of peace with oneself and with others, but also of peace with God.

The spiritual significance of forgiveness is multi-faceted. First, by forgiving others, the individual can seek his or her own forgiveness from God. Several scriptural references make the link between the two quite explicit: "For if you forgive others the wrongdoing they have done, your heavenly Father will also forgive you; but if you do not forgive others, then your Father will not forgive the wrongs that you have done" (Matthew 6:14–15). Second, by forgiving, the individual has the opportunity to live a religiously based life. Central to Judaism, for example, is the duty to imitate the divine (Newman, 1987). Those who follow in God's ways by offering compassion even to their enemies, then, are expressing an essential part of their identity. Third, by forgiving, the individual can seek out greater intimacy with other people and the divine. Forgiveness is, as Patton (1985) describes it, "a quality of the Kingdom to be discovered" (p. 175). In the process of forgiving, the individual can strive to attain a sense of spiritual fellowship, a sense that as children of God we all require forgiveness and we all need to be forgiving, of ourselves, of each other, and of God. The creation of a more peaceful, loving community, one suffused with spiritual presence, is in the minds of many religious thinkers, the heart and soul of forgiving (e.g., Calian, 1981; Patton, 1985).

Models and Methods of Religious Forgiving

The religious literature contains stories of extraordinary figures who were able to transcend their own considerable pain and reach out to others in the spirit of compassion. The family in turmoil can model the example of Joseph, who was able to forgive his brothers in spite of their jealousy, hatred, and willingness to sell him into slavery. The betrayed spouse can look to the story of Hosea, who forgave his wife in spite of her shameless philandering. The victim of a crime can try to follow in the steps of Jesus Christ, who forgave his persecutors in the most extreme of moments.

More concretely, victims of wrongdoing can draw on a variety of religious methods (including elements of other religious coping methods) to activate the four ingredients of forgiving described earlier.

1. Religion can assist in the expression of anger and pain to the offender. "Turning the other cheek" to mistreatment has often been

associated with religiousness, particularly Christianity. There is, however, a long tradition in religious circles of challenge, confrontation, and reproval of offenders. Even God did not escape the anger of Job for his trials.

2. Religion can assist in the decision to forgive. Taking the risk of letting go of negativity can be framed as a "leap of faith." There can be no guarantee the outcome will be positive, just as there can be no absolute assurance of God's existence. Conceptualized as a matter of faith, however, the act of forgiveness is placed in a spiritual context of hope, trust, and good will.

3. Religion can facilitate the humanization of the offender. Compassionate understandings of offensive acts are not hard to find in the religious literature. The final words of Jesus Christ represent perhaps the best known illustration: "Father, forgive them; for they know not what they do" (Luke 23:34). Here Jesus is attributing the acts of his executioners to ignorance rather than malice. Religious literature also contains reminders of everyone's fallibility (e.g., "He that is without sin among you, let him cast a stone at her," John 8:7). Participation in purification rituals can serve as a further reminder that victims, like offenders, need forgiveness. Several writers suggest that forgiveness to others ultimately grows out of forgiveness from God (Pingleton, 1989; Walters, 1983).

4. Finally, religion can promote acts of forgiving. The individual is able to appeal to God for help in forgiveness through prayer. The religious community can encourage people to put their anger and hurt aside in stressful times (see Kinens, 1989). It is important to add that the act of forgiveness, viewed from religious eyes, may involve more than personal choice and effort. It can be experienced as a revelation or a gift. Take the story of Corrie Ten Boom (1971) who, after she was freed from imprisonment in a concentration camp, encountered one of her former SS guards at a church service. When he came up to shake her hand after the service, she felt frozen, unable to respond. Ten Boom then prayed to Jesus for the strength to forgive him. She described the following: "From my shoulder along my arm and through my hand a current seemed to pass from me to him, while into my heart sprang a love for this stranger that almost overwhelmed me" (p. 238). The forgiveness she perceived was empowered by God: "And so I discovered that it is not on our forgiveness any more than on our goodness that the world's healing hinges, but on His. When he tells us to love our enemies, He gives, along with the command, the love itself" (p. 238).

In short, forgiving can be rooted in religious values, models, and methods. How often forgiving is, in fact, religiously based, and whether religious forgiving is more effective than a forgiveness disconnected from religion are a few of the many questions about this topic that have not been answered.

Hard Questions about Forgiving

Many readers might be highly skeptical of the experience described by Ten Boom and by theoretical accounts of forgiveness more generally, and rightly so. Much of this writing is highly prescriptive; clearly, forgiveness is a central value for many of these authors. But how accurate are these accounts? How well do they capture the experience of people struggling to come to terms with injustice? Unfortunately, we do not know. Perhaps because forgiveness is so laden with religious significance, few researchers have engaged in serious study of this topic. Thus, we are left with some important yet unanswered questions.

How Common is Forgiving?

Corrie Ten Boom's story is not unique. The religious and clinical literature contain striking illustrations of forgiving by people in the most extraordinary situations. Critics, however, might warn against taking self-reports of forgiving at face value. The old phrase "easier said than done" may be especially applicable here. A few studies aimed at promoting acts of forgiveness have yielded promising results (e.g., Freedman & Enright, 1995; McCullough & Worthington, 1995). Working with a small group of adult incest survivors, Freedman and Enright (1996) found that participation in a forgiveness-oriented treatment was associated with gains in self-esteem and hope, declines in depression and anxiety, and increases in positive affect to the perpetrator. Their treatment lasted 14 months, on average. The question remains though, how often do people forgive others following serious mistreatment (without the benefit of clinical intervention)? To give up anger and resentment that are so well deserved seems to be an almost saint-like act. Is forgiving a realistic possibility or is it an unattainable ideal? Naturalistic studies of people grappling with personal violations are needed to answer this question. The challenge of this research will be to distinguish forgiveness in the profound, transformational sense used here from other acts, such as denying, minimizing, or simply forgetting about the injustice with the passage of time.

Two related questions have also been largely unexplored: Who is more likely to forgive, and when is forgiveness more likely to occur? A few studies suggest forgiving may be a more available and more compelling form of coping among those who tend to be empathic, altruistic, and humble rather than self-righteous and egoistic (see McCullough,

1995), in those relationships that are well established and highly valued (Rowe et al., 1989), and in those situations in which the offense was not judged to be intentional, the offense was not repeated, and the perpetrator showed remorse (Darby & Schlenker, 1982; Kremer & Stephens, 1983; Weiner, Graham, Peters, & Zmuidinas, 1991).

Are There Times Not to Forgive?

In a book with parallels to the story of Corrie Ten Boom, Simon Wiesenthal (1976) raises a provocative question that grew out of his own experience in a concentration camp. From 1943 to 1945, Wiesenthal had suffered through personal cruelties and the loss of many family members and friends. One day he was assigned to serve as a laborer in a hospital. There he was asked to go to the bedside of an SS soldier who had been fatally wounded and wanted to speak to a Jew before he died. The soldier recounted the story of his life to Wiesenthal. As a young boy, he said, he was caught up in the excitement of the times. He joined the Hitler Youth Movement and later the SS without serious thought or deliberation about these groups or the meaning of his own actions. Sparing none of the gruesome details, the Nazi soldier described his participation in atrocities committed against the Jews in the war, most notably the firebombing of a house filled with over 150 Jewish men, women, and children. Throughout the telling of his story, the soldier expressed a great deal of remorse and contrition. In the final moments of his life, he was confessing his sins and looking to a Jewish concentration camp inmate for forgiveness. The question Wiesenthal asks is simple: What would you have done in response to the soldier's plea?

Wiesenthal posed this question to a variety of renowned theologians, philosophers, and artists, and their responses are included in his book. There was no consensus. Forgive him, was the sentiment voiced by several people. "If hate is met with hate, where will it all end?" asked one (p. 113). "If I expect the Compassionate One to have compassion on me, I must act with compassion toward others," said another (p. 160). In contrast, several respondents said they would not forgive the SS soldier. They presented different rationales: The soldier's repentance was cheap and insincere; Wiesenthal was in no position to forgive the sins committed against other people and God; forgiveness would remove the onus of atonement from the offender; and forgiveness would interfere with the pursuit of justice. (Wiesenthal himself walked away from the SS soldier without a word of response, although the incident continued to gnaw at him over the years.)

From some religious perspectives, forgiving is an unconditional value, an act of love and compassion to be offered to anyone regardless of circumstances (e.g., Phillips, 1986). Others, however, see forgiveness more conditionally. When danger is still imminent, when the perpetrator has not shown sincere remorse, when the violation is too severe, or when the wounds from the personal assault are too fresh, forgiveness is said to be inappropriate, even foolish (e.g., Friedlander, 1986; McCullough & Worthington, 1994a). From this latter perspective, there is a potential downside to forgiveness. Used at the wrong time, in the wrong place, by the wrong person, forgiveness may result in further personal and social damage.

There is no easy answer to questions about the conditionality of forgiveness. Positions on this issue can be deeply grounded in theology and, as a result, may be unlikely to change. Nevertheless, the debate could be informed by further research. Does forgiveness, for instance, increase the risk of further abuse? Does it lead to self-blame? What are the effects of forgiveness on the perpetrator? Does it encourage self-examination and growth as proponents suggest, or does it reinforce the offender for his or her misconduct, as critics might argue? Empirical studies on these questions could shed some light on the benefits and potential limitations of forgiving as a way of coping with serious interpersonal problems.

But I am getting ahead of myself here. The question of the helpfulness or harmfulness of various methods of religious coping is terribly important and deserves much closer attention. We will examine this question in the following chapter.

In this section we have considered religious forgiving as another method of transformational coping. Admittedly, it is one of the more controversial coping methods. At this point in time, there seem to be more questions about forgiving than answers. Nevertheless, forgiving does represent one potentially powerful response to mistreatment and injustice. Some have even suggested that it is the only alternative to a life consumed by bitterness and hatred. This stretches the point too far.

Baures (1996) interviewed 20 famous survivors of extreme trauma who had transcended bitterness and hatred. Several had struggled to forgive their offender, but not all. Rather than letting go of their pain, a few survivors used it as a springboard for creative projects and social action. Their pain was not relieved; it was instead revisited, reworked, and shared with others so they, too, could learn and grow from the experience of injustice. To speak on behalf of those who have suffered and to move the world to greater justice and compassion became the new organizing force for their lives. In some sense, they had responded to their trauma with changes akin to a universal conversion. For them, the commitment to a better world represented a solution to the problem of pain more compelling than forgiveness, but one no less transformational.

CONCLUSIONS

In the early part of this century, George Coe (1916) spoke of the power of religious transformation: "Possibly the chief thing in religion, considered functionally," he said, "is the progressive discovery and reorganization of values" (p. 65). Since that time, relatively few have taken Coe's words to heart. Religion has been seen more as a force for conservation than transformation; the roles of religion in the "discovery and reorganization of values" have gone largely unexamined. Yet, as noted in this chapter, religion has an important part to play in periods of transition, confusion, and loss. Through ritual, the individual may be encouraged to "let go" of old objects of significance. Through prayer, the disorientation that accompanies threat and loss may be replaced with new purpose. Through relationships with others in the religious community or through mystical experience, new visions may be generated in the place of shattered dreams. Through religious models and methods, anger and resentment may give way to peace and goodwill. In short, religion may assist as much in the transformation of significance as in its conservation.

The story does not end with transformation. Once significance has been transformed, coping shifts back to attempts to conserve the new set of values. With respect to religious conversion, Starbuck (1899) writes, the individual adopts a "new determination" to live according to the fresh religious identity. Threats to the now-changed self will be followed by conservational efforts as strong or stronger than the attempts to preserve the identity of old. Coping will likely continue to be defined by conservational mechanisms until the altered identity can no longer be sustained, at which point we may witness transformations of a different kind. And the cycle continues. Of course, the cycle does not always operate in simple, clear-cut fashion. There is no single trajectory to change, religious or otherwise (McFadden, in press). Simultaneously, the individual may be trying to conserve some objects of significance while transforming others. At any point in time, both sets of coping mechanisms may be at work. Preservation and reconstruction, re-valuation and re-creation—the extraordinary power of religion in coping lies not in its power to conserve or transform significance, but in its ability to do both: to make and remake the world, to preserve and protect each new creation.

In the last two chapters, I have reviewed some of the religious mechanisms of conservation and transformation. This review has not been exhaustive. The coping methods of children and of nontraditional religious groups represent particularly fertile ground for further study. Here I have only tried to illustrate some of the rich ways religion may function in coping. This review has also steered away from evaluative issues. To this point, the question of the efficacy of religious coping has only been hinted at. Undoubtedly, many readers have been forming their own judgments of the helpfulness or harmfulness of various religious approaches to coping. But because the evaluative question is so thorny, so complex, and so important, I have saved it for a section of its own. I turn now to the issue of the efficacy of religious coping.

Part Four

EVALUATIVE AND PRACTICAL IMPLICATIONS

Chapter Ten

DOES IT WORK?
Religion and the
Outcomes of Coping

... the conclusion seems inescapable that religiosity is, on almost every conceivable count, opposed to the normal goals of mental health ... on the whole religious piety and dogma do much more harm than good; and the beneficent behaviors that they sometimes abet would most likely be more frequent and profound without their influence.
—ELLIS (1986, pp. 42–43)

A world without God would be a flat, monochromatic world, a world without color or texture, a world in which all days would be the same. Marriage would be a matter of biology, not fidelity. Old age would be seen as a time of weakness, not of wisdom. In a world like that, we would cast about desperately for any sort of diversion, for any distraction from the emptiness of our lives, because we would never have learned the magic of making some days and some hours special.
—KUSHNER (1989, p. 206)

Few people take a neutral position when it comes to religion. Some, such as psychologist Albert Ellis, view religion in a harshly critical light. Religion, it is argued, represents the antithesis of the human struggle for freedom, actualization, and growth. In placing superstition and magical thinking above the powers of rationality and reason, religion contributes to pathology rather than health. Others, such as Rabbi Harold Kushner, see religion as essential to the search for significance. Only by looking beyond oneself, it is said, can the individual reach out to find intimacy,

275

purpose, and some sense of comfort in living. Only with the help of the sacred can the incomprehensible be understood, the unmanageable managed, and the unbearable endured.

In the accounts of people in crisis, we also come across very different assessments of religion. One parent of a young child with a significant developmental delay says:

> I really feel that my faith and my trust in God have been the stronghold of being able to deal with all of this—I can't be mad at Him because He's given me a less than perfect child, health-wise. . . . Cathy just being the way she is is evidence that God does work miracles, that He does answer prayer. He maybe asks a lot of us, but He gives us tremendous blessings in the end. (cited in Weisner, Belzer, & Stolze, 1991, p. 659)

Another parent of a young child faced with similar problems has a different reaction: "[Everyone says] God only gives special children to special people; and I say, 'I'm not so special . . . I don't want any more problems!' and I'm kind of to the point where I'm bitter, I'm angry right now" (cited in Weisner, Belzer, & Stolze, 1991, p. 659).

What is the value of religion? This is a terribly important question, for how we evaluate religion shapes the way we behave toward it. Just imagine the different reactions Ellis and Kushner would have to the client who raises spiritual issues in counseling.

In this chapter and the following one, I evaluate the role of religion in coping. From the outset, it needs to be emphasized that this evaluation will not be based on the ultimate truth of any religious creed. For this reason, many of those from the religious world may find these chapters deficient; the value of religion for them may have everything to do with its veracity. But psychologists can have little to say about the truth of religious claims. Our methods cannot determine whether biblical accounts of miracles are accurate, whether there is a God, or what happens to people after they die. Instead, we must rely on what we can observe, what we can measure. In this chapter, religion will be evaluated from a pragmatic perspective. I will consider whether religion produces results, and if so, whether they are helpful to people or harmful. In the tradition of William James (1902), I will evaluate religion by counting its fruits, bitter and sweet.

This is not the first pragmatic evaluation of religion. Many other researchers have assessed religion from this perspective (see Schumaker, 1992, for review), but their reviews have not focused on times of crisis. Instead, they have examined the relationships between global measures of religious beliefs and practices and general measures of mental health and psychopathology that are disconnected from the specifics of any situation. In contrast, this evaluation will focus on what people do with their religion in stressful circumstances. To answer the question "Does religion work?", I zero in on the most concrete expressions of religion in coping and study the end results.

Although this chapter will have more of an empirical research focus than earlier chapters, I have placed summary information and more technical details about particular studies in tables and reserved the body of the chapter for a review and discussion of the central findings in this literature. I hope that the final result will be of interest not only to researchers but to clinicians and members of religious communities as well.

SELF-EVALUATIONS OF THE EFFICACY OF RELIGIOUS COPING

Is religion helpful? Is it harmful? Is it irrelevant? At first glance, these questions would not seem to be too hard to answer. All we need to do is ask people how helpful they feel their religion is to them in coping. Many researchers have done just that. Judging from the results of their studies, most people appear to find religion helpful in times of trouble.

Let us consider a few examples. In an investigation of over 7,000 combat veterans from four theaters of operation in World War II, 57–83% of the veterans reported that prayer helped them a lot "when the going was tough" (Stouffer et al., 1965). In another study of patients 1 day before they underwent cardiac surgery, 73% reported that prayer was extremely helpful to them in preparing for surgery (Saudia, Kinney, Brown, & Young-Ward, 1991). Among parents of children with a variety of physical handicaps, 85% indicated that religion was helpful to them in their adjustment (Barsch, 1968). Researchers have studied many other groups as well, from women with breast cancer (David, Ladd, & Spilka, 1992) and wives of POWs and MIAs from the Vietnam war (Hunter et al., 1974) to physically abused spouses (Horton, Wilkins, & Wright, 1988) and mastectomy patients (Johnson & Spilka, 1991). The percentage of people who found religion helpful in coping in these studies ranged from approximately 50% to 85%.

The answer seems to be obvious. However, before we jump too quickly to a conclusion, it is important to note that the participants in this research were asked directly how helpful religion was to them in coping. There is reason to treat their responses with some skepticism. What if the participants in these studies were reluctant to make a less-than-favorable judgment about their faith and, in the process, admit something socially undesirable—that their religion had not been helpful? Perhaps the relatively high percentages of self-reported religious helpfulness in these studies were a result of the pointed way the question was asked. Given a more open-ended question about what helps in coping, would people mention religion *spontaneously?*

In fact, many do. Although this open-ended methodology yields somewhat lower percentages, we still find that significant numbers of people mention religion spontaneously when asked what helped them cope with crisis. In one study of parents of retarded children, 42% spoke of religion in response to an open-ended question about the greatest source of help and support in dealing with the challenges of raising a disabled child (Abbott & Meredith, 1986). Fifty nine percent of a sample of widows and widowers responded to open-ended interviews by stating that their religious beliefs had been a major source of comfort to them (Glick, Weiss, & Parkes, 1974). Similar results have been found in other studies of adults coping with cancer and chronic illness (Raleigh, 1992), parents of children with leukemia (Binger et al., 1969), elderly men and women dealing with medical problems (Conway, 1985–1986), terminally ill people (Baugher, Burger, Smith, & Wallston, 1989–1990), and adults faced with unhappy periods (Veroff, Douvan, & Kulka, 1981): 18–69% of these samples spontaneously mentioned that religion was helpful to them in coping.

On the face of it, these results seem to provide a clear answer to the question of the helpfulness of religion. For many, if not the majority, of these people, religion appears to be a source of support in coping. But once again we have to be cautious. People may report that religion was helpful to them because, in fact, it was. Knowing what we know about conservation, however, suggests another possibility. Favorable comments may reflect a desire to "keep the faith," whether or not it was helpful to them in the particular situation. After all, to suggest that religion was not a source of support might in itself be threatening. Better to evaluate the faith favorably than consider the alternative and the possibility that religion may in some sense be diminished.

It is also important to note that these findings may be colored by a not-so-implicit bias in the question itself. Typically, the participant is presented with the question "How helpful was religion to you in coping?" and asked to respond on a scale ranging from extremely helpful to not at all helpful. But what about the darker side of religion? The form of the question and response scale do not allow for the possibility that it may be harmful in coping. In one exception to this rule, Horton et al. (1988) asked physically abused spouses whether they were helped and/or hurt by religion. Forty-seven percent reported that they were helped by religion. However, 27% indicated that religion hurt. Also interesting was the finding that 26% of the sample felt religion both helped and hurt, suggesting that the positive and negative effects of religious life may not be exclusive of each other.

As we take a closer look at the straightforward questions we started with, we find that they cannot be answered so easily. To evaluate the efficacy of religion in coping, we need stronger tests that rely less on the individual's summary judgments of religion and that permit consideration of harmful or neutral religious effects as well as positive ones. Rather than evaluate religious helpfulness or harmfulness in one final assessment, it makes more sense to measure religious involvement in coping separately from its end result and examine the relationship between the two. Through statistical analyses we can then determine whether religion is a positive force, a negative force, or simply irrelevant to the outcomes of coping.

RELIGIOUS ORIENTATIONS AND THE OUTCOMES OF NEGATIVE LIFE EVENTS

In the spring of 1972, 91 men were trapped in an underground fire and died in the Sunshine Mine of Kellogg, Idaho. Seventy-seven of these men left widows behind. Some of these widows had a strong sense of personal religiousness; others did not. Some of these widows were deeply involved in the social and spiritual lives of their churches; others were not. What, if any, relationship was there between the widows' different orientations to religion and their psychological adjustment? Did religion cushion the blow of the disaster? Did it make matters worse? Or was it of little consequence? Six months after the fire, Bahr and Harvey (1979b) interviewed 44 of the miners' widows who could be located and who were willing to talk about their experiences. The widows were asked to assess their own religiousness, whether they belonged to a church, their usual frequency of church attendance, and whether they participated in church social events. They were also asked to assess the quality of their lives 5 years earlier and the quality of their lives presently. Widows who rated themselves as more religious on each of these indicators reported more stability in the quality of their lives over the past years than widows who were less religiously involved. Religion apparently helped many widows sustain themselves through their losses. Are these results typical of the literature or are they unusual in some respect?

I begin this review by focusing on macroanalytic studies of religion. In these studies, religion is measured as a global, stable, personal disposition—a part of the individual's orienting system. Faith in God, long-standing religious beliefs, regular church attendance, and the commitment to live by a religious set of ideals are some of the ways religion can express itself in the orienting system. In this section I consider whether people who are more generally oriented to religion fare better or worse in crisis than their less religious counterparts.

Appendix C summarizes the results of 46 studies that examined the relationship between four facets of religious orientations and the outcomes of negative life events.[1] One set of studies focuses on personal expressions of religion as they relate to the outcomes of negative events. Here religion is measured in terms of belief, faith, religious commitment, religious salience, and the frequency of prayer. The second set shifts from personal to organizational religious expressions. Here religion is measured in terms of level of participation in church services or other congregational activities. The third set of studies focuses on the standard measures of religious orientation in the field: intrinsic, extrinsic, quest, and indiscriminate proreligious orientations. A fourth and smaller set of studies assesses religion by "mixed-measures," that is, measures made up of both personal and organizational religious expressions.

A quick review of Appendix C shows that the studies cover a broad spectrum of groups faced with a number of different critical life events, such as terminal illness, chronic disease, abortion, organ transplants, war, surgery, or the death of a child, spouse, parent, or friend. The measures of outcome in these studies and those that follow in this chapter assess different aspects of psychological and physical functioning, ranging from psychopathology and psychological well-being to measures of physical health, pain, and mortality. Several studies also examine spiritual outcomes, such as changes in relationship to God and spiritual well-being. Some criteria, however, are largely missing from this literature. For example, we know little about the impact of religion on the well-being of *other* people. And we know little about how religion helps or hinders people in the search for significance as they themselves define it.

Scanning Appendix C, we find that several studies paint a positive picture of religion. Among caregivers of people with Alzheimer's disease or cancer, the strength of the caregivers' religious beliefs was associated with better affect 2 years later (Rabins, Fitting, Eastham, & Zabora, 1990). In another study of mostly African-Americans who had been on dialysis for at least 6 months, participation in formal religious services over the previous year was tied to several positive outcomes: more compliance with the treatment regime, a higher amount and better quality of social interaction, and less alienation from others (O'Brien, 1982).[2] Among older women recovering from surgery for broken hips, higher scores on a mixed measure of religiousness were associated with less depression at the time of discharge and with better ambulatory status as assessed by each patient's physical therapist (Pressman, Lyons, Larson, & Strain, 1990).

If we were to focus on these results alone, we might conclude that a religious lifestyle facilitates adjustment to negative situations. However, Appendix C also presents a number of studies in which religion is unrelated to outcome. For example, in an investigation of undergraduates who were coping with the death of a close friend, Park and Cohen (1993) found that adherence to orthodox religious beliefs was unrelated to several measures of adjustment. Similarly, among women who had suffered a neonatal death, frequency of church attendance was unrelated to the grief they felt at 2 months and at 2 years after the loss (Lasker, Lohmann, & Toedter, 1989). And Harris and Spilka (1990) also reported no relationship between intrinsic and extrinsic religious orientations and the success of alcohol abusers in abstaining from drinking.

Many, if not most of the studies in Appendix C show a checkered pattern of results within the same investigation; that is, some (but not all) aspects of religion are significantly tied to some (but not all) aspects of outcome. For example, Gass (1987) interviewed older women who had been widowed 1–12 months earlier. Women with stronger religious beliefs reported fewer behavioral symptoms of psychological and social dysfunction. However, religious beliefs were unrelated to a measure of physical dysfunction. Acklin, Brown, and Mauger (1983) studied patients with cancer and patients receiving treatment for other acute but nonthreatening illnesses. While those who attended church more often reported less social isolation and less anger–hostility than less frequent attenders, church attendance was unrelated to several other measures of grieving, including feelings of despair, depersonalization, and death anxiety.

In short, most of the studies in Appendix C describe either positive or nonsignificant relationships between the various dimensions of religious orientation and the outcomes of negative events. What about the negative side of religion? In only a few instances is religion associated with poorer outcomes. Most of these cases involve the extrinsic orientation (recall that in this orientation religion represents a peripheral part of life, occasionally called upon to help the individual attain personal or social goals). Across several studies, extrinsicness is associated with greater grief and depression among widows and widowers (Rosik, 1989), poorer adjustment among terminally ill patients (Carey, 1974), and depression among single middle-aged men and women (Rutledge & Spilka, 1993). Even here, however, the results are not totally consistent. Other studies yield either no relationship between extrinsic religion and outcomes (e.g., Gibbs & Achterberg-Lawlis, 1978; Park & Cohen, 1993) or, in some instances, *positive* relationships (Acklin et al., 1983; Pargament, Olsen, et al., 1992a; Videka-Sherman, 1982).

To provide a more systematic tally of these findings, each of the statistical relationships in the studies from Appendix C was sorted into one of three relationship categories: significant positive, significant negative, and nonsignificant. The results of this tally are presented in Table 10.1. They provide only modest evidence for the value of religion in stressful situations. In slightly over one-third of the cases, religion is found to have a positive connection to adjustment. This is not an insignificant percentage; it is far greater than what we might expect by chance. Only rarely do examples appear of a negative tie between religiousness and adjustment. Thus, when significant effects are found, they are likely to be positive, with higher levels of personal religious

TABLE 10.1. A Tally of the Results of Research on the Statistical Relationship between Measures of Religious Orientation and the Outcomes of Negative Events

	Significant positive relationships	Significant negative relationships	Nonsignificant relationships
I. Personal religious expressions (religious beliefs, religious salience, frequency of prayer, religious faith)	34% (47)	1% (1)	65% (88)
II. Organizational religious expressions (participation in worship services and other congregational activities)	37% (52)	1% (2)	62% (85)
III. Standard religious orientation measures (intrinsic, extrinsic, quest, indiscriminate proreligious)	29% (27)	11% (10)	60% (55)
IV. Mixed personal and organizational expression measures	40% (4)	10% (1)	50% (5)
TOTAL	34% (130)	4% (14)	62% (233)

Note. Numbers of relationships are enclosed in parentheses following percentages.

belief, faith, and salience; higher levels of church involvement; and a more intrinsic religious commitment tied to beneficial outcomes. Nevertheless, recalling the high percentage of people who report that religion is helpful to them in coping, the numbers of positive results seems to fall short of what we might have expected to find. In fact, most of the time (62% of the cases), religion appears to be *unrelated* to the outcomes of negative events. Moreover, this pattern of results seems to hold true regardless of which aspects of religious orientation are being studied.

How can the relatively modest nature of these findings be explained? Perhaps the findings are inaccurate, the result of methodological flaws in these studies, such as inadequacies in the ways religious orientations and adjustment are measured or unsuspected variables that obscure the association between the two. For instance, eyebrows might be raised about how well a few questions about beliefs and practices truly capture the way religion is personally experienced and expressed. Perhaps different results would follow from improvements in methodology. Some of the studies in this area do make use of stronger measures and provide controls for potentially confounding variables. Even these studies, however, yield mixed findings (e.g., Kass, Friedman, Leserman, Zuttermeister, & Benson, 1991). Furthermore, the sheer number of studies and the consistency of the results across the different dimensions of religious orientation argue against dismissing these findings out of hand.

The alternative is to take these findings seriously and try to make sense of them. Coping theory offers one explanation. Recall that the orienting system is a general guide, a frame of reference that serves as an anchor through unsettling periods. Important as it is, the orienting system is generic, one step removed from the specific coping methods the individual uses in particular situations. For example, knowing that religious faith is a central part of one person's orienting system tells us something important about the individual, but it does not tell us how that faith comes to life in specific encounters. To understand that, we have to focus more sharply on what people do with their religion in the midst of crisis. It is not that the orienting system is unimportant in coping. The orienting system plays a key role in the choice of specific coping activities. However, the outcomes of coping have more to do with what the person does in the specific situation to maximize significance than with his or her general orienting system. To put it another way, situation-specific coping activities serve as bridges or mediators between the orienting system and the outcomes of negative situations (see Figure 10.1). If this way of thinking is correct, then we would expect measures of religious coping to predict the outcomes of coping more consistently than measures of general religious orienta-

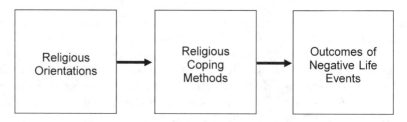

FIGURE 10.1. Religious coping methods as mediators of the relationship between religious orientations and the outcomes of negative life events.

tion. In the following section, I focus on microanalytic studies of the relationship between specific religious coping methods and adjustment to negative life events.

RELIGIOUS COPING AND THE OUTCOMES OF NEGATIVE LIFE EVENTS

Over the last 15 years, literally hundreds of studies have been conducted on the coping process. Religion, however, has received little more than a passing nod in the large majority of these studies. An item or two about prayer or church attendance may be included in measures of coping. But these items are often grouped into subscales with other nonreligious items and, as a result, the specific contributions religion may make to coping are obscured.

Fortunately, there have been some exceptions to this general rule. Several microanalytic investigations have examined the relationships between specific religious strategies for coping with stressful situations and the outcomes of these events. In contrast to the macroanalytic approach in which religion is measured as a global variable removed from any particular life event, these microanalytic studies assess specific, functionally oriented expressions of religion in stressful situations. The results, in some instances, have been striking. For example, even after controlling for confounding variables, aspects of religious coping have been tied to reduced risks of mortality from open heart surgery over the following 6 months (Oxman, Freeman, & Manheimer, 1995), reductions in depression among elderly hospitalized men over a 6-month period (Koenig et al., 1992), and better physical functioning and treatment compliance among heart transplant patients in the following year (Harris et al., 1993).

How commonplace are findings such as these? Table 10.2 presents a tally of the results of 40 such studies. While the total number of studies is not particularly large, most of these investigations include more than one measure of religious coping and more than one measure of outcome. As a result, the number of statistical relationships that have been tallied is not insubstantial (468). Once again, the literature in this area cuts across a variety of groups, confronting a wide range of stressors. The measures of religious coping and adjustment are just as diverse.

Ignoring the distinctions among types of religious coping for the moment, the overall tally in Table 10.2 reveals significant relationships between religious coping and outcomes in 53% of the cases. This figure is larger than the 38% significance rate reported between the measures of religious orientation and outcomes. Interestingly, the increase in significant results is due not only to the relatively high proportions of positive results for some religious coping methods (e.g., spiritual support,

TABLE 10.2. A Tally of the Results of Research on the Statistical Relationship between Measures of Religious Coping and the Outcomes of Negative Events

	Significant positive relationships	Significant negative relationships	Nonsignificant relationships
I. Spiritual coping			
Spiritual support	46% (43)	2% (2)	52% (48)
Spiritual discontent	0% (0)	56% (5)	44% (4)
II. Congregational coping			
Congregational support	37% (16)	2% (1)	60% (26)
Congregational discontent	0% (0)	54% (26)	46% (22)
III. Religious reframing			
God's will and love	53% (19)	0% (0)	47% (17)
God's punishment	0% (0)	52% (11)	48% (10)
IV. Approaches to religious control			
Self-directing	4% (1)	31% (7)	65% (15)
Collaborative	46% (11)	8% (2)	46% (11)
Deferring	28% (9)	6% (2)	66% (21)
Pleading	19% (7)	59% (22)	22% (8)
V. Rituals			
Religious rituals	40% (30)	23% (17)	37% (28)
VI. Patterns of religious coping	56%(15)	11% (3)	33% (9)
TOTAL	32% (151)	21% (98)	47% (219)

Note. Numbers of relationships are enclosed in parentheses following percentages.

benevolent religious reframing), but a high proportion of negative results for some coping methods (e.g., God's punishment, pleading for divine intercession). More will be said about this later.

Of course, comparisons across different studies must be made cautiously. Adding further weight to these conclusions, however, are the results of several studies in which the predictive power of religious orientation and religious coping measures have been compared more directly. Working with several samples of people experiencing different life crises, my colleagues and I had participants complete both types of measures. For example, in the Project on Religion and Coping (Pargament, Ensing, et al., 1990), church members responded to a number of questions about religious coping. To be fair to the traditional approach to measuring religion, we also sampled comprehensively from the menu of religious orientation measures, including scales of loving images of God, intrinsic, extrinsic, quest, doctrinal orthodoxy, religious experience, and average frequencies of church attendance, prayer, and Bible reading. Through statistical analyses, we were able to assess the unique predictive power of the religious coping measures (after controlling for the effects of religious orientation measures) and the unique predictive power of the religious orientation measures (after controlling for the effects of religious coping measures). In comparison to the religious orientation measures, the religious coping measures were much stronger predictors of outcomes. As can be seen in Table 10.3, similar results have emerged from other studies.

Thus, religious coping variables appear to be more consistently and more strongly related to outcomes than are general orientation variables. This pattern of results fits with the idea that religious coping acts as a mediator or bridge between general religious orientations and the outcomes of negative life events.[3] More often than not, what people specifically do with their religion in times of trouble has important implications for how well things turn out. But the results are not always positive.

Let us return to the question "Is religion helpful, harmful, or irrelevant in coping?" The answer is yes. Religious coping is all of the above.

Unfortunately, this is not a particularly satisfying answer. But perhaps the fault lies less with the answer than with the question—whether religion is helpful in coping with stress seems to assume that religion is one thing. We have already noted that religion takes a variety of forms in the coping process. Maybe the question needs to be rephrased. A better question may be "What forms of religious coping are helpful, harmful, or irrelevant?" To go a little further, we might ask whether religious coping is equally effective for all kinds of people? In

TABLE 10.3. The Unique Statistical Effects of Religious Coping and Religious Orientation Measures

Study	Sample	Adjustment measure	Unique effects of religious coping[a] (ΔR^2)	Unique effects of generalized religious measures[b] (ΔR^2)
Pargament, Ensing, et al. (1990)	586 church members coping with a major life event	General Health Questionnaire	.09	N.S.[c]
		Event-Specific Outcome	.26	N.S.
		Religious Outcome	.21	.03
Pargament et al. (1994)	215 college students coping with Persian Gulf war prior to Allied invasion of Kuwait	Positive Affectivity	.06	N.S.
		Negative Affectivity	.11	N.S.
		General Health Questionnaire	.07	N.S.
Pargament, Smith, & Brant (1995)	225 Midwesterners coping with 1993 floods	Positive Affectivity	.16	N.S.
		Negative Affectivity	.22	N.S.
		Physical Health	.12	N.S.
		General Health Questionnaire	.15	N.S.
		Religious Outcome	.17	N.S.
Brant & Pargament (1995)	150 African-American college students coping with racist encounter and negative life events	Positive Affectivity	.15	N.S.
		Negative Affectivity	.25	N.S.
		General Health Questionnaire	.13	N.S.
		Religious Outcome	.28	.18

Note. All R^2 < .05 unless indicated.

[a]Unique effects of religious coping represent incremental R^2 after demographic and generalized religious orientation measures have been entered into the regression analysis.

[b]Unique effects of generalized religious orientation measures represent incremental R^2 after demographic and religious coping measures have been entered into the regression analysis.

[c]N.S., nonsignificant.

all kinds of situations? And is religious coping as effective as other forms of coping? In the sections below, I examine these questions and find that a richer picture of religion emerges when it is studied in a more refined way.

WHAT TYPES OF RELIGIOUS COPING ARE HELPFUL? WHAT TYPES ARE HARMFUL?

Returning to Table 10.2, the microanalytic research on religious coping and adjustment has been broken down according to six types of religious coping: spiritual, congregational, religious reframing, religious approaches to agency and control, religious rituals, and combinations of religious coping methods.[4] We have to be careful in comparing the percentages associated with the different methods of religious coping because several have not received a great deal of attention and the percentages may be unstable. Nevertheless, some of the differences are striking. In 46% of the statistical relationships, spiritual support is tied to better adjustment; on the other hand, spiritual discontent is never tied to better outcomes. Attributing the negative event to God's will or God's love is never associated with poorer outcomes; reframing the event as a punishment from God, however, is tied to poorer outcomes 52% of the time. All forms of religious coping may not be equally effective, these results suggest.

In Appendix D I present a summary of investigations of particular religious coping methods and adjustment.[5] These findings are highlighted in the following sections. Conclusions will be drawn cautiously. This is a developing area of research and, although several studies are well done methodologically, others are more limited. Additional research with strong designs and measures will be needed before we can reach more definitive conclusions about the efficacy of particular religious methods of coping.

Helpful Forms of Religious Coping

Spiritual Support and Collaborative Religious Coping

Perceptions of support and guidance by God in times of trouble appear to be a helpful form of religious coping. The results indicate that those who report a greater sense of spiritual support often experience more positive outcomes. One study of caregivers of Alzheimer's patients provides a nice example (Wright, Pratt, & Schmall, 1985). Caregiving, they note, is extraordinarily stressful. To learn more about how caregivers manage to keep themselves together through their ordeal, Wright et al. distributed questionnaires to 240 caregivers. The questionnaires included a measure of caregiver burden and a measure of coping strategies, one of which was the degree to which the caregivers made use of spiritual support. Of all the coping strategies, spiritual support was most strongly tied to lower burden scores.

Other studies have yielded similar results. In the Project on Religion and Coping, we assessed spiritual support through a more comprehensive spiritually based coping activities scale (Pargament, Ensing, et al., 1990). Items on the scale reflected several components of support: emotional reassurance ("trusted that God would not let anything terrible happen to me"), a close spiritual relationship ("sought God's love and care"), and guidance in problem solving ("God showed me how to deal with the situation") (see Chapter 7). People who reported more spiritually based coping also reported better adjustment to life crises. In fact, of all the methods of religious coping, spiritually based coping emerged as the strongest predictor of outcomes.

Closely related to spiritual support is the collaborative form of religious coping in which the individual and the divine work together to solve problems. The results in Appendix D suggest that the perception of partnership with God in stressful times is oftentimes helpful.

Congregational Support

As noted earlier, significant numbers of people look to their church or synagogue for support in times of crisis, more so than to any other professional (Chalfant et al., 1990; Veroff et al., 1981). Some congregations have been described as second families to those who no longer have kin or friends available to care for them (Steinitz, 1981). One recent widow described how her church became her mainstay: "That very day my husband died, one of the members sent over a huge pot-roast and practically a whole dinner. For two weeks, practically every day somebody would call up and say, 'Expect your dinner at such-and-such a time.' . . . When I returned to Laketown [from a visit] a couple from the church picked me up, and the minister called me up regularly to see how I was doing" (Steinitz, 1981, p. 45).

Empirical studies that have looked into the helpfulness of clergy, leaders, and members during stressful times find that support from the congregation is beneficial to its members. The 37% significant positive-relationships figure for congregational support studies in Table 10.2 may be misleadingly low, for the overall percentage was strongly influenced by one study of people struggling with the type of negative situation that is problematic for many religious institutions—neonatal or fetal deaths, many of which occurred through abortion (Lasker et al., 1989). Generally, the support members derive from their congregation appears to work in tandem with the spiritual support they derive from their faith, both contributing to positive outcomes in stressful times.

Benevolent Religious Reframing

The research suggests that negative events are easier to bear when understood within a benevolent religious framework. Attributions of death, illness, and other major losses to the will of God or to a loving God are generally tied to better outcomes. For instance, Jenkins and Pargament (1988) asked patients with various kinds of cancer how much they felt God was in control of their illnesses. Those who attributed more control over their illnesses to God also reported higher self-esteem and better adjustment according to the ratings of their nurses.

Harmful Forms of Religious Coping

By looking more closely at specific forms of religious coping in times of crisis, it becomes clearer that religion is not necessarily helpful. Some religious coping methods are, in fact, tied to poorer resolutions. How and why religion becomes harmful in coping is a serious question, one I will reserve for a chapter of its own. Below I briefly note some of these apparently hazardous forms of coping.

Discontent with Congregation and God

When people do speak negatively of religion, many of their sharpest remarks are reserved for the members of their congregation or clergy who, they feel, let them down or deserted them in their times of greatest need. Listen to what some battered women had to say about their congregations:

- "The feeling I got from our church was that I was to suffer in silence."
- "When I left my husband years ago, I met with great opposition about my decision to divorce him . . . from church leaders."
- "A clergyman suggested that maybe I wasn't pleasing my husband in bed; and that was why he beat me." (Bowker, 1988, pp. 232–233)

Occasionally people will also express negative feelings toward God in dealing with a traumatic event, as we hear in the painful questioning of one adolescent:

I wonder if God really loves us like people say he does. Then why does he let people hurt so much, why are people homeless, why are people being murdered, and why is the world so screwed up . . . the only time that I have felt that I've experienced God was when I was suicidal. How can a true God desert me through most of my life and only intervene when I want nothing more than to be side by side with him? I don't believe that this world is what God had in mind. Where did he go? (Kooistra, 1990, pp. 89–90)

The feeling that the congregation or God has somehow abandoned or disappointed people in their worst moments seems to be accompanied by other powerful feelings as well: hopelessness, despair, and resentment. Turning to the empirical studies in Table 10.2, we see that expressions of religious discontent with congregation and God are often tied to poorer outcomes. Those who report greater dissatisfaction with clergy, congregation members, and the deity also report poorer mental health status, more negative mood, and a poorer resolution to the negative life event.

Of course, anger toward religion could be merely a first reaction or initial stage in coping. As we saw earlier, religious anger is not commonplace, and when it is expressed it is often time-limited (see Croog & Levine, 1972). What we do not know is whether the effects of religious discontent are long lasting. Perhaps the effects of "railing against the gods" are as short-lived as the railing itself. Or perhaps expressions of religious anger should be understood as a "positive disintegration" (cf. Dabrowski, 1964), an initial, cathartic, yet painful step in the process of constructive change. More longitudinal studies of religious coping are needed to clarify these issues.

Negative Religious Reframing: God's Punishment

Earlier, I noted that people are generally reluctant to view negative events as punishments from God. The cost in terms of guilt and fear might be quite steep. The research in Appendix D seems to bear this out. In several studies, attributions to a punishing God are related to negative mood and negative assessments of how well the events have been resolved. However, as was the case with religious anger, it is unclear whether the negative effects of this type of attribution are short-term or long lasting. To the extent that the punishment from God is seen as just and deserved rather than capricious, the individual may feel reassured that grace can be regained by a change of heart or behavior. Again, longitudinal research is needed to study the longer-term effects of explanations that involve a punishing God.

Forms of Religious Coping with Mixed Implications

Not all forms of religious coping fall so easily into good and bad camps. In Table 10.2, we see that several religious coping methods were associated with positive outcomes in some instances and negative outcomes in others.

Religious Rituals in Response to Crisis

Mixed results are characteristic of studies of religious rituals in times of crisis. According to the tally, religious rituals are helpful in 40% of the statistical relationships and harmful in 23% of the cases. To illustrate one study in which rituals were positively related to outcomes, Morris (1982) worked with physically ill men and women from England who went on a pilgrimage to Lourdes, France, in search of physical and emotional relief. The site of visions of the Virgin Mary by Marie Bernarde Soubirous in 1858, Lourdes has since become an important destination for many sick people seeking a cure for their conditions. The participants in Morris's study completed measures of anxiety and depression one month before, 1 month after, and 10 months after their pilgrimage. Morris reports significant declines in both anxiety and depression 1 month after the pilgrimage. The lower levels of distress were sustained over the following 10-month period. Whether these changes were due to the ritualistic nature of the pilgrimage or to other factors, such as the expectancy of change, companionship, or simply getting away, could not be determined in this study. Morris admits that the lack of a control group (if one could even be found) makes it difficult to form definitive conclusions, but feels that the visit was indeed helpful to the pilgrims: "With one exception [they did] feel that the visit had been beneficial, in that it had strengthened their religious faith, and had made them more relaxed, more content, and more able to accept their physical disabilities" (p. 294).

On the other hand, Zeidner and Hammer (1992), who examined the coping strategies of Israelis in the midst of missile attacks during the Persian Gulf war, found that increased involvement in religious activities in response to the missile attacks was associated with *more* physical symptoms and *greater* anxiety.

How do we explain these mixed findings? One explanation may have to do with differences in the design of the research. While the Morris study was longitudinal, Zeidner and Hammer made use of a cross-sectional design. In the cross-sectional case, it is harder to say whether religious rituals are the *cause* or the *effect* of anxiety and depression. Religious rituals may lead to distress, but they may also be mobilized by distress, and the benefits of ritual practice might not become clear until some time down the road. If the latter "religious coping mobilization" explanation is correct, then we would expect both positive relationships between rituals and measures of distress in cross-sectional studies and negative relationships between rituals and distress in longitudinal research.

There is another, not so complicated explanation for the mixed findings. Quite clearly, very different types of rituals, activities, and groups are being compared in the preceding two studies and in Appendix D. Some types of religious rituals and activities may, in fact, be more helpful than others. Religious rituals may also be more helpful to some groups than others.

Self-Directing, Deferring, and Pleading Religious Coping

Religion provides its adherents with many methods to attain a sense of power and control in coping. Control can be *centered in the self,* growing out of the belief that God gives people the tools and resources to solve problems for themselves. Control can be *centered in God.* Believing that the ultimate responsibility for one's life rests in the divine, the individual may passively defer to God in troubled times. Control can also be *centered in efforts to work through God.* The individual may attempt to influence God and the course of events through pleas for divine intercession. Finally, control can be *centered in the relationship between the individual and God.* The individual may feel a sense of partnership with God, one in which the responsibility for coping is neither the individual's alone nor God's alone, but rather shared.

In an earlier chapter, I described research in which my colleagues and I (Hathaway & Pargament, 1990; Pargament et al., 1988) assessed three of these approaches to religious agency (self-directing, deferring, and collaborative) and their relationship to psychosocial competence. Competence refers to the level of psychological and social resourcefulness the person generally brings to life situations. It includes positive attitudes toward oneself, positive attitudes toward others, and active problem-solving skills (see Tyler, 1978).

Not surprisingly, our studies showed that the self-directing and deferring approaches were related to higher and lower levels of competence, respectively. These findings were consistent with an extensive literature that points to the mental health benefits of an internal locus of control and the mental health disadvantages of an external locus of control (see Lefcourt, 1976). Interestingly, however, the self-directing approach is not the only one with positive implications. Collaborative coping was also associated with higher levels of competence. Later studies provided further evidence for the benefits of this problem-solving style. Fewer symptoms of illness (McIntosh & Spilka, 1990), less anxiety (Schaefer & Gorsuch, 1991), and a greater sense of guilt, but, at the same time, grace and forgiveness for one's sins (Kaiser, 1991) were associated with collaborative religious coping. Intriguing as these results were, we cautioned against jumping to the conclusion that the self-directing and collaborative approaches were healthier forms of coping than the deferring style. Instead, we suggested that the value of these styles might vary from situation to situation.

The picture does indeed become more complicated when we focus on the relationship of these religious coping approaches to the outcomes of specific negative events. Apart from one study of alcohol abusers in which self-directing coping was related to more success in abstaining from drinking (Harris & Spilka, 1990), the significant findings involving self-direction fall in the *negative* category. Self-directing coping is tied to poorer outcomes. With one exception, the significant results having to do with deferring religious coping fall in the *positive* direction. Deferring coping is related to better outcomes.

When we put together the results from the competence and coping research, a consistent pattern of findings emerges only for collaborative religious coping. The shared sense of power and control embodied in this approach seems to bode well for both general mental health and the outcomes of specific negative situations. The other religious approaches to agency have some tradeoffs. Self-directing coping appears to be part of a generally competent way of life, but it is associated with poorer outcomes among some groups in certain situations. Perhaps these are the situations when the individual has, in fact, very little control. In these instances, the most appropriate thing to do may be to give up (see Burger, 1989). But give up to what? In the deferring religious coping style, the individual surrenders not to hopelessness nor to foreign powers. The responsibility for problem solving is delegated to what most see as an omnipotent but benign Being. Considering the alternatives when personal control is no longer possible, this may be one of the more empowering choices. Unlike the forces of chance and fate, God can still be approached, addressed, and perhaps influenced in times of stress. Maybe this is why the deferring coping style is helpful in certain situations, even though it may not be a generally competent way to solve problems. Lacking this benign source of external support, however, the self-directing coping style may leave the individual vulnerable to uncontrollable situations.

A similar explanation could account for the mixed results associated with pleas for divine intervention. While pleading for a miracle may not be effective for dealing with controllable situations, in situations that fall outside of the person's own powers, pleading may offer a way to achieve a sense of vicarious control and mastery through God. The 1990–1991 Persian Gulf war represented just this type of situation. In the days that preceded the Allied military assault to recapture Kuwait, many people felt a great deal of fear and uncertainty. Dire predictions were being made about the potential toll of the assault in human lives. There was little people could do to take direct control over the situations. In our study of college students, religious pleading at the peak of the crisis was predictive of increases in positive affect after the crisis had passed (Pargament et al., 1994). To those who had pleaded for divine interces- sion, the quick resolution of the Gulf war at the cost of few Allied lives may have indeed seemed miraculous. Overall, these findings suggest that the value of some religious approaches to control and agency will depend on the situation.[6]

Religious Conversion and Religious Switching

Of all the religious coping methods, conversion has probably received the most mixed reactions from psychologists and other social scientists. As noted in the previous chapter, some have extolled the benefits of conversion. Conversion has been said to lead to a unification of character (Pratt, 1946), new truths and a new state of assurance (James, 1902), spiritual insight, deeper motives, and a life on a higher plane (Starbuck, 1899). On the other hand, some have likened religious conversion to a drug addiction (Simmonds, 1977), a schizophrenic decompensation (Wooton & Allen, 1983), or brainwashing (Sargant, 1957). How is it that conversion can elicit such different reactions? Empirical evaluations shed some light on this controversial subject, but raise other questions as well.[7]

One way to assess the value of religious conversion is to compare converts and nonconverts on measures of mental health. A few studies have taken this tack, but the results have not been totally consistent. Galanter et al. (1979) found that converts or switchers to the Unification Church scored significantly lower on a measure of emotional well-being than a comparison group of adults of similar age and gender. Spellman, Baskett, and Byrne (1971) reported that church members who had experienced a sudden religious conversion scored higher on a measure of anxiety than a group of church-going nonconverts and a nonreligious group. On the other hand, members of the Rajneeshpuram movement, followers of the Bhagwan Shree Rajneesh in Oregon, scored higher on measures of social support and self-esteem and lower on a measure of depression than other community samples (Latkin, Hagan, Littman, & Sundberg, 1987). Similarly, higher levels of purpose in life (Paloutzian, 1981) and lower levels of loneliness (Shaver, Lenauer, & Sadd, 1980) were reported by those who had experienced a religious conversion than by those who had not. These results are not easy to interpret. Because mental health was not measured *prior* to conversion, we cannot be confident that the differences between groups are truly a *result* of conversion. Perhaps the groups differed in their mental health before conversion as well as after it.

To measure the effects of religious conversion more directly, several investigators have interviewed people after they experienced a religious conversion and asked them to evaluate its impact. The results are pretty clear. Following conversion, people consistently report psychological, social, and behavioral changes for the better. For example, Nicholi (1974) interviewed 17 college students who had experienced a religious conversion while undergraduates. The students felt that their religious change had resulted in increased self-esteem, a greater sense of joy, fewer feelings of despair, and more sensitivity and closeness to family and friends. Sixteen of the 17 students also reportedly stopped using alcohol, drugs, and cigarettes. Wilson (1972) presents similar findings from his study of white Protestant adults who had had a salvation experience. After their experience, the large majority of participants described a number of positive changes, among them less depression, less fear, less confusion, less emptiness, and less shame. They also reported several behavioral changes, including an end to promiscuity, quitting drinking, and fewer fights and arguments. Similar benefits have been described by those who have converted or switched to nonconventional religious groups (Galanter, Rabkin, Rabkin, & Deutsch, 1979; Levine & Salter, 1976) and traditional groups as well (Ullman, 1988).

On the face of it, these studies suggest that many people experience psychological and behavioral relief after a conversion. However, the studies have an important limitation; they are retrospective in design. In essence, the converts are asked to tell a story, to look back on their lives before and after conversion and evaluate the effects of the religious experience. In the process of telling their tale, it may be all too easy for the converts to exaggerate the troubles they had before conversion and exaggerate the happiness they experienced after. This kind of story reflects favorably not only on religious conversion, but on the individual's strength and resilience. Whether the story is accurate is another issue. Longitudinal studies of people pre- and postconversion would help answer this question, but identifying potential converts beforehand is a difficult task, so research of this kind has not been conducted as yet.

Even if we accept the findings that many people experience a "relief effect" (cf. Galanter, 1982) following their conversions, it is important to know whether the benefits are long lasting or short-lived. Recall that a large proportion of those who join nonconventional religious groups leave within a few years (Melton, 1986). But what of those who remain? Unfortunately, there have been few follow-up studies of group converts or spiritual converts. Starbuck's (1899) early work remains an exception. He examined the postconversion autobiographical accounts of 100 Christians and found that 93% of the females and 77% of the males reported some type of personal struggle following their conversion. The struggles included periods of religious inactivity and indifference, storm and stress, struggles to attain an ideal, and struggles with old habits. Starbuck notes that life continues to have its ups and downs for most people, even after they experience a conversion. Only 6% of the converts, however, suffered a complete relapse; almost all continued to identify with their religious experience. Starbuck reaches a favorable conclusion about the long-term implications of conversion: "The effect of conversion is to bring with it a changed attitude toward life which is fairly constant and permanent, although the feelings fluctuate" (p. 360).

Others, however, question this conclusion. Witztum et al. (1990) compared converts to ultra-Orthodox Judaism (baalei teshuva) with nonconverts in terms of their rates of referral to a mental health center in Israel and their psychiatric diagnoses. It was estimated that 66% of the baalei teshuva were "psychiatrically unwell" prior to their religious change. The converts were also overrepresented in the clinic. While only 0.4% of the adult Jewish population in Israel are converts to ultra-Orthodoxy, 12.6% of the referrals to the mental health center came from this group. Compared to the nonconverts, the baalei teshuva manifested more serious psychiatric diagnoses, such as major depressive, schizophrenic, and paranoid disorders. Interestingly, however, the baalei teshuva were not recent converts. On average, their conversion had occurred 5 years earlier.

With some appropriate caution, Witztum et al. (1990) suggest that the baalei teshuva may have become involved in orthodox Judaism in search of greater psychological stability. But, they add, "once the glow of arrival has abated, chronic problems reemerge" (p. 40). This does not mean that conversion *led* to psychological difficulties. The religious change may have diminished or delayed the onset of serious problems. Nevertheless, these findings do raise questions about the power of religious conversion to effect permanent change. In a similar vein, other mental health professionals have also presented accounts of individuals who experienced dramatic improvements in their psychological status following conversion, only to suffer serious setbacks some time later (Bragan, 1977; Levin & Zegans, 1974).

All in all, the research suggests that many people find at least some immediate relief from their problems through religious conversion. How pervasive and durable these changes remain over a longer period of time is still a question mark. While some may experience wholesale change, others may backslide, and still others may suffer disastrous consequences as witnessed in the tragic deaths of members of the People's Temple,

Branch Davidians, and Heaven's Gate. Focused, longitudinal empirical research is sorely needed in this controversial area. Studies of religious conversion have not distinguished sharply between spiritual and group conversion, between group switching and group conversion, nor between conversion to different types of religious groups (for an exception, see Ullman, 1988). Yet distinctions among kinds of religious conversion may be the only way to account for its diverse results. Conversions to a benevolent God are likely to have implications far different from conversions to despotic religious leaders or malevolent religious movements. Ultimately, the value of a conversion may depend on whether the person is converting to a life-serving or a life-negating force (Brenner, 1985).

Patterns of Positive and Negative Religious Coping

Up to this point, I have looked at particular religious coping methods and their implications for adjustment to negative life events. By examining these methods so closely, I may have left the impression that each is used singly or in isolation from the others. This does not appear to be the case. My colleagues and I have found modest to moderately high intercorrelations among the various religious coping scales. Thus, people seem to make use of religious coping methods in some combination with each other.

What are these combinations? To answer this question, my colleagues and I created a brief measure of religious coping (Pargament, Smith, & Koenig, 1996). In developing the Brief RCOPE, we assessed a wide variety of religious coping methods rather than a few coping methods in more detail. Breadth rather than depth was the guide here. We also tried to be sensitive to both potentially harmful and helpful forms of religious coping.

On the basis of the research reviewed above, we expected to find two patterns of religious coping: one made up of the helpful religious coping methods (e.g., spiritual support, collaborative, benevolent religious reframing) and one made up of the harmful religious coping methods (e.g., discontent with congregation, negative religious reframing).

The tragedy of the Oklahoma City bombing provided the context for this study. Six weeks after the blast, 310 members of one Baptist and one Disciples of Christ church located near the site of the explosion completed the Brief RCOPE, a measure of posttraumatic stress, and measures of adjustment to the tragedy. Almost all of the members had been personally exposed to or affected by the blast in some way.

A factor analysis of the 34 items of the Brief RCOPE resulted in two factors that were consistent with our predictions (see Table 10.4).

The first factor, labeled Positive Religious Coping, consisted of items that included spiritual support, collaborative religious coping, and benevolent religious reframing. The second factor, Negative Religious Coping, was made up of items that embody religious pain, turmoil, and frustration. Items on this subscale reflect discontent with the church and God, reframing of the blast as a punishment from God, and prayers for divine retribution. The average score on the Positive Religious Coping subscale was considerably higher than the average score on the Negative Religious Coping subscale. Thus, these church members were far more likely to make use of the benevolent religious coping methods.

What were the implications of these patterns of religious coping for

TABLE 10.4. Positive and Negative Religious Coping Subscales from the Brief RCOPE: Results from Members of Churches Near the Oklahoma City Bombing

Positive Religious Coping subscale items
 1. Thought about how my life is part of a larger spiritual force
 2. Worked together with God as partners to get through this hard time
 3. Looked to God for strength, support, and guidance in this crisis
 4. Thought about sacrificing my own well-being and living only for God
 5. Tried to find the lesson from God in this crisis
 6. Prayed for those who were killed in the bombing and for the well-being of their families and friends
 7. Looked for spiritual support from my church in this crisis
 8. Tried to give spiritual strength to other people
 9. Confessed my sins and asked for God's forgiveness
 10. Asked God to help me find a new purpose in living
 11. Reminded myself that the victims of the bombing are now at peace with God in heaven
 12. Prayed for the spiritual salvation of those who committed this bombing

Negative Religious Coping subscale items
 1. Disagreed with the way my church wanted me to understand and handle this situation
 2. Felt that the bombing was God's way of punishing me for my sins and lack of spirituality
 3. Wondered whether God had abandoned us
 4. Felt that God was punishing the victims of the bombing for their sins and lack of spirituality
 5. Tried to make sense of the situation and decided what to do without relying on God
 6. Questioned whether God really exists
 7. Prayed to God to send those who were responsible for the bombing to Hell
 8. Expressed anger at God for letting such a terrible thing happen
 9. Thought about turning away from God and living for myself alone

the adjustment of the church members to the bombing? To answer this question, we conducted a path analysis. The results of this analysis suggested that higher levels of posttraumatic stress trigger both positive and negative religious coping. Apparently, at least part of what the church members were coping with was their own traumatic reactions to the tragedy. However, the two patterns of religious coping were associated with different outcomes. People who reported more use of the positive methods of religious coping also reportedly grew more as a result of the blast, spiritually and psychologically. Negative religious coping, on the other hand, was associated with reports of greater callousness to others.

Whether these short-term differences in adjustment hold up over a longer period of time is an open question. Perhaps the negative patterns of religious coping reflect a process of religious struggle that ultimately holds more beneficial implications for the individual. Or perhaps the positive patterns of religious coping produce only short-term relief (or even longer-term problems). These results are only preliminary. Before reaching definitive conclusions about the helpfulness or harmfulness of these patterns of religious coping methods, we need to extend these findings to other groups over a longer period of time.

It does seem clear, however, that people do not use religious coping methods singly. Instead, they are applied in patterns or configurations with each other (see also Boudreaux, Catz, Ryan, Amaral-Melendez, & Brantley, 1995). These patterns may lend added power to the role of religion in the coping process. Studies of particular coping methods and studies of coping patterns are both needed to gain more insight into the workings of religion in stressful times.

In this section, we have seen that the specifics of what people do with their religion often makes a difference to the outcomes of coping. Specific forms of religious coping that, singly or in combination, appear to have helpful, harmful, or mixed implications for adjustment have been tentatively identified. I have, however, glossed over some variables that are potentially relevant to this microanalysis, such as who is doing the coping and what the individual is coping with. Questions remain as to whether religion is equally helpful to all people, in all situations, and in all ways.

IS RELIGION MORE HELPFUL TO SOME PEOPLE THAN OTHERS IN TIMES OF STRESS?

Only a few studies have compared the helpfulness of religion to different groups of people faced with negative life situations. They do, however, suggest that religion is more helpful to some people than others. As part of one national survey of adult black Americans, participants were asked to indicate the one coping response that helped them the most in dealing with a serious personal problem (Neighbors, Jackson, Bowman, & Gurin, 1983). Overall, 44% said that prayer was the one coping response that helped them the most. A higher proportion of lower income (50.3%) than higher income (34.9%) people found prayer to be the most helpful coping response. Prayer was described as more helpful to females (50.7%) than males (30.2%), and more helpful to the older group (64.3%) than the middle-age (46.6%) or younger (32.2%) groups. In another national study of Americans in 1957 and 1976, Veroff, Douvan, and Kulka (1981) asked their sample what helped them to face unhappy periods in their lives. Prayer was mentioned by 42% of the sample in 1957 and 31% of the sample in 1976. As in the study by Neighbors et al. (1983), prayer was more helpful to the poorer, older, and female participants. In addition, prayer was reportedly more helpful to those who were black, less educated, widowed, churchgoers, and fundamentalists. Other researchers have reported similar results (Bijur, Wallston, Smith, Lifrak, & Friedman, 1993; Conway, 1985–1986; Ellison, 1991; Ferraro & Koch, 1994; Pollner, 1989).

Elderly, poorer, less educated, blacks, widowed, women—why should religion be more helpful to these groups in coping? What do they have in common? In general, these groups have less access to secular resources and power in our culture. Religion, for them, represents an alternative, a resource that can be accessed more easily. It may be no coincidence that the groups that find religion more helpful are the same groups that report higher levels of personal religiousness and more frequent use of religion in coping (see Chapter 6). For them, religion has become a larger part of their orienting system, a framework more frequently called upon for coping with major crises. It appears that those who invest more in their religion gain more from it in coping (Dufton & Perlman, 1986; Elkins, Anchor, & Sandler, 1979; Horton et al., 1988; Lasker et al., 1989). For example, in their study of men and women who had experienced a pregnancy loss, Lasker et al. (1989) compared the relationship between various measures of religiousness and grief for groups who rated themselves to be more religious and less religious. Among the more religious people, higher levels of faith, church attendance, and support from the church were associated with better outcomes. Among the less religious group, the same measures of religiousness were generally unrelated to grief outcomes.

In short, the groups that profit most from religion in the coping process seem to be the groups that involve religion most deeply in their lives.[8] We suspect that the religious orienting system for these groups is better equipped to assimilate and respond to crisis. Drawing on a more deeply established system of religious beliefs, practices, feelings, and relationships, the individual may be in a better position to find compelling religious solutions (e.g., spiritual and congregational support, benevolent religious reframing) to fundamentally disturbing problems. Unfortunately, there is not a great deal of research on this topic. One exception, however, is a study by McIntosh et al. (1993) of parents who had lost a child to sudden infant death syndrome. They found that those who felt religion to be more important to them also engaged in more cognitive processing about the baby and his or her death. Greater cognitive processing was, in turn, associated with greater well-being and less psychological distress 18 months later. McIntosh et al. suggest that the more religious parents had a more developed religious cognitive framework or schema that facilitated their efforts to come to terms with their loss.

This is not to say that other demographic groups and less religious people do not find religion helpful to them at times. I recall a conversation with an ostensibly nonreligious colleague who somewhat sheepishly admitted that after his father died, he went to synagogue regularly to say Kaddish (the prayer for the dead) and has since followed the Jewish custom of lighting a "Yahrzeit" candle on the anniversary of his father's death. "You know it's funny. I'm not religious," he said, "but doing those things really meant something to me." Generally, however, empirical studies suggest that those who benefit the most from religion in times of stress are those who have invested more of themselves into religion.

IS RELIGION MORE HELPFUL IN SOME SITUATIONS THAN OTHERS?

In an earlier chapter, we saw that, although religious practices and beliefs are not reserved for times of loss and pain, people are more likely to turn to religion for help as situations become increasingly stressful. Stressful experience, it was said, mobilizes religious resources. Is this mobilization successful? Is religion *more effective* in more difficult times? Some would say yes. Sociologist Talcott Parsons once wrote: "Religion has its greatest relevance to the points of maximum strain and tension in human life" (cited in Fichter, 1981, p. 21). Many of the religious mechanisms of coping, as noted earlier, do seem to be specifically designed to help people through their most disturbing periods of life, when significance is at greatest risk. Perhaps, then, it would not be altogether surprising to find that religion is particularly helpful in moments of greatest stress.

But keep this in mind—to say religion is more helpful in more stressful times also means religion is *less* helpful in *less* stressful times. Is it really the case that religion is less valuable to people when their stressors are less severe? Or is the efficacy of religion unconditional? Does the value of religion hold true regardless of whether the negative situation confronting the individual is major or minor?

These two arguments can be restated in more scientific terms (see Wheaton, 1985). Implicit in each argument is a distinctive model of the relationship between the stressfulness of situations, religious coping, and the outcomes of negative events. The first argument holds that religion is a moderator of the relationship between stressfulness and outcomes: At different levels of religious coping the relationship between stressfulness and outcomes changes. This model, the *religious stress moderator,* is depicted in Figure 10.2. As can be seen, for those who make little use of religion in coping, increased stress results in poorer outcomes. Without the protective cushion of religion, the individual is more vulnerable to the effects of crisis. On the other hand, higher levels of stress do not have the same negative impact for those who are more involved in religious coping. For this group, religious coping serves as a buffer from the effects of stress. To put it another way, as stress levels increase, those who cope religiously are more protected from the detrimental effects of stress than their less religious counterparts. But religious coping holds no advantage for the individual at lower levels of stress.

According to the second argument, religion is as helpful to people in more difficult situations as it is in less difficult ones; regardless of the level of stress, religion proves to be beneficial. This second model, the *religious stress deterrent,* is also shown in Figure 10.2. As can be seen, higher levels of religious coping are associated with better outcomes in less stressful situations as well as more stressful ones. Clearly, stress exerts its own negative effects on outcomes, but religion works in the opposite direction, acting consistently as a deterrent to stress whether the situation is large or small.

Even though the two models have been presented as if they were mutually exclusive, it is possible to find support for both. In the *combined religious moderator–deterrent* model of Figure 10.2, religious coping is associated with better outcomes at all levels of stress (consistent with the stress deterrent model), *and* the benefits of religious coping increase as stress intensifies (consistent with the stress moderator model).

Several investigators have tested these models of religious involvement in coping. Appendix E presents a summary of 30 of these tests.

A. The Religious Stress Moderator Model

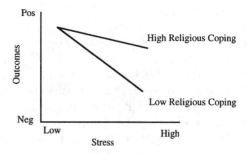

B. The Religious Stress Deterrent Model

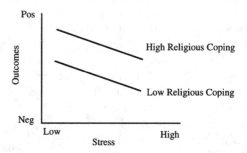

C. The Combined Religious Moderator-Deterrent Model

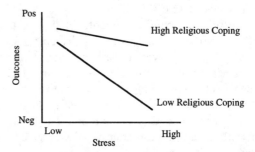

FIGURE 10.2. Three models of the relationship between stress, religious coping, and outcomes of negative life events.

Evidence for the Religious Stress Moderator Model

Seventy-three percent of the studies offer at least partial support for the religious stress moderator model. In an early test, Stouffer et al. (1965)

found that prayer was reportedly more helpful to World War II combat soldiers who had faced more stressful situations. Seventy-two percent of the soldiers who described themselves as frightened in battle felt that prayer was helpful to them in comparison to 42% of the soldiers who felt less battle fear. Similarly, soldiers who had seen combat rated prayer as more valuable to them than those who had not. Soldiers who had seen close friends killed or wounded in action were also more likely to find prayer helpful than those who had not.

Relying as it did on self-reports of religious helpfulness, the Stouffer study did not provide a very strong test of the religious stress moderator model. But several more sophisticated studies have yielded similar results. For example, working with a sample of elderly poor Protestants and Catholics, Zuckerman, Kasl, and Ostfeld (1984) reported that a general measure of religiousness (e.g., self-rated religiousness and church attendance) moderated the effects of illness on mortality over the next 2 years. The mortality rates for healthier males and females did not differ by religion. However, among the more sickly participants in the study, mortality rates were lower for religious males (19%) and females (11%) than for less religious males (42%) and females (20%).

Some studies also suggest that the buffering effects of religion may be fairly selective; that is, for any group, only certain types of religious coping may offer protection against the effects of stress. A study of members of religious and nonreligious kibbutzim in Israel by Anson, Carmel, Bonneh, Levenson, and Maoz (1990) illustrates the point. Membership in the religious kibbutz offered some protection against the effects of negative life events on psychological distress and physical symptomatology, while membership in the nonreligious kibbutz did not. On the other hand, higher levels of personal religiousness such as private prayer and self-rated religiousness did not buffer the effects of stress in this sample. Thus, for the Israelis, it was the social rather than the personal forms of religious expression that offered some protection against stress. These results may reflect the special importance of communal religious involvement within Israeli society.

But we have to be careful not to overgeneralize from the Israeli case. The types of religion that buffer the effects of stress in one group may be quite different from those that buffer stress in another. In fact, measures of personal religiousness have emerged as stress buffers in other groups. For example, Park, Cohen, and Herb (1990) found that intrinsic religiousness buffered the effects of uncontrollable life events on subsequent levels of depression for Protestant college students. Interestingly, intrinsic religiousness did not serve the same function for the Roman Catholic students in their sample. For them, religious coping buffered the negative effects of *controllable* rather than uncontrollable life stressors. The authors suggest that Protestants and Catholics draw on different types of religious stress buffering mechanisms. Protestants may find that their intrinsic orientation provides a particularly important framework of meaning when confronted with uncontrollable life events. In contrast, Roman Catholics may find guilt-reducing religious beliefs and practices to be particularly helpful for resolving the distress associated with controllable negative events. Thus, specific forms of religious coping may be particularly effective stress buffers for particular groups faced with particular kinds of problems.

Finally, a close analysis of this literature reveals an important difference in findings depending on the way adjustment is defined and measured. When adjustment is defined in terms of a negative indicator (e.g., depression, physical symptomatology), at least partial support for religiousness as a stress moderator emerges in 89% of the studies. When adjustment is defined by positive indicators such as life satisfaction or self-esteem, partial support for religiousness as a moderator emerges in only 50% of the studies. Preliminary as this analysis is, it suggests that religion operates more consistently as a cushion against the negative effects of stress than as a force for enhancing positive functioning as stress increases.

Overall, many people do appear to find religion most helpful in times of maximum tension and strain, as Parsons asserted. Does that mean that religious coping is of little value in less stressful circumstances? Not necessarily.

Evidence for the Religious Stress Deterrent Model and the Combined Model

Returning to the results of Appendix E, 66% of the studies also yield at least partial support for the religious stress deterrent model. For instance, in one study of elderly black Americans, higher levels of involvement in the church were associated with greater self-esteem, and higher levels of personal religiousness were associated with feelings of greater personal control and mastery *regardless* of the numbers of negative life events they had experienced in the past month (Krause & Van Tran, 1989). In another national survey of adults, people who reported a close relationship with the divine also reported greater happiness and satisfaction in living, irrespective of whether they had recently experienced up to four major life events (Pollner, 1989). Both of these studies supported the religious stress deterrent model and not the religious stress moderator model.

But the majority of studies (72%) that found evidence for the religious stress deterrent model also yielded some support for the religious stress moderator model. For example, working with a sample of recently bereaved parents (higher stress) and parents who had lost a child more than 2 years ago (lower stress), Maton (1989b) found that spiritual support was related to lower levels of depression for both groups. This finding is consistent with the stress deterrent model. However, consistent with the stress moderator model, Maton also found that spiritual support was related to depression and self-esteem more strongly for the recently bereaved group of parents than those who had lost a child more than 2 years ago. Thus, Maton's study offers support for the combined moderator–deterrent model.

Overall, the findings on the relationship between religion, stressors, and adjustment suggest that there is a grain of truth to each of the three models. It is true that religion can be of greatest help in times of greatest stress. Does this mean that religion has little value outside of crisis? No, for it is also true that higher levels of religiousness can be more helpful than lower levels of religiousness regardless of how much stress the individual is under. Religion demonstrates a capacity to buffer the effects of higher stress, to deter the effects of stress at higher and lower levels, and to do both. But, the word "capacity" should be underlined. Religion does not always act as a stress moderator, stress deterrent, or stress moderator–deterrent. As yet, the research does not offer a clear answer to the question of when religion will take on (or fail to take on) these roles. However, we do know that the relationship between religious coping, stress, and adjustment seems to depend on the type of religious coping, the type of group, the type of outcome, and the type of problem under study.[9] Finally, remembering that some forms of religious coping are more harmful than helpful, we might also guess that religion has the capacity to exacerbate the effects of stress—to make bad matters even worse (see Park et al., 1990). These effects may be less evident in the religious stress moderator/stress deterrent research because most of the studies in this literature focus on aspects of religious orientation (e.g., average frequency of prayer or church attendance) rather than specific forms of religious coping, which have been shown to hurt as well as help in the coping process.

In prior sections, we have seen that the helpfulness of religion in the coping process depends on the particular religious coping mechanism and the person who is doing the coping. To this list, we should now add the nature of the situation. Religion can be of greatest help in times of greatest stress (for at least some groups and some types of religious coping). Why should this be so? Let me suggest that these are the situations that push people to the limits of their personal capacities or beyond them. To put it another way, in the face of the most difficult circumstances, people are confronted most directly with their own insufficiency. Religion is perhaps uniquely equipped to respond to those times when people are faced with the limits of their own power, as I discuss in the following sections.

How Helpful is Religious Coping in Comparison to Other Forms of Coping?

Perhaps the easiest way to compare religious and nonreligious coping is to see whether those who cope religiously with negative events fare any better or worse than those who cope through nonreligious methods. Only a few researchers have taken this *between-groups approach.* In three instances, few differences were found between religious and nonreligious copers in their adjustment to stressful situations. Weisner et al. (1991) compared the adjustment of religious and nonreligious families who were coping with a young child with a significant developmental delay of uncertain cause. The religious parents coped differently than the nonreligious parents: They were more likely to value family togetherness and nurturance, more likely to see their child as an opportunity rather than as a burden, and more likely to see their religious convictions as helpful to them in coping. However, the interviewers who rated the adjustment of the families found no differences between the two groups. Moreover, religious and nonreligious parents did not differ in the degree to which they accepted the child, their peace of mind about the child's present and future, and their own feelings of disappointment, concern, or depression. Similarly, Dufton and Perlman (1986) compared groups of conservative believers, nonconservative believers, and nonbelievers in the ways they coped with loneliness. While the two religious groups clearly conceptualized and dealt with their loneliness from a religious framework, they did not differ from the nonbelievers in their level of loneliness. Finally, Koenig, Siegler, and George (1989) compared a group of elderly persons who made use of religion in coping with a stressful event with those who did not and found no significant differences between them on 12 measures of coping and adaptation. They did, however, find that a small subgroup of those who reported the highest frequency of religious coping ranked highest on 9 of the 12 measures of coping and adaptation.

Two other experimental studies of Christian groups comparing the relative efficacy of relaxation training with prayer (Elkins, Anchor, & Sandler, 1979) and with devotional meditation (Carlson, Bacaseta, & Simanton, 1988) yielded discrepant results. In the Elkins et al. (1979) study, relaxation training produced more physiological and subjective tension reduction than a control condition; however, prayer did not. On the other hand, Carlson et al. (1988) found that devotional meditation was more effective than progressive relaxation in reducing muscle tension, anger, and anxiety.

Overall, these studies do not show that religious copers experience more benefits than their nonreligious counterparts. On the face of it, people appear to be able cope as effectively without religion as with it. Before we accept this conclusion though, it is important to consider some limitations of this literature. First, these studies generally gloss over potentially important differences in *types* of religious coping. As we found earlier, some religious coping methods appear to be more helpful than others. It may also be true that certain kinds of religious coping are more effective than certain kinds of nonreligious coping, and vice versa. Second, it is unclear how well this literature covers those times when we might find religion to be maximally effective, namely, situations of greatest stress, such as the death of a loved one, when people feel the least sense of personal control. Finally, and perhaps most importantly, between-group studies rest on what may be an artificial dichotomy between religious coping and nonreligious coping. Few of us are completely enveloped in the religious world. When problems arise, religious coping is rarely used to the exclusion of other forms of problems solving. For example, in the Dufton and Perlman (1986) study, religious copers used as many nonreligious coping strategies as did the nonreligious copers. Furthermore, many situations call for both religious and nonreligious coping. How well do the two approaches compare when *both* are being used by the same person?

Here we shift from between-group to *within-group* studies. When asked to compare religion to other coping strategies, many people give religion more favorable ratings. For example, asked to indicate the one thing they did that helped them most in coping with a serious personal problem, prayer was mentioned by African-Americans most often, more frequently than facing the problem squarely, doing something about the problem, keeping busy, and staying relaxed (Neighbors, Jackson, Bowman, & Gurin, 1983). Similarly, "faith" was ranked the most effective of 27 coping mechanisms by a sample of elderly community residents coping with a loss, threat, or challenge (McCrae & Costa, 1986).

Even these studies, however, create what may be an artificial rivalry between religious and nonreligious forms of coping. Earlier I noted that the two approaches to coping have been consistently intercorrelated in the empirical literature. To ask "Which works best, religious or nonreligious coping?" may only distort the coping process by forcing these two allies into head-to-head competition. The better question may be whether religious coping adds something *distinctive* to the coping process.

Several researchers have put this question to test. In research terms, they have examined whether religious coping predicts adjustment to negative life events above and beyond the effects of nonreligious coping. The results are clear: Religion does appear to add a unique dimension to the coping process. For instance, measures of spiritual support have predicted adjustment above and beyond the effects of general measures of social support (Kirkpatrick, 1993b; Maton, 1989b). In a similar fashion, greater social involvement in the church has been tied to lower levels of loneliness (Johnson & Mullins, 1989) and greater life satisfaction (Ellison, Gay, & Glass, 1989), even after the effects of other social relationships are controlled. In research with my colleagues (see Table 10.5), I have found that both religious and nonreligious measures of coping add something unique to the prediction of outcomes to stressful life experiences.

What does the religious dimension add to the coping process? In earlier chapters, we described some of the specific religious coping mechanisms and the specific ways they may conserve or transform significance. But, certainly, nonreligious coping methods can serve some of these same purposes. What are the distinctive contributions of religion to the coping process? I believe religion offers a response to the problem of human insufficiency. Try as we might to maximize significance through our own insights and experiences or through those of others, we remain human, finite, and limited. At any time we may be pushed beyond our immediate resources, exposing our basic vulnerability to ourselves and the world. To this most basic of existential crises, religion holds out solutions. The solutions may come in the form of spiritual support when other forms of social support are lacking, explanations when no other explanations seem convincing, a sense of ultimate control through the sacred when life seems out of control, or new objects of significance when old ones are no longer compelling. In any case, religion complements nonreligious coping, with its emphasis on personal control, by offering responses to the limits of personal powers. Perhaps that is why the powers of the sacred become most compelling for many when human powers are put to their greatest test. Johnson (1959) sums it up more eloquently:

> It is because man is a finite person with infinite possibilities that he ventures upon the religious quest. He is naturally finite, yet he learns of infinite possibilities which he cannot reach alone. Thus, he will never be content to endure the finite loneliness of self-sufficient isolation. . . . Religious learning is the discovery of ultimate resources to meet infinite longings of the finite spirit. (pp. 64–65)

TABLE 10.5. The Unique Statistical Effects of Religious Coping and Nonreligious Coping

Study	Sample	Adjustment measure	Unique effects of religious coping[a] (ΔR²)	Unique effects of non-religious coping[b] (ΔR²)
Pargament, Ensing, et al. (1990)	586 church members coping with a major life event	General Health Questionnaire	.03	.04
		Event-Specific Outcome	.07	.09
		Religious Outcome	.26	N.S.[c]
Pargament et al. (1994)	215 college students coping with Gulf war prior to Allied invasion of Kuwait	Positive Affectivity	.08	.13
		Negative Affectivity	N.S.	.11
		General Health Questionnaire	.06	N.S.
VandeCreek et al. (1995)	150 people in hospital waiting room awaiting outcome of cardiac surgery of loved one	Beck Anxiety	.06	.14
		Beck Depression	.07	.16
		Event-Specific Outcome	.13	.06
		Religious Outcome	.44	N.S.
Pargament et al. (1995)	225 Midwesterners coping with 1993 floods	Positive Affectivity	N.S.	.08
		Negative Affectivity	.09	.11
		Physical Health	N.S.	.09
		General Health Questionnaire	.08	.12
		Religious Outcome	.43	N.S.
Brant & Pargament (1995)	150 African-American college students coping with racist encounter and negative life events	Positive Affectivity	.08	.05
		Negative Affectivity	.19	N.S.
		General Health Questionnaire	.12	N.S.
		Religious Outcome	.41	N.S.

Note. All R^2 < .05 unless indicated.

[a]Unique effects of religious coping represent incremental R^2 after demographic and nonreligious coping measures have been entered into the regression analysis.

[b]Unique effects of nonreligious coping represent incremental R^2 after demographic and religious coping measures have been entered into the regression analysis.

[c]N.S., nonsignificant.

CONCLUSIONS

I have covered a lot of territory in this chapter. The seemingly straightforward question, "Does religion work," could not be answered with a simple "yes" or "no." Instead, the answer depends on the kind of religion one is talking about, who is doing the religious coping, and the situation the person is coping with. Depending on the interplay among these variables, religion can be helpful, harmful, or irrelevant to the coping process. Religious coping variables predict the outcomes of negative life events more strongly than traditional, generic measures of religious orientation. The specific mechanisms of religious coping represent critical mediators or bridges between the general religious orientation of the individual and the outcomes of negative events. A closer look at the effects of these specific mechanisms reveals that not all forms of religious coping are alike: Empirical studies suggest that some are helpful (spiritual support, collaborative religious coping, benevolent religious reframing, and congregational support), some are harmful (expressions of discontent with congregation and God, and negative religious reframing), and some have mixed implications (religious rituals, self-directing and deferring religious coping, and religious conversion). Several other conclusions are also warranted: (1) Religious coping seems especially helpful to more religious people, (2) religion can moderate or deter the effects of life stress, or both, and (3) religious coping adds a unique dimension to the coping process.

Although the religious role in coping was the focus here, the magnitude of these findings should not be overstated. The sizes of the religious effects in most of the research studies are fairly modest. They indicate that religion is only one of many forces shaping the outcomes of coping. Even so, given psychology's historical neglect of the religious dimension, we may be more likely to underestimate than overestimate the importance of religion in coping. In the majority of studies, across diverse groups dealing with diverse problems, religious coping emerges as an important predictor of adjustment. Adjustment here is not limited to psychological well-being, although most studies have focused on psychological measures of outcome. Religious coping has also been shown to have short-term and longer-term implications for physical health, mortality, and spiritual well-being. Admittedly, these investigations vary in their quality. However, even in the more tightly controlled studies that apply more sophisticated measures and statistical analyses, religious coping has proven to be an important predictor of adjustment. Clearly, religion deserves greater recognition and attention than it has received in the coping literature. Detailed microanalytic studies of the specific ways religion expresses itself in times of crisis represent an important direction for religious study.

Research in this area could be advanced in several ways. First, more longitudinal studies are needed to clarify and distinguish among the mobilization of religious coping under stress, the short-term effects of religious coping on adjustment, and the longer-term effects of religious coping. Second, improved measures are needed that do justice to the richness and diversity of religious coping methods. Measures of individual religious coping methods and measures of patterns of religious coping both have an important place in coping research. In developing these measures, particular care should be taken to avoid confounding coping efforts (attempts to attain significance) with coping outcomes (the success or failure of these attempts). Third, much of the literature in this area has focused on conservational methods of religious coping and their ability to preserve psychological well-being, physical health, social intimacy, or the sense of meaning in stressful times. We need to learn more about transformational types of religious coping (e.g., rites of passage, religious forgiveness) and the ability of these mechanisms to create new sources of significance when old ones are threatened or lost. Fourth, studies of the ways children involve religion in coping are sorely needed. Finally, researchers should attend carefully to the criteria of successful or unsuccessful coping. It is important to consider how religious coping impacts on the full range of human functioning—physical, social, psychological, and spiritual. The effects of religious coping on the immunological system, on the individual's *own* objects of significance, and on the well-being of *other* people represent three uncharted but valuable areas for study. Still in its infancy, the study of religious coping has a lot of room for growth.

Up to this point our approach to the question of religious efficacy in coping has been unabashedly pragmatic. The pros and cons of religion have been evaluated by its end results. This is not an unusual approach. Much of the psychology of religion, and psychology in general, comes out of this mold. There are, however, some important limitations to pragmatism. For one, it assumes that whatever works is good. However, some positive results may be fortuitous, as in the case of Mircea and Tabita Bricci (*"She defies court's order . . . ,"* 1993). Far along in pregnancy, Ms. Bricci was told by doctors that her fetus was not getting enough oxygen or nutrients from the placenta. Unless she received a caesarean section, they said, her child was almost certain to die or suffer mental retardation. The Briccis refused, saying that they would place their baby's health in the hands of the Lord. Following natural childbirth, their son was born, apparently normal. Does the happy ending to this story reflect well on the Briccis way of coping? I would say no. All of the available information indicated that their baby was heading for trouble. Rather than solve what appeared to be a solvable problem themselves, they deferred the responsibility to God, and in the process, put their son at great risk. In this case, positive results occurred *in spite of,* rather than because of the way the situation was handled.

The pragmatic approach also assumes that what does not work is not good. But if it is true that some positive results are fortuitous, it is just as true that some negative results are inevitable. Death and a certain degree of pain, suffering, and loss in life are unavoidable, regardless of how well we cope. In short, the relationship between action and results is not perfect, and because of that, pragmatic evaluations can be misleading. There is value to certain pathways and destinations in the search for significance, whether or not the search proves to be successful. This is the essence of the process approach. From this perspective, the key to coping lies not in a particular act nor in a particular outcome, but rather in the integration among the pieces of the coping process.

In the following chapter, I examine the efficacy of religious coping from this process perspective, with an added twist. The focus will shift to the darker side of religion, to the times when religion plays a destructive role in coping. Though they may be the exception rather than the rule, failures of religion in coping can have calamitous consequences. They have to be taken seriously. The process perspective offers one source of insight into what happens when religion fails.

Chapter Eleven

WHEN RELIGION FAILS
Problems of Integration
in the Process of Coping

WOMAN CLAIMS, "I WAS IMPREGNATED BY THE
DEVIL!"

RELIGIOUS SCAMS TOTAL $450 MILLION: CON
ARTISTS STEALING IN THE NAME OF GOD!

HINDUS ON RAMPAGE KILL 5000 SIKHS AFTER
MURDER OF INDIRA GANDHI!

A critic of religion does not have to search long or hard to find material
to draw on. Scan the television channels or browse through the newspapers and sensational headlines such as those above often stand out,
attesting to the association of religion with the odd and the extreme. But
the media are not the only ones who tie the religious to the pathological.
Mental health professionals often make the same connection (see
Richardson, 1993).

The accuracy of this antireligious view, however, is questionable. In
the last chapter, the review of empirical studies indicated that religious
forms of coping are more often helpful to people than harmful. Does
this mean that religion is *entirely* benign? No. The links between religion
and personal and social pathology can be all too real. No evaluation of
religion and coping would be complete without a closer look into this
connection.

This will not be an easy job. Of the many things that are hard to understand about religion, perhaps the hardest is how it can be associated with such diametrically opposed behaviors. The force that has produced many of the world's greatest models of courage, compassion, and composure in the face of adversity has also been implicated in violence, self-destruction, and emotional turmoil. How do we reconcile such different religious personalities? In this chapter, we look at what happens when religion goes wrong.

It is important, though, to keep this evaluation in a proper perspective, one balanced by the recognition that we tend to sensationalize and overexaggerate what has been called "the seamy side" of religious life (Pruyser, 1977).

Again, it must be stressed that the psychologist cannot evaluate the absolute truth of religious claims. However, religion can be evaluated on different psychological grounds. In the last chapter, I approached the question of whether religion works from a pragmatic point of view. In essence, I dissected the coping process, searching for specific types of coping that were defined as healthy or unhealthy by virtue of their end results. Yet, as was asserted earlier in the book, coping is a dynamic *process,* one that involves many elements—personal, situational, and social— interacting and evolving over time. The nature of this process has as much to do with the efficacy of coping as any one coping activity and its outcomes. At its best, the coping process is well integrated, with each of the parts operating in smooth, coordinated fashion with the others. There are times, however, when the system loses its balance, its synchrony. The fault here lies not with any one element of the process, but with the system itself.

In this chapter, I will examine how religion becomes involved in problems of integration in the coping process. There are many forms of "dis-integration" (physicists have noted that there are far more varieties of disordered states than ordered ones). Therefore, the evaluation has to be selective. First, I will focus on religious involvement in three types of problems in the process of coping: problems of ends, problems of means, and problems of fit between the individual and the social system. Later in the chapter, I will try to account for these problems by focusing on some of the general, dispositional characteristics of religion that weaken the orienting system and leave the individual vulnerable to trouble in coping.

Be forewarned that this evaluation will be just that—value-laden. The reader will encounter terms not usually associated with science, such as effective and ineffective, good and bad, right and wrong. However, value issues cannot be avoided in scientific study, and the psychology of religion and coping is no exception to this rule. Values, in this chapter, will be made very explicit, so they can be considered, debated, affirmed, or rejected in favor of other values.

THE WRONG DIRECTION: PROBLEMS OF ENDS

Several years ago, I saw a man in psychotherapy who admitted that he had been having an affair with a married woman, a mother of five. A husband and father of a large family, he described himself as a successful businessman, respected in his community, and a leader in the church where he had met his lover. Asked why he was coming to counseling, he quietly spoke of the distress his extramarital affair was causing him. I asked him to tell me more about his feelings (expecting that he would describe his own guilt, ambivalence, and pain), but he surprised me. He was not upset with himself. He was upset with his lover; it seems that she had begun to have some second thoughts about their affair and was no longer willing to see him on a weekly basis. What became clear in this first meeting was that my client was not having any qualms about his behavior. He wanted to rekindle the affair, and he wanted my help in this process. I would not help my client get to where he wanted to go. Where he wanted to go was, in fact, a big part of the problem.

Is the individual heading in a good direction? This is one of the questions basic to how we evaluate the coping process. "It makes a great deal of difference to a man," James (1902) wrote, "whether one set of his ideas, or another, be the center of his energy" (p. 193). It is hard to argue with this sentiment. But *evaluating* the merits of these various "centers of energy" is another matter. Is one guiding force inherently better or worse than another? James, for one, said no. Who is to say that the search for meaning is more worthwhile than the search for intimacy or the search for a better world? He spoke instead of the importance of a harmonious balance among the competing, sometimes warring, interests that make up the "hot place" in consciousness. Pluralist that he was, James saw room for many viable "teleological unions" that could motivate and direct behavior. Problems, he said, are likely to arise only when the individual is unable to achieve an integration among purposes. In the following sections I consider two ways religion can be involved in the "dis-integration" of the ends of coping.

Religious One-Sidedness

Ours has been called the age of anxiety, when traditional values are breaking down and people are desperately grasping for direction. In changing times, simple solutions to the problems of significance can be particularly tempting. But the simple solution of any kind—be it drugs, food, and wealth or relationships, meaning, and self-development—becomes destructive, even daimonic, as May (1970) said, when it takes over the whole person. The problem here lies not so much in the strength of the desire as in its one-sidedness. As James (1902) noted, devotion to any significant end unbalanced by other values can cause trouble. The client above was dedicated to his own pleasures exclusively, ignoring their impact on others around him. As a result, he engaged in activities that were destructive to himself, his family, and even his lover.

One-sidedness can also be rooted in the religious world. In their clinical work with elderly women who had experienced the death of an adult child, one group of researchers (Goodman, Rubinstein, Alexander, & Luborsky, 1991) noted that the Jewish mothers appeared to be having more trouble coming to terms with the loss than the non-Jewish mothers. They put their observations to test by interviewing and surveying a group of elderly bereaved Jewish and Christian mothers. Consistent with their observations, the Jewish mothers reported higher levels of depression and loneliness, and lower levels of positive affect, mastery, and control in their lives than the non-Jewish mothers. Interviews with the two groups also indicated that the Jewish women seemed "stuck" in their lives, unable to go beyond their loss and grief, while the Christian women were able to view their loss more philosophically and move on to new interests.

What accounted for the difference? The authors believe that the reactions of each of the two groups were embedded in their cultures. Devotion to the nurturance of their children was, for many Jewish mothers, the focal point of their existence. Significance for them was very much tied to the perpetuation of their own families, and the survival of the Jewish people more generally. The authors suggest that "the extreme glorification given to the begetting and raising of children in Jewish culture places bereaved Jewish mothers in double jeopardy. Having invested in the survival of Judaism by instilling their beliefs in their children, the loss of a child denies them, not only their own generativity, but the generativity of their culture" (p. S323).

In the words of one grieving Jewish woman, we can hear how the loss of her primary source of significance left her without purpose and direction:

INTERVIEWER: Would you say there is a main purpose or task in life?

MRS. GROSS: Now? I really don't have a purpose or task.

INTERVIEWER: What was your purpose?

MRS. GROSS: To see my daughter . . . since she died . . . I don't seem to want to give to anybody else. It seems that I've given my all . . . I have no purpose. I just float now.

INTERVIEWER: You wouldn't say you have any goals?

MRS. GROSS: No, not at all. I don't want a goal anymore. No. All that has left me . . . my daughter's gone . . . my future is gone because of her . . . our children are our future. And that's finished. And that's why I feel when I die there'll be nobody here. (p. S325)

In contrast to Jewish culture, the authors assert, American Christian culture places greater emphasis on autonomy and self-reliance of children from their families. Less contact and more emotional distance characterize the relationship between the generations, and both parents and children feel greater freedom to pursue their own independent lives. Painful as it is, the loss of a child presents less of a blow to significance because significance itself is more multifaceted. Contrast the interview above with the response of one 69-year-old Quaker woman to the death of her 29-year-old son:

MRS. HOWARD: After my son Paul's death, it was a Godsend that I was already teaching. That I had many, many, many adult students in whom I could invest. And from whom I got the kind of response that that brings.

INTERVIEWER: Was there anybody in any sense that took the place of your son . . . ?

MRS. HOWARD: Just my whole class, classes of students.

INTERVIEWER: Can you elaborate on that, what do you mean, there was an emptiness that had to be filled through contact with younger people . . . ?

MRS. HOWARD: Yeah, there was a big place to be filled, a big part of me that was emotionally unemployed. . . . I have this very close network of extended family that feel like my own kids and kin. (p. S325)

The elderly Christian women whose generativity was not so closely intertwined with their children's lives could turn to other sources of meaning and satisfaction. They may have been able to derive additional solace from their belief in a life after death, unlike their Jewish counterparts, who focus more on the rewards and punishments of this world than of the hereafter.

Certainly, the Jewish mothers in this sample should not be faulted for their commitment to their children. By most yardsticks, Jewish children flourish in the protective, nurturant environment of the Jewish home. It is the *exclusiveness* of the devotion to their offspring that made these Jewish mothers especially vulnerable to the loss of a child.

Any end, even the most virtuous, can become problematic when pursued to the exclusion of other values. From a religious perspective, the attempt to expand personal powers without an appreciation of human limitations is especially arrogant and misguided. "To fancy one's self one's own creator, or to place death within the power of the will," Bakan (1968) said, "are the real sins of mankind" (p. 128). Similarly, theologian Paul Tillich (1951) wrote that "the elevation of preliminary concerns to ultimacy" is the essence of idolatry. "Something essentially conditioned is taken as unconditional, something essentially partial is boosted into universality, and something essentially finite is given infinite significance" (p. 13).

One-sided solutions could be viewed as forms of false worship, failed attempts to find viable substitutes for the sacred. But, religious devotion itself is not exempt from the danger of one-sidedness. It too can become unbalanced. The religions of the world have occasionally underscored the primacy of the spiritual ends of life by *demeaning* the worldly. The purity of the sacred is pitted against the vulgarity of the profane, and the individual is asked to choose between the two irreconcilable alternatives—the earthly city characterized by "love of self, even to the contempt of God" or the city of God marked by "the love of God, even to the contempt of self" (Saint Augustine, 1950, p. 477). Every religious group offers illustrations of people who have tried to elevate the spiritual by degrading the human. In one of his steps in his search for truth, Siddhartha Gautama, the man who was to become Buddha, joined a group of ascetics and experimented with a variety of bodily punishments before rejecting this approach. James (1902) catalogued other striking examples. One was Saint John of the Cross, a 16th-century mystic, who offered this spiritual prescription:

> The radical remedy lies in the mortification of the four great natural passions, joy, hope, fear, and grief. You must seek to deprive these of every satisfaction and leave them as it were in the darkness and the void. Let your soul therefore turn always:
>
> Not to what is most easy, but to what is hardest;
> Not to what tastes best, but to what is most distasteful;
> Not to what most pleases, but to what disgusts. . . . (p. 299)

Modern-day examples may be less striking, but equally problematic.

Consider Mrs. Abbott, a 37-year-old woman who, finding her own congregation unsatisfying, joined a new church that quickly became the sole focus of her life (Tarjanyi, 1990, p. 18). "Every single thing I did was church-related. Any type of social activity was church-related." As the church increased in importance, other interests and relationships were cut off: She stopped bowling because of her uneasiness with the "sinners" at the alley; old friends withdrew, uncomfortable with her religious arguments; and she became fearful of a world where everything "was evil and only God was good." Life, for Mrs. Abbott, became "disconnected and out of balance." She felt that she had turned from a "human being into a zombie."

The schism between the spiritual and the human is apparent here. Only by devaluing the human can the spiritual be reached. This is the authoritarian religion Fromm (1950) described so critically, a religion that at its heart involves "despising everything in oneself, of the submission of the mind overwhelmed by its own poverty" (p. 36). It should be emphasized, however, that the problem in these cases is not excessive religious enthusiasm. For many people, a strong, overarching spiritual center, one that incorporates human needs, is the organizing force for a life of tremendous satisfaction and value. Problems arise when that spirituality is defined narrowly, in a way that excludes other balancing personal and social values. James (1902) put it best: "If the balance exists, no one faculty can possibly be too strong—we only get the stronger all-round character. . . . Spiritual excitement takes pathological forms whenever other interests are too few and the intellect too narrow" (p. 333).

Unfortunately, one-sidedness is not always recognized as a problem in itself. When the search for significance goes awry, rather than broaden their vision, some people jump from one imbalanced set of ends to another, including religious ones. A life devoted to drugs or sex may prove to be empty, and the transition to a life of spiritual devotion may provide immediate relief. However, unless a way can be found to integrate spiritual needs with personal and social ones, the religious solution is likely to fail and the cycle is likely to continue as the individual jumps to yet another one-sided solution.

Religious Deception

One-sidedness becomes an even greater problem when it is accompanied by religious deception, when unsavory ends are cloaked in religious garb. The problem here is not simply that of one-sidedness, but of subterfuge—the concealment of one's true motives. Religion provides the mask of piety that allows antisocial ends to be pursued without fear of detection (James, 1902). Masquerading in the guise of virtue, spiritual ideals, or scriptural authority, any set of ends, even those that promote the well-being of the group or individual at the expense of others, gains greater legitimacy and power.

In some instances, religious deception is quite deliberate. Swindlers in Utah, claiming that they were connected to the Mormon hierarchy, reportedly fleeced 10,000 unsuspecting investors out of over $200 million ("Religious scams . . . ," 1989). In another story, the treasurer of one of the largest churches in Alabama bilked 193 investors (including a U.S. congressman) out of $19 million. Even though the money he received was never invested, he regularly mailed false account statements with a Bible verse at the bottom.

Not all cases of religious deception are deliberate. At times, religious subterfuge may be more a matter of self-deception than anything else. Unaware of their true motivation and equally unaware of how religion has been called on to conceal these motives, those who engage in religious deception may feel quite convinced of the rightness of their positions and defend them with tremendous fervor.

The lack of consciousness to religious deception does not make it any less problematic. Whether deliberate or hidden from awareness, spiritual justification and religious rationale have been offered to justify social oppression with great effect. Listen, for example, how Alexander Stephens, the Vice President of the Confederacy, defended the institution of slavery:

> To maintain that slavery is in itself sinful, in the face of all that is said and written in the Bible upon the subject, with so many sanctions of the relation by the Deity himself, does not seem to be little short of blasphemous! It is a direct imputation upon the wisdom and justice, as well as the declared ordinances of God. . . . (Seldes, 1985, p. 399)

Or consider the story of one Polish immigrant's education prior to World War II:

> Some people asked the priest whether it was all right to boycott the Jewish stores. The priest put all our consciences at ease. "Although God wants us to love all fellow men, He does not say that we should not love some of them more than others. Therefore, it is all right to love Poles more than Jews and to patronize Polish businesses only." (Allport, 1954, p. 446)

Twisted and distorted as it was, this kind of religious deception provided sanction and support for prejudice and bigotry, and helped to set the stage for the genocide that was to come.

A more recent case in point comes from El Salvador, where the membership in Pentecostal and fundamentalist churches grew by about one-fourth during the civil war in the 1980s. Psychologist Ignacio Martin-Baró (1990) argues that the movement toward the evangelical churches was, at least in part, the result of "psychological warfare" by the Salvadoran Armed Forces. Threatened by progressive, social justice-oriented sectors of the Catholic and Protestant church, the military leaders engaged in systematic persecution of these groups. More to the point of religious deception, the government also offered invitations to evangelical churches in North America to engage in missionary work in their country. Many churches accepted and began working in El Salvador and other South American countries. Martin-Baró maintains that the recruiting efforts of the regime were not based on sincere religious interest. They were, instead, self-serving attempts to boost support of the populace for the political order. Theologically, the evangelical churches posed far less threat to the regime, for they hold that the solution to oppressive social conditions lies in religious faith rather than in social change. His conclusion is that these missionary efforts were not what they appeared to be. In reality, they were used as "part of the ideological offensive against Central American revolutionary movements and, more concretely, as part of the psychological war carried out in the 'low-intensity conflict' strategy of the military" (p. 104). In a sad postscript, one that only lends further weight to his analysis, Martin-Baró was killed by a military death squad in El Salvador in 1989.

This is the kind of religion that gives religion a bad name. Complaints of religious hypocrisy are, in fact, among the most common reasons people give for their lack of religious involvement (see Moberg, 1987). However, perhaps no one finds these kinds of religious misuses more offensive than religious people themselves. Johnson (1984) asked a sample of students and community residents to serve as a mock-jury to a videotaped child abuse trial. In one condition, religion was used as a defense to justify the child abuse; specifically, the mock jury was told that the defendant was "a fine Christian man who follows the word of God as stated in the Bible in all of his family affairs and thus, must be a good father" (p. 215). No mention of religion was made in the other condition. The religious defense backfired. The sample as a whole was more likely to find the defendant guilty in the religious defense condition than in the nonreligious condition. Moreover, mock-jurists who held a more right-wing Christian orientation recommended stricter sentences in the religious defense condition than did their less right-wing Christian counterparts. Thus, the conservative Christians appeared to be especially offended by the attempt to justify child abuse through professed religiousness.

Allport (1954) once wrote that religion becomes involved in prejudice when it stands for more than just faith. In a sense, this is true, but, in a sense, it is not. Because religion is a matter of the human as well as the spiritual, it always stands for more than just faith. However, there are important distinctions to be made among the various personal and social values religion upholds. Religion runs into trouble when it is aligned with one-sided ends of any kind. The trouble only increases when religion is used to conceal these ends from oneself or from others. The central point here is not that one motive is inherently better than another. Instead, it is the integration among motives that holds one key to good coping. Johnson (1959) summed it up this way: "Purity of motives is often lauded as if superior to mixed motives. But all motives are mixed; the only purity is not simplicity but harmony of many coordinating motives in symphonic chords of ongoing purpose" (p. 214).

THE WRONG ROAD: PROBLEMS OF MEANS

It is almost impossible to catalogue all of the definitions that have been offered of positive mental health. One theme common to these diverse definitions, however, is the importance of being in contact with reality (see Jahoda, 1958). Effective functioning is said to rest on an accurate appraisal of life situations, one's personal and social resources, and the tasks necessary to maximize significance. Faulty appraisals, on the other hand, can be costly. After all, how can people anticipate and plan for the future if they fail to size up their situations and themselves with some degree of accuracy? The problem may be a failure to take a threatening situation seriously or, conversely, obsessive worry over situations that could be safely ignored. It may be unwarranted confidence in one's abilities to solve a problem or just as unwarranted doubts about one's skills. Or it may involve errors in judgment about the steps needed to resolve a crisis. In any case, the problem lies not in a particular kind of appraisal or coping method in and of itself, but rather in the lack of integration between an appraisal, a method of coping, and the world, oneself, and one's goals.[1] To put it another way, the road taken may be poorly suited to the weather or poorly suited to the condition of the traveler. On top of that, the road may not take the traveler where he or she wants to go.

While religious groups have traditionally encouraged their members to take the "right road," they do not always succeed. In some instances, their members take a wrong turn. Whether religion is directly responsible for the wrong turn is not always easy to tell. Clearly, however, poorly integrated appraisals and coping methods can be wrapped in religious beliefs and practices. In the following sections, I consider religion and three problems of integration in the means of coping.

Errors of Religious Explanation

In the 1980s and 1990s, a flurry of spectacular accounts was reported in the media. Activities ranging from grave desecrations, animal mutilations, and occult messages hidden in rock music to ritual abuse, the abduction of children, and human sacrifice were described, all purportedly planned and carried out by nationally organized, clandestine, Satanic cults (Bromley, 1991). For instance, according to one popular estimate, anywhere from 50,000 to 60,000 innocent people were being ritually sacrificed annually. Mental health professionals contributed in their own way to the scare. Reports were made of thousands of patients who had recovered memories of satanic abuse as children. Workshops sprang up to train other professionals to deal with the "growing problem" of Satanic trauma (Mulhern, 1991).

The Satanic alarm, however, appears to have been overblown. Evidence in support of these accounts proved to be thin. Unexplained animal deaths were, upon further investigation, almost invariably attributable to disease, trapping, poisoning, or road kills (Bromley, 1991). Equally unconvincing were the claims of human sacrifice by Satanic groups. One FBI investigator was unable to identify a single documented satanic murder in the United States and concluded that, if these murders have occurred, they are few in number (Bromley, 1991). Similar questions were raised about psychotherapist's accounts of Satanic ritual abuse. In a survey of over 2,000 practicing psychologists, Bottoms, Shaver, Goodman, and Qin (1995) found that 70% of the clinicians had not seen any cases of ritualistic abuse. Of those who did report ritual cases, the large majority of incidents came from a few clinicians who reported more than 100 cases each. One clinician reportedly saw 2,000 cases of ritualistic abuse! Bottoms et al. noted that clinicians who attended workshops on ritual abuse were more likely to report cases of religious abuse, a finding which suggests that training seminars on this topic may have legitimated Satanic rumors and fears

The Satanic scare represents an error of explanation, one in which religion of a particular form is seen as the cause of phenomena whose roots lie elsewhere. It might be tempting to dismiss the scare as an emotional overreaction of little consequence, but its impact has been quite real. A great deal of fear has been spawned in many communities. The lives of teachers, parents, ministers, and daycare workers have been seriously disrupted as the result of allegations that they were involved in Satanic activities. As importantly, the attention devoted to the Satanic has diverted attention from where much of it more properly belongs: the social, psychological, and cultural conditions that set the rumors and panic in motion in the first place. Errors of explanation can be quite costly.

But how do we tell whether an error of religious explanation has occurred? The question is even harder to answer when it comes to explanations that invoke God or the devil, rather than a religious group, as the causal agent. Consider, for instance, one explanation for the AIDS epidemic. It is no accident that the largest proportion of people with AIDS are homosexual, Chilton (1987) writes. Homosexuals, he states, have willfully chosen to engage in behavior that God "utterly hates and detests" (p. 37). The disease is a punishment visited on homosexuals for their violation of God's laws. AIDS is, in this sense, an "immorality" disease, a divine judgment homosexuals have brought on themselves by their choice to participate in "unhygienic, perverse, and violent practices" (p. 17). Although not all AIDS victims are homosexual, Chilton acknowledges, they, too, pay the price for the moral depravity of a society that tolerates such abominations. The perceived solution to the AIDS epidemic follows from the perceived cause. "The answer is not condoms, 'rubber dams,' and so-called 'safe sex' " (p. 72). These solutions only "make the world safe for perversion" (p. 43). Instead, "the answer is, as God commands, simply obedience to His Word" (p. 72).

Many readers might find something very wrong here. But what? Is the problem that Chilton is using a religious frame of reference to make sense of AIDS? No. In previous chapters, I reviewed research indicating that many people interpret negative life events from a religious perspective, and that some religious explanations (especially benevolent ones) are associated with positive outcomes. Is the problem that Chilton uses a particular *type* of religious interpretation? Perhaps. Attributions to a punishing deity, empirical studies have shown, tend to be tied to poorer outcomes of negative life events. However, before we dismiss beliefs in punitive spiritual forces or outside evils too quickly, it is important to remember that the threat of ultimate punishments may have some value as well. Like a strict parent, the punitive God or the devil who is active in the world may discourage people from acting out destructive impulses. Furthermore, beliefs in punitive forces (as long as they operate fairly) provide some reassurance that the world is ultimately orderly, just, and controllable; to avoid divine retribution, simply avoid transgressing against the spiritual order.

From the process perspective, there is nothing necessarily wrong with punitive religious appraisals nor any other appraisal or coping method for that matter. Instead, the problem lies in the use of religious explanations *to the exclusion of* other explanations. Whether an event is, in actuality, divinely or demonically inspired cannot be determined through empirical methods. However, it is possible to demonstrate empirical connections between life events and other potential causal factors. There is, for example, compelling evidence that AIDS is caused by a virus that suppresses the operation of the immunological system. The evidence is also compelling that virtually anyone, heterosexual or homosexual, can contract the virus. The flaw in Chilton's account lies not so much in the fact that he made a religious appraisal, nor in the fact that his appraisals involved the forces of sinfulness and a punishing God. The error lies in the use of religious explanations that leave no room for other interpretations, including those that are well grounded empirically. Defined simply as an "immorality" disease, the biological, psychological, and social roots of the AIDS epidemic are shortchanged. The end result is a nasty form of religious scapegoating. Already burdened by illness, the person with AIDS is asked to bear the brunt of the blame for his or her condition. This is not to say that the individual is not responsible for choices that may have been made to engage in risky practices. It is, however, inaccurate and unfair to explain the illness solely in terms of morality. Physiological, psychological, social, and cultural forces have also converged to create the epidemic.

Other people are not the only ones who suffer the consequences of errors of religious explanation. Inappropriate religious guilt can also follow from misinterpretations of negative life events. Knox (1985) illustrates this point in the case of Mrs. B., a 34-year-old woman who came to a mental health clinic because of depression. In the past 2 months she had lost her savings and her mother had died. In addition, her husband was unemployed and an alcoholic. Her explanation for these events made them all the more painful. She believed that she was being punished by God for her past sins, the biggest of which had been a pregnancy before she was married, followed by an abortion.

Most clinicians have come across cases like Mrs. B. Some might see the problem as one of religious guilt. Once again, however, from the process point of view, there is nothing necessarily wrong with punitive religious appraisals, even when the individual him- or herself is viewed as the guilty party. The problem arises when religious guilt *precludes* other relevant causal factors. In viewing her current predicament solely as a divine retribution for her earlier pregnancy and abortion, Mrs. B. relieved her husband of the responsibility for his abuse of alcohol and the economy of the responsibility for the couple's financial problems. She also ignored the more immediate causes of the illness that led to her mother's death. Undoubtedly, Mrs. B. shared some of the responsibility for her circumstances, but by focusing exclusively on her own moral failures, she scapegoated herself for her plight.

Errors of religious explanation point the finger of blame for negative life events to punitive deities, other people, or oneself. Other important roots to crises in living are overlooked. The result may be the victimization of people already struggling with misfortune.

There is one more drawback to misperceptions of the cause of problems—they interfere with the solution to problems. Failing to explain the negative situation accurately, the individual may also fail to identify the most appropriate resources for coping with the problem.

Errors of Religious Control

On May 28, 1994, 9-month-old Allyson Bergman became ill (Hughes, 1990). Her symptoms included a stiff neck, a distended belly, and lethargy. Allyson's parents, members of a faith healing sect that explains illness as the work of the devil and a direct result of disobedience to God, responded by reading the Bible to their daughter, fasting, and holding a prayer vigil. They did not take her temperature, nor did they seek out medical care. Allyson died 10 days later as the result of a respiratory infection that developed into pneumonia and meningitis. Had it been treated earlier, the illness could have been cured. The parents were charged with reckless homicide and neglect. At the trial, Allyson's mother said that she had not realized how serious the illness was. She went on to voice her belief that, even had she "feared and doubted God" by seeking medical help, the outcome would have been the same.

The Bergmans made a critical error of religious explanation. Their religious appraisals of Allyson's illness led them to reject the relevance of other causal agents. But, unfortunately, the problem went well beyond a simple misunderstanding, for not only did the Bergmans reject other ways to explain Allyson's condition, they also rejected alternative solutions that could have saved her life. Prayer, Bible reading, and fasting were the *only* viable solutions from their point of view. The idea of seeking medical help would have been antithetical to their beliefs. Therein lies the problem.

As noted in the previous chapter, religious forms of coping that involve prayer and Bible reading are often helpful to people in times of stress. Difficulties arise, however, when religious resources are used to the exclusion of other resources in coping. Like religious explanations that leave no room for other interpretations, religious solutions to problems that allow for no other solutions may lead to serious trouble, particularly in situations that are, in some sense, controllable. Some problems cannot be solved by prayer alone; they require other tools as well. As Johnson (1959) wrote:

Prayer does not work as a substitute for a steel chisel or the wing of an airplane. It does not replace muscular action in walking or faithful study in meeting an examination. These are not the proper uses of prayer. But prayer may help to calm the nerves when one is using a chisel in bone surgery or bringing an airplane to a landing. Prayer may guide one in choosing a destination to walk toward, and strengthen one's purpose to prepare thoroughly for an examination. (pp. 142–143)

Errors of control grow out of a misreading of the demands posed by life crises and, in turn, a misreading of the resources that are required to meet these demands. Consider, for example, the case of a man charged in the death of his son, who died from starvation ("Father views starving death . . . ," 1989). The man had lost his job and was in financial trouble. His reading of the situation was exclusively religious. God, he felt, was testing his faith "to the utmost—like when God asked Abraham to sacrifice his son" (p. 1). The answer to his family's plight, in turn, would also come from God. "We always thought that God would reveal himself in our situation and provide for our means" (p. 1). The much hoped for religious solution in this case precluded all other solutions. Not only did the man reject government assistance or help from charity, he and his wife also had over $3,500 in cash and bank accounts at the time of their son's death. This money, however, had been reserved as a tithe for God and, he felt, could not be used for food. The man firmly believed that God would be "the source of all food" for the family (p. 1).

The tragedy in this case should not be attributed to the appraisal of the financial problem as a spiritual test. This was, in fact, a positive reframing of a difficult situation, one that has proven helpful to many people. Even the decision to abandon human initiative and defer the control to God might have been appropriate in a truly uncontrollable situation. The tragedy was in the renunciation of personal control in conditions that called for it. To rely exclusively on religious resources in circumstances that require some degree of human initiative represents an error of religious control, or religious overcontrol, to be more specific.

It is important to point out that errors of control occur on the other side as well. The attempt to take personal control over events that are uncontrollable may be as dysfunctional as the deferral of control to God when the problem can be resolved through personal action. The former might be described as errors of personal overcontrol (or religious undercontrol) as opposed to errors of religious overcontrol. A study by Bickel and his colleagues (in press) is relevant here. Working with Presbyterian church members, they examined whether self-directing and collaborative forms of religious coping were a help or hindrance to people dealing with situations they perceived to be controllable and uncontrollable. Among church members faced with uncontrollable events, a more self-directing coping style was associated with *greater* depression. In striking contrast, a more collaborative coping style was associated with significant *reductions* in depression among those dealing with uncontrollable events. Neither coping style was related to depression for members in controllable situations. Friedel and Pargament (1995) reported similar findings in a study of emergency medical care professionals coping with stressful work-related situations.

These results are preliminary. We do not know whether similar findings would emerge from longitudinal research designs that permit stronger conclusions. Nevertheless, the findings are provocative. They seem to suggest that personal control and self-direction are counterproductive when people struggle with unmanageable events. Accepting the limits of personal power may be the more adaptive alternative in these situations. Is this the same as giving up? Not necessarily. Many in Bickel's sample were engaged in what they perceived to be a partnership with God in problem solving. In that partnership, they maintained some degree of active involvement for themselves, while looking to God for assistance. Power and responsibility were shared, and this collaborative approach appeared to be the more helpful style of coping with uncontrollable situations.

Whether it is an error of religious overcontrol or an error of personal overcontrol, the failure to read the demands of the situation accurately and draw upon the most appropriate resources can have unfortunate consequences, for when religious resources are not properly coordinated with the situation and with other resources, the coping process begins to disintegrate. Of course, this is not exactly a new idea. The Serenity Prayer, recited by members of 12-Step groups for many years, makes the same point, only more eloquently: "God grant me the serenity to accept things I cannot change, Courage to change things I can, and wisdom to know the difference."

Errors of Religious Moderation

It were better for sun and moon to drop from heaven, for the earth to fall, and for all the millions who are upon it to die of starvation in the extremist agony, so far as temporary affliction goes, than that one soul . . . should commit one single venial sin, should tell one willful untruth. (Cardinal Newman, 1833, cited in Seldes, 1985, p. 307)

Religion, with all the fervor and passion it is capable of generating, occasionally falls prey to excess. In some instances, the excess is merely rhetorical, as we hear in the words of Cardinal Newman. In other cases, the excess has more serious repercussions. Listen to a part of the rationale offered by one man who murdered his wife, three children, and mother:

> With [my daughter] being so determined to get into acting I was also fearful as to what that might do to her continuing to be a Christian. . . .
>
> Also, with [my wife] not going to church I knew that this would harm the children eventually. . . .
>
> At least I'm certain that all have gone to heaven now. If things had gone on who knows if this would be the case. . . .
>
> It may seem cowardly to have always shot from behind, but I didn't want any of them to know even at the last second that I had to do this. . . .
>
> I'm only concerned with making my peace with God and of this I am assured because of Christ dying even for me. ("Memorandum . . . ," 1990, p. 25)

Certainly, this is a dramatic, unusual case. Yet it remains true that excessive acts of all kinds, including violence toward one's own family, can be justified in the name of religion.

In a book entitled *Spare the Child: The Religious Roots of Punishment and the Psychological Impact of Physical Abuse*, Greven (1991) describes how certain religious writings, beliefs, and interpretations have provided legitimation for the physical discipline of children and, beyond that, child abuse (also see Capps, 1992). Physical violence, he notes, is far from a stranger to the world's major religions. Illustrations of vengeance, violence, sacrifice, and slaughter run throughout the great religious stories. In these same texts, the reader can also find religious advice that condones and even encourages corporal punishment (e.g., "Withhold not correction from the child; for if thou beatest him with the rod, he shall not die. Thou shalt beat him with the rod, and shalt deliver his soul from hell" (Proverbs 23:13–14)). According to some religious perspectives, it is the parents' duty to "break the will of the child," to turn the child away from his or her own natural inclinations to a life of devotion to God. While this "breaking of the will" may be restricted to appropriate forms of discipline, it may also cross the line between discipline and abuse.

Greven (1991) illustrates this point through the child-rearing advice of some modern-day religious advocates of corporal punishment. Some writers encourage parents to begin physical punishment while their children are still "in the cradle." Parents are told not to be troubled too greatly by minor injuries suffered through physical discipline. "Some children have very sensitive skin that will welt or even bruise quite easily. Parents should not be overly concerned if such minor injuries do result from their chastisement as it is perfectly normal" (Fugate 1980, cited in Greven, 1991, p. 80). Parents are warned not to take their child's tears too seriously. If anything, crying may be a cause for further punishment. "Real crying usually lasts two minutes or less, but may continue for five. After that point, the child is merely complaining, and the change can be recognized in the tone and intensity of the voice. I would require him to stop the protest crying, usually by offering him a little more of whatever caused the original tears" (Christenson, 1970, cited in Greven, 1991, p. 78). At times, this advice seems to go beyond the point of acceptable levels of discipline.

To be fair to the authors of these child-rearing manuals, it should be noted that most contain warnings to parents about the dangers of going too far in their use of physical punishment (see Bartkowski, 1995). Further, it is important to add, empirical studies have not addressed the question of whether religious involvement actually fosters child abuse. Although studies have shown that conservative Protestants (particularly those who believe in the literal truth of scriptures) are more likely to favor and use physical punishment with children (Ellison, Bartkowski, & Segal, 1996; Ellison & Sherkat, 1993; Grasmick, Bursik, & Kimpel, 1991), physical discipline has to be distinguished from physical abuse.

Do certain forms of religiousness, in fact, encourage child abuse? More research is needed to test Greven's (1991) controversial thesis. Even so, I believe he has made an important point. Religion should be called to task to the extent it has created a breeding ground in which the abuse of children is permitted.

In one sense, the type of religious excessiveness described by Greven can be viewed as another case of religious one-sidedness, of devotion to ends so great no room is left for anything else, including the feelings, values, and well-being of others.[2] "The problem," Wiesel (1992) writes, "is exaggerated love, fanatical love, which turns religion into a personal battlefield that is dangerous to others and demeaning to the very faith it professes to cherish" (p. 21). But the distortion here has as much to do with means as it does with ends. In the single-minded pursuit of an end, other people are not only devalued, they come to be seen as obstacles that must be manipulated, overcome, or eliminated. The goal is so important that any and all means are justifiable, even if they include violence to one's own family, even if they call for the extirpation of other religious groups that hold a different worldview, even if the means themselves undermine the goals that are so desperately desired, as in the case of the right-to-life proponent who murders an abortionist.

What we have here are excessive responses of systems under threat. In an effort to protect its values, the individual or group goes beyond marking its immediate boundaries to attacking others outside its circle. An experimental study by Dor-Shav, Friedman, and Tcherbonogura (1978) illustrates this process. They worked with two groups of female Israeli college students: One group defined itself as religious, the other as secular. The students were informed that they were participating in a study to determine "the level of general knowledge" of religious and irreligious people, as well as to determine "the effects of punishment in stamping out incorrect responses" (p. 219). The students listened to the responses of the religious and secular learners to religious and secular-content questions. The students were told that they could control the severity of the shocks they administered to the learners when they gave incorrect responses to the questions. Unbeknownst to the students, the learners were, in fact, confederates. No shocks were actually given.

Dor-Shav et al. predicted that the religious students would administer higher levels of shock following wrong answers to religious questions than to secular questions. This prediction was confirmed. The researchers believe that the wrong answers to the religious questions posed a threat to the values of the religious students and stimulated, in turn, aggressiveness to the learners. Interestingly, the researchers also found that the secular students (unlike their religious counterparts) administered stronger shocks to religious learners than to secular learners, irrespective of the content of the errors. Perhaps the religiousness of the learners represented a threat to the secular subjects, eliciting greater aggressiveness on their part. These latter findings are noteworthy, for they suggest that any group, religious or nonreligious, can go overboard in its response when significance is threatened.

Dramatic as it may be, fanaticism is only one error of religious moderation. Religion is as capable of apathy as it is of excess. Campbell and Pettigrew (1959) documented one particularly salient example of religious apathy—the response of clergy to the 1957 Little Rock crisis over the integration of black students into Central High School. Interviewing a cross-section of 29 clergy in this community, they found that only five of the sample were avowed segregationists. Even though the remainder were supportive of racial integration, most did not take an active role in promoting their beliefs as a religious imperative. For instance, on the Sunday before schools opened, only two of the clergy used their pulpit to voice their support for integration.

What accounted for the clergy's inaction at this crucial time? Campbell and Pettigrew cite a number of factors, most notably, the fears among the clergy of dissension in the church and criticism from their superiors. To have taken a more vocal stance, they believed, would have placed their ministries at risk. Given that the clergy were serving segregationist churches, their fears were likely quite realistic. Feedback from their own superiors in the church hierarchy only amplified these concerns. One administrator warned the clergy in his jurisdiction: "It's OK to be liberal, boys; just don't stick your neck out" (p. 514). And few did. In spite of the moral nature of this crisis, the clergy were largely silent.

Religious apathy represents a failure to mobilize the resources necessary to reach a goal. The cost of the effort may be perceived to be too great, the obstacles too many, the likelihood of success too remote. In any case, the individual or group remains where it is, unmoved. Instead of confronting a changing world, the system responds, in essence, by defending *against* change, even though other people and the system itself may suffer as a result.

Be it excess or apathy, problems arise when means are disproportionate to ends in coping. Solutions are likely to be effective only to the degree they are modulated to the demands of the situation and the goals of the individual. To the extent that religion is involved in disproportionate solutions, it contributes to problems of integration in coping. The same holds true for religion's involvement in faulty explanations and misused resources. Earlier in the book I noted that helping people stay on the right path is very much a religious concern. But, as we have seen here, religion itself occasionally accompanies people down the wrong road.

AGAINST THE WIND: PROBLEMS OF FIT

The search for significance takes place amidst social systemic forces that have pushes and pulls of their own. Families, organizations, and communities (like individuals) have their own preferred ways of thinking and acting as well as their own objects of value. Differences in these patterns of means and ends are what make systems, not just individuals, unique. We may fail to notice that our social systems have their own goals and preferred ways to reach them, but this does not mean that social systems are insignificant. Instead, it is an indication of social integration, a sign that our means and ends are meshing so nicely with those of the system that we pay no attention to the system. The search for significance goes more smoothly in these instances.

There are times, however, when people fall out of harmony with their groups, when individual purposes and methods for dealing with the world clash with those prescribed by social systems. What we search for in times of stress may be inconsistent with the system's goals of greatest value. What we would like from our social system in terms of coping assistance may conflict with what the social system is willing and able to provide. For instance, parents of children with physical and mental handicaps are often given religious inspirational literature by family and friends to help them cope with their situation. To some, however, the message in the literature may be far from particularly inspirational. Felker (1990) distributed one such inspirational poem to mothers of handicapped children and solicited their responses. In the poem, the handicapped child is described as a "special child" and the parents are cast as specially selected by the Lord to care for their "gift from Heaven." In essence, the situation is reframed from one of loss to one of religious opportunity. How did the parents respond?

The initial reactions to the poem were negative for a majority (58%) of the women. At the time of the interview, 40% of the women continued to feel negatively toward the poem. To some it suggested that God was not benevolent. "It's just stupid to say that—God helps me get through the rough days," one woman said, "he didn't give [the rough days] to me." Other women felt the poem minimized their pain and loss. As one mother put it, "They don't realize that it's worse than death. Not only is this not the baby you expected, but you are faced with what looks at the time like an overwhelming burden. Then someone says, you shouldn't feel bad because God did it" (p. 8). Not all women responded negatively to the poem. Those who felt comforted by it, however, were more likely to agree with its basic tenet, that God determines the shape of their lives.

There was nothing necessarily wrong with the message in this poem. Nor was there anything necessarily wrong with the negative reaction of many of the women. The problem was simply one of fit; designed to be inspirational for all, the message in fact clashed with the spiritual needs of many.

Problems of fit are not unusual in the religious realm. Religious social systems can run counter to where the individual wants to go and how he or she wants to get there. And when individual and social system rub against each other, friction and strain often result.

Several years ago, Elizabeth, a devout Christian woman, came to my office complaining of tension and anxiety. Eighteen months earlier, her young daughter had died in an accident. At first I thought her emotional troubles were connected directly to her daughter's death. But this was not the case. While she missed her daughter a great deal, Elizabeth spoke with great feeling about the comfort she drew from the knowledge that her daughter was in heaven with the angels, looking out for the well-being of the family. Was this belief a problem in and of itself? I did not think so. Many Christians (and members of other religious traditions) hold that this life is followed by a heavenly afterlife, and many people believe in angels as well. Elizabeth herself appeared to be functioning quite adequately in life, beliefs and all. I learned that her problems had more to do with the reactions of her extended family than her beliefs. It seemed that Elizabeth wanted her family to acknowledge her daughter's spiritual presence. She asked them to celebrate her daughter's birthday, visit her grave, and talk about her from time to time. The family, on the other hand, felt Elizabeth was "being weird about the whole thing." They had attended the funeral and helped Elizabeth through the first few months after, but what she was asking for was too much. From the family's perspective, it was time for Elizabeth to put the death behind her. They refused her requests, questioned her sanity, and encouraged her to get counseling. The tension and anxiety Elizabeth was experiencing was rooted not in pathological religious beliefs and practices, but in the contrasting visions held by Elizabeth and her family of how she should come to terms with her daughter's life and death.

Researchers have also found that tension and dissatisfaction often accompany a lack of fit between the individual and his or her religious system. For example, within the Church of Jesus Christ of Latter-Day Saints, a group that emphasizes the importance of marriage and family relationships, many single adults reportedly feel like second-class citizens; those that do appear to be at higher risk for depression (Rutledge & Spilka, 1993). Similarly, Roman Catholic women report more guilt and depression following an abortion than non-Catholics (Osofsky & Osofsky, 1972; Payne, Kravitz, Notman, & Anderson, 1976).

The consequences of misfit, in its milder forms, may be limited to feelings of strain and demoralization. Misfit, in some instances, may even have some advantages. For example, in one study of churches and synagogues, we asked clergy to nominate members who fit well in their congregation (i.e., those who basically shared or identified with the congregation's values, beliefs, and practices) and members who fit less well (Pargament, Tyler, & Steele, 1979b). The congregation members completed a battery of measures of psychosocial competence. "Nonfitters" reported less satisfaction with their congregations than "fitters." However, nonfitters also reported more active problem-solving skills, greater personal control, and higher self-efficacy than fitters. While marginal status in the congregation may have been uncomfortable for the nonfitters, it may have also encouraged greater independence and a more active coping orientation.

Problems of fit can have more serious implications for the individual when they are exacerbated by intolerance on the part of the system. Members of minority religious groups are especially vulnerable to pressures to conform to the dominant religious system. If they do not, they may face negative sanctions in the form of prejudice, scapegoating, and fanaticism. Rosenberg (1962) illustrates this point in a study comparing Protestant, Roman Catholic, and Jewish high school students who were reared in religiously consonant neighborhoods (75% or more coreligionists) with those raised in religiously dissonant neighborhoods (25% or less coreligionists). Protestants, Catholics, and Jews raised in a dissonant neighborhood were more likely to have lower self-esteem, greater depression, and more psychosomatic symptoms than their counterparts who grew up in religiously consonant environments. The explanation, Rosenberg believes, lies in the diminution of the values, traits, and behaviors of the religious minority by the dominant neighborhood group. In support of this interpretation, he goes on to note that the religiously dissonant students were more likely than others to report being teased, left out of things, or called names because of their religion. Those who experienced this type of bigotry, in turn, reported more psychosomatic symptoms, more depression, and lower self-esteem. Rosenberg concludes, the "qualities which may be accepted or admired in one's own group may be rejected by members of another group. Hence, there is a real likelihood that one will feel different when in a dissonant social context, and this sense of difference may lead the individual to question himself, doubt himself, wonder whether he is unworthy" (p. 9).

There are many worthwhile destinations in coping and many roads to reach them. The problems of fit we have considered so far arise when there is no room for differences, when individual or system cannot tolerate the assortment of means and ends that make up viable approaches to coping. But what happens when an individual or system's approach to significance is, in fact, flawed? Here we have to be more careful in applying the criterion of fit to coping.

A Time and Place for Not Fitting

Consider the individual who is on the right track in a system that is seriously misguided. Is it best for the person to adjust to a dysfunctional system, such as a totalitarian state? A case could be made for *misfit* in these types of settings as the better alternative. In his interviews with 27 Christians who risked their lives to rescue Jews from the Nazis in World War II, London (1970) notes that social marginality was one of the rescuers' characteristic features. One man had grown up in Prussia with a mother who spoke a dialect different from others in the area, refused to go to church, and had no political affiliation. On top of that, he had a problem with stuttering that set him further apart from his community. Yet he helped organize an underground network responsible for saving several hundred people in Russia and Western Europe. London suggests that the experience of marginality (misfit) enabled this rescuer and others to persist in their heroic efforts despite the accompanying social isolation and threats to their own survival.

On the face of it, misfit would seem preferable to the kind of adjustment in which individual and system walk hand in hand to their destruction. Perhaps that would be true if these were the only two choices. But there is an alternative to unending alienation or acquiescence. The system itself can be transformed. Rather than "go with the flow," the answer may be to redirect the stream. In fact, this is just what the rescuers of the Jews tried to do. They did not settle for a passive marginality; their actions represented a challenge to the system. In effect, they helped create a world more fitting with their own ideals.

Fit with what? The evaluation of individual–systems fit cannot be fully separated from the evaluation of pathways and destinations (Pargament, Johnson, Echemendia, & Silverman, 1985). Misfit may have considerable value if it is accompanied by efforts to turn dysfunctional systems into systems worth fitting. To be sure, this type of active marginality has its costs. Just consider the price many rescuers paid for opposing the Nazis. But, the alternative, to acquiesce to a system gone awry, has terrible consequences of its own, consequences that extend beyond individual lives to the integrity of society as a whole.

NO SINGLE BEST WAY TO COPE

I have illustrated some of the ways religion fails in the coping process. The focus has not been on specific beliefs or practices that are harmful in and of themselves; instead, attention has been focused on problems of integration among the dimensions of coping. From this perspective, *there is no single right road, no single right direction, but rather many potentially worthwhile destinations and pathways to reach them.* People run into trouble in coping not because they have failed to discover the only solution to their problems, but because the process itself is out of kilter. When ends become unbalanced, when means become disconnected from ends and from the demands of life situations, and when individual and system work against each other, the flow of coping is disrupted. As we have seen, religion can contribute to these problems. Occasionally, religion accompanies people or even leads them down the wrong road.

The critical question that remains unanswered is "Why?" How do we account for the failures of religion in coping? An answer to this question would require a book in itself. But I will offer a few tentative thoughts before concluding this chapter.

ACCOUNTING FOR THE FAILURES
OF RELIGION IN COPING

Several years ago, I received one of those late night phone calls we all dread. A friend of mine, Ruth, had killed herself. I knew that Ruth had been depressed over a series of recent losses: Her husband had left her for another woman, her mother had died, and work was difficult. Even so, the news came as a terrible shock to me. Ruth was a wonderful, loving person. She seemed to have so many things going for her—a child she cared about deeply, the friendship of many people, a history of bouncing back from adversity, and the help of a psychotherapist. I had thought that Ruth had turned the corner of her depression and was well on her way to rebuilding her life. And, perhaps she had. But on the night of her suicide, I later learned, she had suffered yet another humiliating rejection from another man.

For a long time after, I struggled to make sense of Ruth's death. Like many others left behind by suicide, I asked myself whether I could have done more to help. My initial reaction was to see Ruth's decision to kill herself as purely impulsive—that the pain of her most recent romantic rejection was so intense and her hopelessness so great, she chose to eliminate her pain by eliminating herself. Ruth did have resources she could have used to help her that night, it seemed to me, and she had other things to strive for besides her relationships with men, but she lost touch with all of that. In one impulsive moment, ending the pain became the only thing that mattered.

However, to see Ruth's suicide only as a single impulsive act essentially removed her death from the context of her life. She had, after all, suffered loss and rejection in the past without attempting to hurt herself. Impulsive as it was, the reality was that Ruth's suicide came only after a succession of losses had depleted her and pushed her past her breaking point. Had her resources been stronger or had she been able to access them more fully, I believe she would have lived. On the other hand, had she experienced less rejection and loss, I believe she also would have survived. Pushed beyond her capacities, she fell apart.

In some sense, Ruth is no different from the rest of us. We all have our breaking points, the point where we can no longer keep ourselves together. What determines where that breaking point is? Two things: the severity of the attack on significance and the ability of the orienting system to withstand these attacks. We are at our most vulnerable when our deepest values are touched by events for which we have the fewest resources and the heaviest burdens (see Figure 11.1). To put it another way, we are more likely to become "disoriented" when the threats, challenges, or losses to significance exceed the capacity of the orienting system.

Conditions of high stress jeopardize not only significance, but also resources for sustaining significance. When that happens, old, formerly successful ways of coping may become unworkable and we may be left completely befuddled, unsure of where to go or how to get there. With sufficient stress, desperate alternatives that never would have been considered become more available and more compelling. I believe this was the case with Ruth. It was also the case with the Doomsday Cult members described by Festinger et al. (1956; see Chapter 6, this volume) who turned to their cataclysmic view of the world only after repeated failures to find significance through mainstream involvements.

A similar process may also help to explain the increased popularity of the occult among Jews in Israel. Psychologist Benjamin Beit-Hallahmi

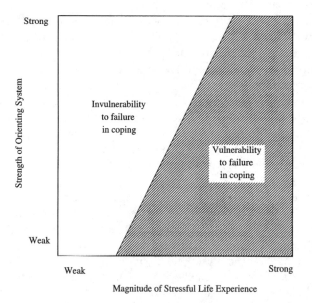

FIGURE 11.1. Vulnerability to failures in coping as a function of the strength of the orienting system and the magnitude of stressful life experiences.

(1992) chronicles the large numbers of Israelis who have become involved in astrology, graphology, numerology, palm reading, even "foot reading" in recent decades. He attributes this and other fundamental changes in Israeli society to the 1973 Yom Kippur war. Until that point, Beit-Hallahmi maintains, Israelis had a feeling of self-confidence, hope, and optimism about their individual and collective futures. And why not? They had met and triumphed against wave after wave of assault by enemy countries. But the Yom Kippur war changed all that. The war took the much admired defense forces by surprise; many were injured, killed, or taken prisoner in the conflict. The confidence in the future of the state was replaced by the feeling that Israel was living on the edge of disaster, and might continue to do so for the foreseeable future. Beit-Hallahmi writes that the Yom Kippur war shattered the "illusion of Israeli invincibility and invulnerability" (p. 133). Terrorism, economic crises, the Lebanon war, and the *intifada* of recent years have only added to this sense of precariousness. All of these stressors, Beit-Hallahmi believes, have led to a crisis of significance. With the Zionist dream so deeply threatened, Israelis have struggled to find new sources of significance. The rise of interest in the occult, which may seem incomprehensible to those who look at Israel from afar, can be understood as one reflection of the desperate lengths people will go to in their search for salvation when the world blocks the realization of old dreams.

The "breaking point" in coping comes not only from attacks on significance, but from limitations in the orienting system. It is an axiom of coping that people are not helpless in the face of life stress. The orienting system of general beliefs, practices, relationships, and emotions can anchor people through stormy times. But, as noted earlier, not all orienting systems are alike. Some are characterized by greater resources and fewer burdens than others. By virtue of its ability to generate well-integrated solutions, the stronger orienting system can withstand considerable pain, loss, and deprivation. Weaker, "disoriented" systems are more likely to generate poorly integrated solutions and, in this sense, prove vulnerable to even slight change. It is these differences in the strength of the orienting system that help to explain why some of us are able to withstand major life stressors, while others seem to crumble at the first sign of trouble.

Religion can add strength to the orienting system or weaken it. Certain forms of general religious commitment and involvement have been tied to resources such as optimism (Sethi & Seligman, 1993), self-esteem (Benson & Spilka, 1973), subjective well-being (Witter, Stock, Okun, & Haring, 1985), psychosocial competence (Pargament et al., 1979), social support (Taylor & Chatters, 1988), and marital satisfaction (Wilson & Filsinger, 1986). But other general, dispositional characteristics of religion appear to be part of an inadequate orienting system, one that may contribute to the specific failures of religion in coping. I consider a few of these religious culprits in the following sections.

Undifferentiated Religion

One of the most basic of all psychological principles is that development proceeds from states of globality to states of greater differentiation. Delivered into a world of continuous experience, the infant begins to create some order. Making distinctions is a central part of this process. Lines have to be drawn (Zerubavel, 1991). Where does the physical self end and the world begin? Where is it that dreams stop and reality starts? Who is a caretaker and who is not? What is good and what is bad? With development comes greater discrimination and more finely tuned response. Watching my sons advance through Little League baseball, I have been amazed at the rapid progression from the comedic ballet of the "peewee" players (who literally throw themselves into every toss of the ball) to the agile acrobatics of "senior" players only 5 years older.

The capacity of the organism to make finely differentiated physiological responses, tailored to particular stressors is a prerequisite for survival. As Hinkle (1974) notes: "An animal which responded to a bacterial infection of its lung by creating inflammation in its left ankle would not live very long" (p. 351).

Differentiation in the psychological and social spheres is just as necessary for survival. Existence depends on the articulation and knowledge of basic differences within the self, life situations, and the world: that the self is capable of some things and incapable of others, that some situations are harmless and others are not, that some people are trustworthy and others are not. Without a differentiated orienting system, the individual would be incapable of understanding or dealing with everyday demands. Life would be an incomprehensible blur and the response to it would be primitive and stereotyped. A more differentiated system, however, equips the person with a broader repertoire of responses, more capable of coping with a wider range of life experiences. In this vein, some empirical research suggests that greater self-differentiation and a larger set of coping options facilitates adjustment to life crises (Collins et al., 1990; Linville, 1987).

Differentiation is also important in the religious realm. In fact, the first acts of creation, according to Judeo-Christian tradition, were acts of division. The separation of light from darkness, the division of water and land, and the days of creation that followed are successive differentiations. Religious traditions are vitally concerned about differences: how virtue differs from sin, what is sacred and what is profane, who is a member and who is not a member of the group, pathways to follow and pathways to avoid. Distinctions such as these are summarized in shorthand form through commandments, catechisms, and codes. But most religious groups do not stop there. Over the centuries, religious leaders and sages have developed rich commentaries and theologies that elaborate further upon these basic distinctions. Killing is said to be generally wrong, but it may be justifiable in some situations. Even though marriage is a sacred covenant, the contract can, in some instances, be nullified or broken. Finer distinctions of this sort make the tradition relevant to a wider range of life demands.

Many people, however, are not aware of the fine distinctions among beliefs, practices, and moral codes that are a part of their faiths. What they know mostly about are the shorthand summaries. A few of the Ten Commandments or a few of the catechisms from Sunday school may be recalled. As an ironic footnote to this, religious education often ends in adolescence, just when the young adult is developing the capacity to engage in and appreciate the more abstract, differentiated thinking of the tradition. What many people take from their religious education are the abbreviated guidelines for living and summaries of doctrine that cannot provide an adequate response to life's multiple challenges. Of course, this is not true of everyone. Certain forms of personal religious orientation have been associated with greater religious differentiation and cognitive complexity (e.g., Batson & Raynor-Prince, 1983; Nielsen & Fultz, 1991). Those who lack a well-differentiated religious orienting system, however, appear to be vulnerable to major life stressors.

The problems with undifferentiated religion often manifest themselves when people encounter pain. The greatest religious minds have struggled with the question of how we understand and come to terms with pain, suffering, and evil for thousands of years, and even they have been unable to arrive at a universally satisfying answer. It seems clear that there are no easy solutions when it comes to the problem of pain. On the contrary, simple solutions to difficult problems, including religious ones, can make matters worse. Let us take a look at a few examples.

Submit to God's Will

According to some traditions, we are duty-bound to submit to whatever we face, including pain and suffering, since everything that happens in the world is part of God's plan. While this belief offers comfort and reassurance that there is an ultimate meaning in all of our encounters, it can lead to errors of explanation and errors of control in coping, unless some role for other causal factors and human agency is differentiated from this general belief. Baider and De-Nour (1987) illustrated this point in an interview study of Arab Muslims who had had a mastectomy. They found that none of the women discovered the lump by touching it, and only 3 of the 10 women reported seeing the lump. Several did not realize they had a problem until symptoms of the disease were advanced (e.g., pain and bleeding), and most of the women did not tell others about the problem until precious months had gone by. Even well after their mastectomies, few of the women had any information about their disease or the operation.

The passivity of the Muslim women in response to their life-threatening illness was embedded in the basic predeterministic belief of their traditional culture. As one woman said: "It is God's will what happens to me, and I am here just to obey God. God is with me and my fate is his." Another spoke more pointedly to the interviewer: "It is not in our power to decide our destiny. You, or doctors, cannot help me because it is beyond human decisions. Illnesses are part of our destiny" (p. 9).

It is important to note that other Muslim groups have demonstrated a more differentiated view of disease and medical treatment (e.g., Ide & Sanli, 1992). The problem experienced by the women in the Baider and De-Nour study was rooted not in Islam, but rather in their undifferentiated approach to Islam. Their lives were jeopardized because they were unable to articulate a role for forces other than the divine in the way they understood and handled their illness.

Ignore the Negative Side of Life

Another response to the problem of pain and suffering in the world is to minimize it, to overlook it, or even to deny that it exists. In its strongest form, this perspective views the negative as an absence of the positive rather than as a reality in itself; evil represents the absence of love, not a force with a palpable quality of its own. This tendency to ignore the negative side of life, James (1902) wrote, is the essence of healthy-minded religion, a religion that refuses to "make much" of the "evil aspects of the universe" (p. 125). James went on to note that, while healthy-minded religion has its advantages, it is ultimately an incomplete orientation: "because the evil facts which it refuses positively to account for are a genuine portion of reality; and they may after all be the best key to life's significance, and possibly the only openers of our eyes to the deepest levels of truth" (p. 160).

A religious frame of reference that fails to face and respond to the negative side of life cannot sustain the individual through the most painful of life's experiences. Several years ago, I counseled a depressed woman who had been abused by her parents for many years. Although the physical abuse had ended after her marriage, the emotional abuse continued. Her parents would greet her on the phone with "Hello, Fatso" and would taunt her for being "big, dumb, and lazy." In spite of the mistreatment, my client kept her feelings to herself and continued to visit her parents weekly. Why, I asked, didn't she confront her parents more directly? She responded by noting that the Bible says to honor thy mother and father. This undifferentiated religious view was not the only reason for my client's predicament, but it was partly to blame for her failure to take better care of herself. Her religious beliefs gave her no room to examine the maliciousness of her parents, nor did they give her room to express her own feelings of pain; anger, from her religious perspective, was sinful. Part of the work of therapy was to encourage a more differentiated religious framework.

Many people, however, are reluctant to take a critical look at their religion. My students and I encountered this problem in our efforts to help churches and synagogues identify their strengths and weaknesses (the Congregation Development Program; Pargament et al., 1991). In completing a very comprehensive survey about church/synagogue life (over 500 items), some members would not make a single critical comment about their congregation. We did not know whether these members were reporting accurately on congregations that were, in fact, exemplary, or whether they were refusing to admit to themselves or outsiders that their congregations had some problems. To try to sort this out, we developed a measure of "indiscriminate proreligiousness" made up of items so extreme that they are, in reality, unlikely to be true (Pargament et al., 1987). We administered this measure to members of three churches and a sample of college students. The number of participants agreeing with these items was surprising to us. For example, one-fourth of adults and students agreed that "I am always inspired by the sermon topics (in my congregation)." Over one-third of the participants agreed that "I always live by my religious beliefs." Almost two-thirds of adults and students agreed that "Differences of opinion are always welcome in (my) congregation." Clearly, many people were unable or unwilling to describe their congregations in less than ideal terms. Indiscriminate proreligiousness is not hard to understand. It protects the faith from threat. Unfortunately, it also protects the faith against the critical scrutiny that is so necessary for religious development and growth. Ignoring the negative side of religion leaves the individual ill-equipped to cope with events that call for religious change.

No Room for Redemption

James (1902) contrasted healthy-minded religion with the religion of the sick-souled. While the former has little stomach for the disagreeable aspects of existence, the latter has trouble seeing beyond suffering and sinfulness. James was respectful of the willingness of the sick-souled to look squarely at the horrors of a world in which "every individual existence goes out in a lonely spasm of helpless agony" (p. 160). However, he also pointed out, the religion of the morbid-minded brings with it self-contempt, dread, and melancholy, and may be incomplete in its own way: "As the healthy-minded enthusiast succeeds in ignoring evil's very existence, so the subject of melancholy is forced in spite of himself to ignore that of all good whatever: For him it may no longer have the least reality" (p. 142).

We get some sense of this total preoccupation with the dark side in John Bunyan's autobiographic account of his religious melancholy: "I was more loathsome in my own eyes than was a toad; and I thought I was so in God's eyes too. Sin and corruption, I said, would as naturally bubble out of my heart as water would bubble out of a fountain. I could have changed heart with anybody, I thought none but the Devil himself could equal me for inward wickedness and pollution of mind" (cited in James, 1902, p. 155). Later in life, Bunyan was to experience a religious conversion. At this point, however, there was no place in his religious orientation for atonement, purification, or redemption. Lacking these elements, Bunyan was ill-equipped to deal with the demands of his life.

Watson, Morris, and Hood (1988) illustrated the same point in a series of empirical studies with Christian college students. From the Christian perspective, they note, those who are unable to see beyond their own sense of personal sinfulness and guilt in the world have succeeded at defining the problem, but have failed to locate the solution—the possibility of forgiveness and grace through God. "Through confession, believers can ease their struggle against personal fallibility by laying claim to divine pardon" (p. 350). Watson et al. tried to quantify this sense of grace through a brief self-report measure made up of items such as "My sins are forgiven" and "Grace entered my life when I was forgiven for my sins." In contrast to a measure of guilt, the grace scale was associated with lower levels of depression, less exploitiveness (Watson, Hood, Foster, & Morris, 1988), lower levels of emotional irresponsibility (Watson, Morris, et al., 1988), and higher levels of self-esteem (Watson et al., 1985). Particularly relevant to this discussion was their finding that when the statistical effects of grace were removed from the analysis, stronger relationships were found between guilt and anxiety and depression (Watson, Morris, et al., 1988). In plainer language, the effects of guilt appeared to be softened by grace. Once this opportunity for resolution was removed from the equation (literally and figuratively), guilt became more problematic.

I have reviewed only a few of the possible forms of religious undifferentiation. Whatever form it takes, an undifferentiated religion leaves the individual vulnerable to challenges, particularly to challenges to the "undifferentiated zone" of the orienting system. A call for personal agency cannot be heard by those who believe they must submit to everything they encounter. A traumatic event cannot by assimilated by those who believe pain is merely illusion. A plea for help cannot be answered by those who feel they are beyond redemption and have nothing to give. The undifferentiated religious system proves to be a burden in coping because it is incapable of generating an adequate repertoire of responses to the full range of life events.

Fragmented Religion

Differentiation does not in itself make for an effective religious orienting system. Not only must distinctions be made in the religious realm, the bits and pieces must be put together into some sort of coherent whole. But this is easier said than done. As religion has become less a cultural given and more a private affair, people have felt greater freedom to pick and choose their own particular pattern of religious beliefs, practices, motivations, and institutional involvements. The end product is not always harmonious. "Religion à la carte," Bibby (1987) argues, has led to religious fragmentation for many people.

Bibby reached his conclusion through a series of large-scale surveys of Canadian adults in the 1970s and 1980s. If the committed Christian is defined by a set of core beliefs, practices, experiences, and knowledge, then only a small proportion of the Canadian population appears to be committed. Although 90% of Canadians are Roman Catholic or Protestant, Bibby found that only 20% of them (1) believe in God, the divinity of Jesus Christ, and an afterlife; (2) engage in private prayer; (3) have had an experience of being in God's presence; and (4) know who the disciple Peter was. In fact, only one in three Christians who call themselves "committed" demonstrated this core of belief, practice, experience, and knowledge. One Anglican housewife commented: "I believe in God but do not believe in the divinity of Jesus." Another science administrator wrote: "I believe in Jesus Christ but have doubts about immortality" (p. 82).

Bibby presents evidence that a mixture of conventional and less conventional beliefs, practices, and experiences appears to be taking the place of adherence to a traditional religious core. For instance, 75% of Canadians report reading their horoscope at least occasionally (more than the 45% who report reading the Bible), about 50% feel they have experienced mental telepathy, and almost 25% believe it is possible to communicate with the dead. Those who attend religious services weekly were only slightly less likely than their less observant counterparts to report beliefs in astrology, extrasensory perception (ESP), and psychic powers.

Fragmentation also appears between organized and personal forms of religious expression. For increasing numbers of people, Bibby reports, the church has become less and less relevant to spiritual life. One mother notes: "I've been through a great deal in life and my faith is very strong. But I believe that one is closer to God in their own home and garden than a church. I see going to church these days as 'keeping up with the Joneses' " (p. 83). This is not to say that religious institutions have been entirely abandoned. Bibby finds that even infrequent attenders expect to participate in various church rites. For example, 90% of inactive Anglicans in the Toronto diocese feel they have the right to church baptisms, marriages, and burials. As one inactive Anglican said: "Just because people don't attend Church doesn't mean they don't believe in God and shouldn't be able to be baptized, married, and buried in a church, which represents God" (p. 77).

It is not that religion has been discarded, Bibby asserts. Instead, it has been transformed. "The gods of old have been neither abandoned nor replaced," he concludes. "Rather, they have been broken into pieces and offered to religious consumers in piecemeal form" (p. 85).

Fragmentation between Religion and the Other Sides of Life

The resulting mosaic is not necessarily well integrated. Clergy speak with frustration of their "C & E's" (Christmas- and Easter-only members), who compartmentalize religion from day-to-day behavior, reserving it exclusively for special occasions. Troubling inconsistencies can grow out of the fractionalization between the religious realm and other aspects of the orienting system. For example, Brutz and Allen (1986) studied the relationship between peace activism, religious commitment, and marital violence among Quaker husbands and wives. They reasoned that commitment to the principles of the Society of Friends should be associated with lower levels of marital violence. For the sample as a whole, this appeared to be the case. Religious participation and commitment were related to less marital violence overall. However, a closer look at their findings revealed an unsuspected result related to peace activism, an important expression of Quaker principles. As expected, Quaker wives who were more involved in peace activism reported lower levels of violence in their marriage. Involvement in peace activism for the Quaker husbands, however, was associated with *higher* levels of marital violence, particularly for husbands who were less committed to the Society of Friends. Brutz and Allen suggest that peace activism is consistent with the societal norms of nonaggressiveness for women. Men, on the other hand, are exposed to norms of aggressiveness, and their involvement in peace activism may be difficult to reconcile with this societal expectation. We are left with a disconcerting sign of fragmentation: men who are involved in religiously based efforts to bring about world peace who are violent to their wives at home.

Fragmentation between Religious Belief and Practice

Fractures can also be found *within* the religious orienting system. Among the most common divisions are those between religious commitments and religious practices. I recall a discussion with a graduate student in psychology who rather forcefully stated that she was not religious. She went on to admit, however, that she planned to send her young daughter to Catholic school. When I asked her about this seeming contradiction, she said that if she happened to be wrong about religion, she did not want her daughter to suffer. "I want my daughter to be covered," she said, "just in case there is a hell." I wondered how she would explain her own religious disaffiliation to her daughter, and how she would help her daughter come to terms with the differences between what she was learning in school and what she was learning at home. Would the daughter see the mother, and perhaps herself, as hypocritical? Would their rituals be hollow? Would the daughter continue the intergenerational progression toward a vestigial form of religion? At that point in time, the graduate student had not given much thought to the inconsistency between her religious beliefs and religious practices, nor to the implications of these contradictions for her daughter or herself.

There is some empirical evidence that these types of belief–behavior discrepancies may be disadvantageous. Several years ago, my colleagues and I (Pargament et al., 1979) examined differences in the levels of psychosocial competence of four groups of church and synagogue members: frequent attenders at religious services who were highly religiously committed, infrequent attenders who reported low religious commitment, infrequent attenders who were highly committed, and frequent attenders who indicated low religious commitment. Of the four groups, only the frequent attenders–low committed revealed less psychosocial competence. Compared to the other three groups, they showed a lower sense of personal control, lower self-esteem, less trust in others, and less active coping skills. How did we interpret this finding? It seemed that whether the individual attended services frequently or infrequently, and whether the individual was more or less religiously committed, was less critical than whether the individual demonstrated *consistency* in practice and commitment. Of the four groups, it was the group of uncommitted–frequent attenders who were the least religiously inte-grated, participating in religious life without religious conviction. We concluded that the congruence between beliefs and practices may be as important for the well-being of the individual as the nature of the beliefs and practices themselves. Other researchers have reported findings that lead to a similar conclusion: An active religious commitment, or no religion at all, may be preferable to religion of the half-hearted kind (Hannay, 1980; Ross, 1990).

Fragmentation between Religious Motivation and Religious Practice

Belief–behavior discrepancies are closely related to another important form of fragmentation within the religious orienting system—rifts be-tween motivation and practice. Religion serves many different legitimate purposes, but certain purposes are not well suited to religious practice. Seeking out business connections, sociability, looking for personal com-fort—these motivations are, in Allport's (1950) word, "extrinsic" to the central purpose of religion. However, while Allport seemed to suggest that these functions are problematic in and of themselves, I would maintain that there is not anything inherently wrong with them. Most of us are motivated to improve our work lives, our personal comfort, and our relationships with others. The problem lies not in these purposes per se, but in their lack of fit with the essential design of religion. Religion is, as it has been defined here, a search for significance in ways related to the *sacred*. The sacred is, in one form or another, the organizing force for religious expression. It is important to recall that any purpose can become spiritualized, a more intrinsic part of religion. But to the extent that they are devoid of any spiritual connection, motivations such as a desire for personal well-being or closeness with others are poorly suited to the most basic purposes of religion—to bring people closer to God.

Guilt and external pressures may be similarly mismatched motivations for religious practice. Along these lines, one group of researchers distin-guished between two types of religious involvement—one based on "Iden-tification" and the other based on "Introjection" (Ryan, Rigby, & King, 1993). In the former approach, the individual feels that his or her religious beliefs, practices, and values are personally chosen. The individual prays and goes to church because they are satisfying acts in and of themselves. In the latter approach, religious involvement is motivated more by guilt, anxiety, and external pressure. The fear of disapproval from others or oneself pushes the person to pray or attend religious services. Ryan et al. developed scales to measure these two religious approaches and administered these scales, along with measures of mental health, to a variety of Christian samples. Scores on the internalized religious measures were consistently associated with better mental health and higher self-esteem. Religious introjection, on the other hand, was consistently tied to poorer mental health and lower self-esteem. Others have reported similar results (Echemendia & Pargament, 1982; O'Connor & Vallerand, 1990). Once again, problems arise with a religion motivated by matters that are divorced from the essential purpose of religion.

In this section, I have considered some of the problems that accompany religious fragmentation. It does not follow that religious systems have to be perfectly unified. Recently, I watched a television interview with two grieving parents who had lost all six of their children in a terrible accident. Noticing their composure in the face of this loss, the interviewer asked them how they managed to make sense out of such a horrendous trauma. The father admitted that he could not understand it. Some things were beyond his ken, he felt. But, he also had faith that God held the answer: "His thoughts are not our thoughts. He has his reasons. We don't have to know his reasons. We have confidence and love in the Lord." The belief that there was an ultimate explanation helped sustain the parents, despite the limits in their religious understanding.

Few people have airtight, comprehensive religious orienting systems capable of responding to each and every exigency of living. Built into most religious perspectives, however, is a tolerance for some inconsistency and fragmentation. People can hold on to themselves and their religions, imperfect orienting systems and all.

But if there are too many holes and inconsistencies—if the religious realm is too disconnected from the secular, if practices are unrelated to beliefs, if motivations have little to do with practices—the orienting system loses its ability to guide the individual through troubled times. The religious beliefs prove empty, the institutions alien, and the rituals hollow. Fragmented as it is, religion becomes another burden in coping, for all it has to offer are piecemeal solutions to complicated problems.

Religious Rigidity

A well-differentiated, unified orienting system is a necessary condition for effective coping, but it is not a sufficient condition. The system must also be flexible.

"He was a simple man who died of complications." So goes the epitaph of one man who apparently preferred to hold on to a simpler way of looking at things when change may have been in order. The capacity to adapt to change, internal and external, is an important resource for coping (e.g., Collins et al., 1990; Wheaton, 1983). Rigidity, on the other hand, increases vulnerability to new, increasingly complex situations.

Religious people have often been accused of rigidity. One of my former students, a member of the Church of Jesus Christ of Latter-Day Saints, spoke to me of an encounter he had with a psychologist who said: "You religious types have difficulty with rigid thinking." My student neatly turned the tables on the psychologist by asking: "Do you see that as a problem with *all* religious types?" As this small encounter illustrates, rigidity is not the exclusive domain of the religious. Neither does it appear to be true that religious people are necessarily rigid. For instance, in a comparative study of members of conservative and mainline Lutheran churches, we found that the conservative members reported higher levels of religious commitment and involvement than mainline members (Pargament, Echemendia, et al., 1987). Contrary to the stereotype about rigidity among religious conservatives, however, the conservative members described their churches as *more* open to change and *more* supportive of member's autonomy than the mainline members. Furthermore, the two groups of members did not differ in their reported tolerance for diversity. We concluded that orthodox beliefs (e.g., the divinity of Jesus Christ, the Second Coming, life after death), the defining feature of religious conservatism, are not necessarily held in a rigid manner. "In fact," we suggested, "the commitment of the members to conservative beliefs may provide them with the security to consider new approaches, ideas, and practices in the congregation" (p. 282). Others have also reported orthodox religious beliefs to be generally unrelated or negatively related to indices of social prejudice (Altemeyer & Hunsberger, 1992; Kirkpatrick, 1993a).

One form of religiousness, however, has been implicated in prejudice—fundamentalism. Working with five samples of college students, Kirkpatrick (1993a) found that religious fundamentalism was associated with more discriminatory attitudes toward blacks, women, homosexuals, and communists. Similarly, Altemeyer and Hunsberger (1992) reported consistent relationships between fundamentalism (as well as lower religious quest) and prejudice toward a wide range of minority groups. Some of their specific findings were particularly disconcerting. Higher fundamentalism and lower quest scale scores were associated with a greater willingness to support the arrest, torture, and execution of political "radicals" and more agreement with the belief that "the AIDS disease currently killing homosexuals is just what they deserve" (p. 123). Although fundamentalism has been studied most often among Christians, Hunsberger (1996) has reported a link between fundamentalism and prejudice toward homosexuals among other religious groups—Hindus, Muslims, and Jews.

These studies do not suggest that fundamentalism is tantamount to aggressiveness and prejudice. The correlations are not *that* strong. Clearly, not all fundamentalists are prejudiced. Nevertheless, the statistical link between the two cannot be dismissed. What is it about fundamentalism that may increase the vulnerability to prejudice? The rigidity of fundamentalists at both personal and social levels may be at least partly to blame.

At the personal level, fundamentalism involves a commitment to an inerrant set of teachings about God and humanity, and to an unchanging set of life practices (Altemeyer & Hunsberger, 1992). This commitment leaves little room for personal interpretation or modifications. Religious leaders or writings are authoritative and are not to be questioned. This unwillingness to question religion may leave the individual vulnerable to a changing, increasingly diverse world. In this vein, lower levels of "religious questing" have been associated with higher levels of prejudice in several studies (see Batson et al., 1993).

Inflexibility is also a part of fundamentalism at the social level. Fundamentalism assumes its adherents have a special relationship with God and must engage in continual battle with evil forces. To maintain this worldview, rigid walls are built against potentially threatening ideas, practices, and people. But fundamentalism does not stop there, for active steps may be taken to protect the faith from contamination. In the fight against evil, lifestyles that go against the teachings of the faith are not necessarily overlooked; they are challenged. If change does not occur, these lifestyles may be discredited or denigrated. Thus, Glock and Stark (1966) found that Christians who see themselves as "singularly possessed of the one true faith" (p. 21) are also more likely to agree that "Jews can never be forgiven for what they did to Jesus until they accept Him as the True Saviour" and "The reason the Jews have so much trouble is because God is punishing them for rejecting Jesus" (pp. 96–97). This is not a process of marking boundaries, but rather an *overmarking* of boundaries. Again, not all fundamentalists are prejudiced. However, fundamentalism does appear to be linked to personal and social rigidity, which, in turn, may leave its adherents vulnerable to errors of religious moderation—attacks against peoples and perspectives that are perceived as threats to the religious tradition.[3]

Of course, it is important to note that a rigid religious orienting system offers its members the benefits of a clear view of the world and a clear sense of direction about how life should and should not be lived. These are powerful incentives for many people, particularly those lacking control and direction in their lives. It should be added that the rigid religious system may be quite effective as long as it operates in a predictable, stable, and homogeneous environment. Diversity and change, however, reveal the flaws in the system. Unable to get along with (or avoid) others who profess or practice a different way of life, the religiously rigid may respond by lashing out. The unfortunate victims of this process may be members of minority groups or other religious traditions, rather than the religiously rigid themselves. But the religiously rigid may also flounder, given enough uncertainty and change. Conway and Siegelman (1982), for instance, assert that individuals who leave cults are vulnerable to psychopathology, particularly those who were more involved in the cult's activities. Acknowledging that these data are controversial, Kirkpatrick, Hood, and Hartz (1991) suggest several reasons why leaving a cult could lead to problems in adjustment, among them the lack of knowledge among cult members about alternate points of view and the difficulty in facing new, contradictory beliefs.

The power of any religious system lies in its ability to offer compelling answers to life's most pressing and profound questions. As these questions change, the religious system must also be able to bend and flex if it is to remain viable. This is not to say we need more wishy-washy religion; as we have seen, undifferentiation and fragmentation in the religious realm create problems of their own. But flexibility and a strong commitment to a well-differentiated, well-integrated religion are not necessarily incompatible. McIntosh and his colleagues identified groups of people who were both religiously flexible (as measured by quest and religious seeking scales) *and* strongly committed to their faith (as evidenced by the intrinsic religiousness scale). Moreover, those who held this flexible/complex/central approach to religion reported fewer physical health symptoms (McIntosh & Spilka, 1990), greater well-being, and better adjustment to an aversive life event (McIntosh, Inglehart, & Pacini, 1990). Thus, flexibility should not be confused with fuzziness. As Zerubavel (1991) notes, "Flexibility need not entail giving up structure altogether. It does imply, however, dynamic, elastic mental structures. Such structures would allow us to break away from the mental cages into which we so often lock ourselves, yet still avoid chaos. With them, we can be creative as well as secure" (p. 122).

Insecure Religious Attachment

True religion, according to the world's theistic faiths, is about God. Not a God divorced from humanity, but a God and a people who embrace each other. From most religious perspectives, whether we believe in God is less important than the nature of our relationship with the divine, and who we become through that relationship. The encounter with the divine has been described in many ways. Assorted expressions of attitudes and feelings toward God fill the religious literature—from awe, fear, anger, and defiance to adoration, love, and devotion. Factor-analytic studies have also pointed to many images of God (Gorsuch, 1968; Spilka, Armatas, & Nussbaum, 1964). "Comforting," "loving," "protective," and "supporting" are terms frequently used to describe God. However, God can also be described as "avenging," "hard," "severe," and "wrathful."

Psychologist Lee Kirkpatrick (1992) has noted how strikingly similar these images of God are to images of parental figures. Drawing on Bowlby's attachment theory, he suggests that it might be useful to think of God as another "attachment figure." Like a parent, God can serve as a haven of comfort in stressful times. Some support for this notion comes from the empirical evidence presented earlier (see Chapter 6) of higher levels of religious coping in periods of tension and transition. But the attachment to God, Kirkpatrick suggests, offers more than a shelter against the world, so reminiscent of Freud's point of view. Like the attachment to a parent, a religious attachment can also provide a secure base for learning, growth, and exploration when it is safe to do so. Armed with the knowledge that protection can always be found in God's loving arms, the religious individual may feel greater confidence venturing out into the world, searching for other forms of significance. Indeed, higher levels of religious commitment have been associated with lower anxiety (e.g., Baker & Gorsuch, 1982; Bergin, Masters, & Richards, 1987; Sturgeon & Hamley, 1979) and greater life satisfaction and well-being (Willits & Crider, 1988; Witter et al., 1985).

Not all attachments to God are secure, though. Kirkpatrick notes that relationships with the divine can be every bit as anxious/ambivalent or avoidant as relationships with one's parents. In fact, he suggests, attachments to parents have important (albeit complex) implications for attachments to God. Extrapolating from Kirkpatrick, four types of relationships between parental and religious attachments can be described (see Figure 11.2). A secure attachment to God can grow out of a secure relationship with parents. Those who developed trusting, loving relationships with their parents may be more likely to develop a view of God that *corresponds positively*. Consistent with this idea, some research has shown correlations between concepts of God and images of the preferred parent (e.g., Nelson & Jones, 1957). On the other hand, a secure attachment to God can *compensate* for insecure parental ties. In essence, God or a religious leader becomes the "good parent" the child never had. Earlier, I reviewed some evidence that children with poor parental relationships are more likely than others to switch to a loving God, particularly under conditions of greater stress (see Chapter 8).

What about the insecure religious attachment? A poorly developed connection to parents may leave the individual unequipped to build strong adult attachments or a secure spiritual relationship. In the search

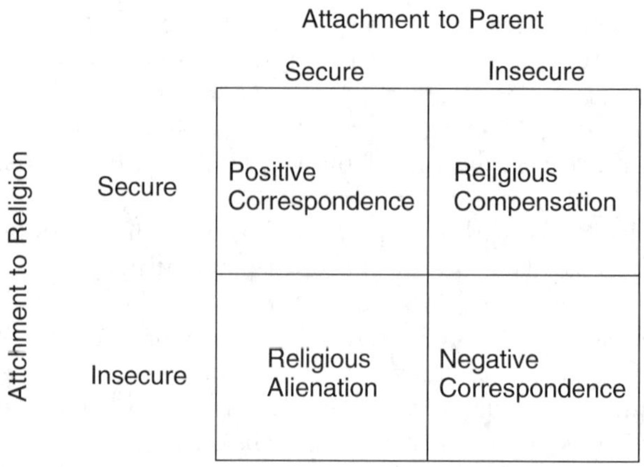

Attachment to Parent

		Secure	Insecure
Attchment to Religion	Secure	Positive Correspondence	Religious Compensation
	Insecure	Religious Alienation	Negative Correspondence

FIGURE 11.2. The relationship between parental and religious attachments.

for stronger ties, the individual may end up switching inadvertently to "false gods," attachment figures that *correspond negatively* to parents. These false gods may take the form of chemical addiction, a codependent relationship, religious dogmatism, or involvement in a dysfunctional cult. For instance, one study of heroin addicts revealed that they were more likely to have experienced premature deaths in their families and family separations as children and adolescents than psychiatric outpatients and normal students (Coleman, Kaplan, & Downing, 1986). Another study of delinquent adolescents found that youths who reported low parental attachment were more likely to be involved in Satanic activities (e.g., ceremonies to worship the devil) (Damphouse & Crouch, 1992). Perhaps least common of all cases are children with secure parental attachments who develop insecure religious ties, a process of religious *alienation*. As we saw in Chapter 8, however, cataclysmic events (e.g., war, natural disaster) can shatter even the most secure social network and, along with it, the sense of trust in a safe, benevolent world. Through this process, the belief in a loving, protective God may become less compelling and less available as well (e.g., Vetter & Green, 1932–1933).

Further research is needed to better understand the development of secure or insecure religious attachments. What is fairly clear at this point in time, however, is that insecure religious attachments (like insecure parental attachments) do not augur well for the individual. In the most direct study on the topic, Kirkpatrick and Shaver (1992) asked adults from the community to select which of three types of attachment best describes their relationship with God (see Table 11.1). Those who saw themselves as having an insecure attachment to God (avoidant or anxious/ambivalent) reported more anxiety, loneliness/depression, poorer physical health, and lower life satisfaction than those who described a secure religious attachment. Furthermore, attachment to God predicted mental health more strongly than did several other measures of religiousness. Other researchers have found similar relationships between measures that parallel secure/insecure religious attachment and measures of health and well-being, such as self-esteem (Benson & Spilka, 1973), purpose in living and medical symptoms (Kass, Friedman, Leserman, Zuttermeister, & Benson, 1991), happiness and life satisfaction (Pollner, 1989), and loneliness (Schwab & Petersen, 1991).

The secure and the insecure attachment to God appear to be associated with quite different orientations to the world. While the former seems part of a generally purposeful and satisfying way of life, the latter is accompanied by general psychological, social, and physical discomfort. Although the relationship between attachment and coping has not been studied yet, we might expect that the secure and insecure religious attachment also translate into distinctive methods of coping with stressful situations. The individual with the secure religious attachment may be more likely to make use of the religious coping methods that tend to be helpful, such as benevolent religious reframing, religious support, and collaborative religious coping. In contrast, the individual with the insecure religious attachment may be more likely to encounter some of the problems in religious coping described earlier in this chapter: falling prey to false Gods (Wrong Direction), interpreting events solely as a spiritual punishment or abandonment (Wrong Road), or difficulty in finding a religious home (Against the Wind). Thus, I tentatively add

TABLE 11.1. Three Styles of Attachment to God

Secure

> God is generally warm and responsive to me. He always seems to know when to be supportive and protective of me, and when to let me make my own mistakes. My relationship with God is always comfortable, and I am very happy and satisfied with it.

Avoidant

> God is generally impersonal, distant, and often seems to have little or no interest in my personal affairs and problems. I frequently have the feeling that He doesn't care very much about me, or that he might not like me.

Anxious/ambivalent

> God seems to be inconsistent in His reactions to me. He sometimes seems very warm and responsive to my needs, but sometimes not. I'm sure that He loves me and cares about me, but sometimes He seems to show it in ways I don't really understand.

Note. From Kirkpatrick and Shaver (1992, p. 270).

insecure religious attachment to the list of burdensome factors that increase the individual's vulnerability to major life stressors. Undifferentiated religion, fragmented religion, religious rigidity, and the insecure religious attachment—these are some of the culprits in the religious orienting system that weaken the larger orienting system and leave the individual open to problems of integration in coping.

CONCLUSIONS

In this chapter, I have taken a look at the failures of religion in coping from a process point of view. The process perspective does not point to methods of religious coping that invariably result in trouble. Neither does it point to methods of religious coping that work well for all people in all situations. It makes a different assumption, one articulated by philosopher Ibn Gabirol: "There is no quality so deplorable that it sometimes serves a use, and no quality so praiseworthy but that it sometimes is lamentable" (cited in Rosten, 1972, p. 159). But if the process perspective rejects the search for universal solutions, it does not accept the relativistic alternative. All ways of coping are not equally worthwhile. A key to coping lies not in particular beliefs or practices, but in the integration among the psychological, social, and situational dimensions that make up the coping process. At its best, the process of coping flows smoothly. At its worst, the process loses all continuity.

I have considered some of the ways religion contributes to problems in coping, and have examined some of the features within the religious orienting system that increase the individual's vulnerability to these difficulties in times of stress. But the focus here on the failures of religion in coping should not overshadow what has been presented in earlier chapters: that religion can play many valuable roles in the conservation and transformation of significance, and that empirical studies have generally shown religion to be more helpful than harmful in coping. Nevertheless, religion does have its darker side and ignoring it will not make it go away. We need to learn more about how and why religion goes wrong (as well as right) in coping. With a deeper understanding of religion's multifaceted character, we will be in a better position to help people struggle toward significance in their most difficult times. In the following and final chapter, I take a look at some of the practical implications of a psychology of religion and coping.

Chapter Twelve

PUTTING RELIGION INTO PRACTICE

CLIENT: *I've been so sad and tired since my wife left me.*

COUNSELOR: *That's a pretty understandable reaction when you think about everything you've been through.*

CLIENT: *Sometimes I feel as though God really has it in for me. What do you think?*

COUNSELOR (**to client**): [*Silence*]

COUNSELOR (**to self**): *What do I do now?*

Most people are familiar with the unsettling feeling in the stomach that comes from not knowing what to do when someone asks for help. Mental health professionals spend many years in training learning how to avoid that sinking sensation. The mention of religion, however, can test the wherewithal of even seasoned helpers. Few professionals come to their jobs well equipped to handle religious issues. Training programs in counseling, even those in religious universities, have not typically provided much practical guidance about religious and spiritual topics (Kelly, 1994; Shafranske & Malony, 1990). How then should the helper respond when religious issues are raised? Are they appropriate topics of conversation? Is it appropriate to draw on religious resources and coping methods in a counseling relationship? Is it appropriate to address problems in religiousness? If so, how does the helper assess and work with religious issues? In short, what do I do now?

The reader will not find any easy answers to these questions here.

But easy answers or cookbook solutions may not be the best response to problems as thorny and complicated as religious ones. Helping requires far more than a bag of techniques. It rests on theoretical frameworks—ways to understand people, problems, and the process of change. Theoretical frameworks are not simply theoretical; they can generate action and, in this sense, have a practical value of their own.

The psychology of religion and coping represents one such action-oriented framework. Not only does it suggest ways to understand and evaluate the roles of religion in stressful times, it also suggests methods of helping people in their search for significance. This concluding chapter examines some of the practical implications and applications of a psychology of religion and coping.

ATTENDING TO THE HELPER'S ORIENTATION TO RELIGION

People seek help when their usual approaches to the world are no longer working for them. They look for someone who can throw them a lifeline in their turbulent struggle. But what keeps the helper from getting caught up and swept away in all of this turmoil? An orienting system. The helper comes to the relationship grounded by a set of basic assumptions about people, life, and helping. Drawing on this orienting system, the helper tries to assist others who have become disoriented and are unable to cope effectively. Helping, in this sense, involves a meeting of worlds.

This meeting is far from a value-free encounter. It comes as no surprise that help seekers have preferred pathways and destinations of significance, but helpers have preferences of their own, too. Embedded within the helper's orienting system are assumptions about what is of ultimate significance and what are the most appropriate methods for attaining significance. These assumptions may be less than apparent to professional counselors and psychotherapists who have incorporated formal theories of personality and methods of psychotherapy into their orienting systems. However, formal theories also rest on values, although they are more often implicit than explicit (see Jones & Wilcox, 1993). The notion that helpers, professional or nonprofessional, can set aside their own values and enter into relationships as "blank slates" does not stand up well to empirical scrutiny. Counselors affect the goals for therapy (Worthington & Scott, 1983), influence their clients' values over the course of counseling (Kelly, 1990), and selectively attend to and overlook what their clients are saying. Even Carl Rogers, the founder of "nondirective" therapy, demonstrated this selective responsivity to his clients (see Truax, 1966).

The value-laden nature of helping is not a cause for alarm. A well-articulated, value-based orienting system provides the necessary "road map" for helping. Without that, the helper would have little to offer people in distress, and might, instead, join them in their pain and confusion. The dangers here lie not in the value-laden nature of helping, but in certain problematic ways of dealing with these values (Bergin, 1980).

The most obvious danger is the arrogant manipulation of a client's values or the coercive imposition of undesired values on the client. The more subtle, but perhaps greater danger is the failure to recognize the impact of one's own orientation on others. I recall a conversation with a clinical psychologist who insisted that she remained neutral in her work as a therapist. Psychotherapy, for her, was a process of helping clients reach whatever goals they defined for themselves. I asked her whether she would work with a concentration camp guard who was coming to therapy to help reduce his work-related anxiety. Much to my surprise, she said she would; after all, it was not up to her to judge her client's goals. She was unable to see how, in the name of neutrality, she would be supporting her client's crimes.

Unaware of the impact of their own orientations, counselors may follow people or lead them in undesirable directions. The risk of this danger seems particularly high in the religious realm. Some surveys have shown that mental health professionals, especially psychologists, are less involved in traditional religious practices and institutions than those they serve (Ragan et al., 1980; Shafranske & Gorsuch, 1984). On the basis of these findings, concerns have been raised that therapists, knowingly or unknowingly, may "convert" their clients to a secular value position (e.g., Tjelveit, 1986). More recent surveys, however, suggest that the "religiosity gap" between therapists and clients may be narrowing (e.g., Bergin & Jensen, 1990; Shafranske & Malony, 1990). Nevertheless, it remains the case that mental health professionals receive little training on religious issues, including the potential impact of their own religious orientations on the helping process. Thus, many helpers may be at least somewhat disoriented themselves when it comes to religion.

Education about religion is an important part of the remedy to these value-related problems. Part of that education should involve self-analysis, an appreciation for the power of the helper's own orientation to religion. Four of these orientations and their implications for the helping process will be examined in this chapter (see Zinnbauer & Pargament, 1996). Table 12.1 contrasts these orientations in terms of their responses to basic ontological questions and questions about the role of religion in helping relationships.

TABLE 12.1. Four Helping Orientations to Religion

	Religious rejectionism	Religious exclusivism	Religious constructivism	Religious pluralism
Is there an absolute reality?	Yes	Yes	No	Yes
Does God really exist?	No	Yes	No	Yes
Is there a single best way to approach reality?	Yes	Yes	No	No
Must the counselor share the individual's religious views?	No	Yes	No	No
Is the counselor respectful of religion?	No	Yes/No	Yes	Yes
Should religious issues be discussed in counseling?	No	Yes	Yes	Yes
Should counselors involve religious resources and coping methods in counseling?	No	Yes	Yes	Yes

Religious Rejectionism

Most notorious of the helping orientations is religious rejectionism. Some religious adherents have charged psychologists with disregard or derogation of religious and spiritual dimensions. Striking examples of religious disparagement can be found in many major schools of psychotherapeutic thought and practice. Freud (1930/1961) viewed religion as a childish response to feelings of insecurity and helplessness. About the reality of a higher power, Freud was clearly dismissive. Religion, he said, works by "distorting the picture of the real world in delusional manner . . . by forcibly fixing [adherents] in a state of psychical infantilism and by drawing them into a mass-delusion" (p. 31–32). Albert Ellis (1986), founder of rational–emotive therapy, has expressed a similar disdain for religious thought and practice. Religion, he argues, supports virtually every major form of irrationality and "is, on almost every conceivable count, directly opposed to the goals of mental health" (p. 12). To support religiousness in psychotherapy then would be counterproductive: "Obviously," Ellis writes, "the sane effective psychotherapist should not . . . go along with the patients' religious orientation and try to help these patients live successfully with their religions, for this is equivalent to trying to help them live successfully with their emotional illness" (p. 15).

The religious rejectionist does not necessarily deny the presence of an absolute reality. What is rejected is the reality of larger forces at play in the universe. How then are expressions of religiousness and spirituality to be understood? From the rejectionist point of view, they cannot be taken at face value; beliefs in God, religious practices, and mystical experiences are signs of a more profound disturbance—the individual's unwillingness to face reality head on. I recall a psychologist who, upon hearing my account of a student who often talked to God while walking to her classes, commented "she must be schizophrenic." Religious matters were, for him, a reflection of deeper psychological problems. To share or respect the individual's religious approach from this rejectionist viewpoint is not only unnecessary, it is counterproductive. The helper's task is to cut through the bulwark of religious defense and encourage a more ego-oriented, rational approach to life.

Religious rejectionism has serious disadvantages as a helping orientation. The first disadvantage is purely pragmatic. It is not unusual to find people who present religious or spiritual issues in counseling (Shafranske & Malony, 1990). Moreover, they appear to be looking for spiritually sensitive helpers. In an earlier chapter, it was noted that mental health professionals are not, in fact, the first choice for help by most people; clergy are (Chalfant et al., 1990; Veroff et al., 1981). The preference for clergy as helpers may be partly explained by concerns that mental health professionals will demean or try to change basic religious beliefs and values (Keating & Fretz, 1990; McLatchie & Draguns, 1984). Religious rejectionism does just that. It seems unlikely, then, that the religious rejectionist would be able to form a strong working relationship with the significant number of help seekers who are religiously committed.

Second, the assumptions of rejectionism are inconsistent with research findings. In earlier chapters I reviewed empirical studies that indicate religion is not merely a defense; it serves many purposes in coping apart from anxiety reduction and does so through many methods other than avoidance, denial, and passivity. Furthermore, a review of the literature pointed to effective as well as ineffective forms of religious coping. Thus, the presumed connection between religion and pathology does not stand up well to empirical scrutiny.

Third, religious rejectionism is problematic on ethical grounds. A helping orientation that rejects religious experience and expression out of hand or reduces it to psychopathology runs counter to recent professional ethical guidelines. According to the "Guidelines for Providers of Psychological Services to Ethnic, Linguistic, and Culturally Diverse Populations" published by the American Psychological Association (1993): "Psychologists respect clients' religious and/or spiritual beliefs and values, including attributions and taboos, since they affect world view, psychosocial functioning, and expressions of distress" (p. 46). The American Psychiatric Association (1990) has issued similar guidelines discouraging the imposition of religious or antireligious belief systems on patients.

In spite of its notoriety, religious rejectionism does not appear to be a common orientation among helpers. As noted earlier, the "religiosity gap" between mental health professionals and their clients may be narrowing. For example, in one survey of therapists from different disciplines, 77% agreed that "I try hard to live my life according to my religious beliefs " (Bergin & Jensen, 1990). In the general population, 84% agree with this statement. Furthermore, many professionals see religious and spiritual issues as relevant to their work. In a national survey of clinical psychologists, 74% disagreed with the item "religious or spiritual issues are outside the scope of psychology" (Shafranske & Malony, 1990, p. 75). Finally, there is little evidence that secular counselors dislike their religious clients more or evaluate religious issues in counseling as more pathological than do religious counselors (Worthington & Scott, 1983).

It may be more accurate to say that many professional helpers are confused and ambivalent about religion and its role in the helping relationship. Take, for example, the results of one survey of marriage and family therapists. While 89% indicated that their religious beliefs have some or significant impact on their therapeutic interventions, 58% of the same sample stated that their religious beliefs should be "completely" separate from their therapy (DiBlasio & Benda, 1991). In another survey, 52% of the clinical psychologist sample reported spirituality to be a relevant part of their professional lives. However, 67% of the same sample agreed that "Psychologists in general do not possess the knowledge of skills to assist individuals in their religious or spiritual development" (Shafranske & Malony, 1990, p. 75).

Because of their ambivalence and uncertainty, many helpers may tiptoe warily around religion, giving the impression of rejectionism, when in fact they just do not know what to do with it. It may seem easier simply to carve religion out from the helping process—if religious issues are raised, change the subject; if they will not go away, call in a religious counselor or chaplain. While preferable to rejectionism, this type of "religious separatism" has problems of its own, for many psychological and religious issues cannot be so easily disentangled from each other. Furthermore, mental health professionals who believe they should stay out of spirituality may be missing important issues and opportunities for change (Prest & Keller, 1993).

Religious Exclusivism

Just as rejectionism is scorned by the religiously committed, so is exclusivism derided by many mental health professionals. Yet, as can be seen in Table 12.1, the two orientations have some interesting parallels.

Both assume an absolute reality and a single best way to approach it. Unlike rejectionism, however, exclusivism insists that God is a central part of that reality and an integral part of the solution to any problem. While the rejectionist reduces religious expressions to physical, psychological, or social problems, the exclusivist elevates all human problems to spiritual concerns (see Wilber, 1995).

Bobgan and Bobgan (1987) illustrate this point. The varieties of human suffering, they say, "are due to separation from God because of the sinful condition of mankind and the presence of sin in the world after the Fall" (p. 207). Similarly, all solutions must address this religious alienation. "Jesus," they write, is "the only means to reestablish relationship between God and man and to enable people to live by faith in God" (p. 207). From the exclusivist point of view, religiously oriented counseling is always the treatment of choice. The exclusivist is respectful of an individual's religion within the limits of the exclusivist's own understanding of reality. When these views diverge, it is part of the exclusivist's task to bring the individual back to the right and true religious path. Other systems of belief and practice can only mislead the individual. Bobgan and Bobgan (1987) write: "Psychological systems of counseling may lead a person along the broad way which leads to destruction. . . . The entrance into new life through faith in Jesus is the small gate" (p. 225).

Religious exclusivism has its drawbacks. On the practical side, the helper's sphere of influence will likely be limited to those who share a similar religious worldview. Those outside of it may have some skepticism and concerns about religious counseling, particularly with someone who holds the exclusivist position. For example, Lewis and Epperson (1993) asked Christian college students to give their perceptions of written descriptions of a nondirective or a Christian counselor. In contrast to the nondirective counselor, the Christian counselor was described as less flexible and more likely to try to influence the client's values, thoughts, and behaviors. While the evangelical Christian students were as willing to see the Christian as the nondirective counselor, the nonevangelical Christian students preferred the nondirective counselor.

Like religious rejectionism, exclusivism raises ethical concerns to the extent that it *imposes* a particular view of significance on the individual. And, like religious rejectionism, exclusivism does not stand on solid empirical ground. Earlier in this volume, studies of coping were reviewed that showed both religious and nonreligious forms of coping have something unique to add to the prediction of adjustment to negative life experiences. These and other findings say that the religious dimension cannot be fully reduced to the psychological level, nor can the psychological dimension be fully elevated to the spiritual.

Just how common is religious exclusivism? Although I am not aware of any data that directly address the question, my own sense is that religious exclusivism, like religious rejectionism, is not very common in our culture. Many religious counselors work within a particular religious tradition, but relatively few might argue theirs is the only meaningful approach to life. Even within a religious tradition, there is little to suggest that helpers have settled on a uniform approach to counseling. Worthington and his colleagues (Worthington, Dupont, Berry, & Duncan, 1988) conducted one study of a small sample of counselors who explicitly identified themselves as Christians. The counselors reported wide differences in their use of therapeutic techniques. Christian therapists, these researchers concluded, are not all alike.

Over the years, heated arguments have arisen between religious adherents who see mental health professionals as rejectionists, and mental health professionals who see religious helpers as exclusivists. In a sense, however, each has tried to justify a position by caricaturizing the views of the other. To be sure, there are rejectionists and exclusivists. But their numbers seem to have been overexaggerated and, as a result, suspicions have been raised about both secular and religious helpers. The other unfortunate effect of this debate has been to obscure an important fact—that there are other, richer orientations helpers can take toward religion.

Religious Constructivism

We do not assume that an industrial psychologist must be a businessman or businesswoman, Strunk (1977) has observed. Nor do we expect child psychologists to be children. Only in the psychology of religion, he notes, is it so widely assumed that the psychologist must be religious. Is it the case that a psychologist or any other helper must share the individual's belief in an absolute reality? Not according to the religious constructivist position.

Constructivism questions the assumption of an absolute reality "out there" waiting to be discovered. Reality is, instead, constructed by the individual on the basis of experiences, relationships, beliefs, values, and the larger sociocultural context (Guba & Lincoln, 1989). Belief in God or disbelief in God, from this perspective, are both constructions; neither is "true" nor "false" in an absolute sense. This is not to say that constructions cannot be evaluated. They can, but their assessment is based on the "quality" of the construction rather than the degree to which it corresponds to an absolute reality. Quality here refers to the internal consistency, differentiation, and flexibility of the construction as well as its capacity to deal with world demands

(Neimeyer, 1995). Symptomatology is one sign of "construct trouble." But the cure to symptoms does not lie in education about the "correct" way of believing and acting. Rather, the helper must enter the individual's uniquely constructed world and repair and strengthen this world from within.

To the extent that the individual constructs the world religiously and to the extent that these constructions are a source of problems or potential solutions, religion becomes an appropriate topic of conversation for the constructivist. The religious constructivist does not have to share the individual's religious views. However, the constructivist must be respectful of religious traditions and familiar with their symbols, imagery, and methods.

> Daie, Witztum, Mark, and Rabinowitz (1992) illustrate a constructivist approach in their work with Rafik, a 19-year-old Israeli Druze soldier who came to treatment because of a deep fear of weapons and an inability to wear a uniform. Rafik's anxiety was tied to his belief that in a prior incarnation he had been a Syrian Druze executed for treason by a shot to the middle of his forehead. The belief in the transmigration of souls, the authors note, is normative within the Druze tradition. Rafik's problem, they felt, was not his belief in the reality of his reincarnation, but the anxiety his beliefs generated. Although the therapists were apparently secular Israeli Jews themselves, they accepted Rafik's understanding of his problems and developed a treatment plan that drew on the resources of his tradition. In this vein, they encouraged Rafik to access the healing powers of an amulet he had received as a child from a Druze *Sheikh*. In addition, they integrated idioms and rituals consistent with Rafik's worldview into the psychotherapy process:

> > The next day "Rafik" arrived at the session in a great state of anxiety and again was hypnotized. The therapist put his finger on Rafik's forehead [where he believed he had been shot] and asked him to announce when he felt a pleasant warm beam emanating from the therapist's fingers. When the patient said that he felt the beam, the therapist explained that the beam had a healing power and would eliminate his fears. The beam's healing powers would join those of the amulet . . . and would be strong enough to prevent him from suffering further fears, bad dreams and nightmares. A few minutes later, he was returned to a waking state. There was a remarkable change in the patient's feelings and anxiety-related complaints. (p. 127)

The willingness to enter different worlds, the ability to help people understand their problems from the perspective of their own orienting systems, and the interest in solutions that are consistent with the methods and metaphors of these orienting systems are the keys to religious constructivism.

In a culture as religiously varied as ours, most helpers are likely to encounter people from religious traditions outside of their own. Religious constructivism represents one orientation that allows helpers, even the most secular, to assist people who come from many religious worlds. With its appreciation for the diverse ways people put their lives together, constructivism would seem to be less vulnerable than rejectionism and exclusivism to the dangers of imposing one particular brand of significance on the individual. Yet some questions can also be raised about constructivism.

First of all, how fully can the helper enter the client's own world and leave his or her own world behind? More specifically, can the secular constructivist, who views religious beliefs as true only in the sense that myths are true, work effectively with the religious client whose God is "really, real?" Spero (1985), for one, has serious doubts. "There is a quantum difference," he states, between the belief that "a patient's fantasies have an 'almost real' quality and the possibility that a 'third party' (God) is present in the relationship. Therapists who reject this distinction eventually will convey this attitude to the patient, resulting in misalliance" (p. 83). One empirical investigation suggests Spero's concerns may be overdrawn. Nonreligious therapists were found to be *more* effective than their religious counterparts in providing a religious form of cognitive-behavioral therapy to Christian clients who were clinically depressed (Propst, Ostrom, Watkins, Dean, & Mashburn, 1992). Apparently, the nonreligious therapists were able to offer help that was sensitive to the religious orientation of their clients. This is, however, only one study. Further research is needed to determine whether secular therapists can work effectively within their clients' religious worlds.

Another, perhaps more unsettling question has to do with the potentially manipulative character of the constructivist approach. Clients might have concerns about the sincerity and trustworthiness of helpers who are themselves secular, yet draw upon sacred symbols and rituals to achieve their ends, as in the case of the therapist above who directed a "healing beam" to Rafik's forehead. Questions of authenticity could also be raised about the religious constructivist who seems to operate in a position of pseudoreligious authority without the formal legitimacy of a religious tradition. That the individual seeking help may be unaware of the helper's own religious position only compounds these concerns about sincerity and authenticity. Thus, even if the constructivist is effective in producing positive outcomes, troubling questions remain about the *process* that has led to change. Additional studies are needed to clarify the merits and potential limitations of the religious constructivist orientation to helping.

Religious Pluralism

Religious pluralism departs from the constructivist's disavowal of an absolute reality. It departs from the rejectionist's assumption that there is no higher power in that reality. And it departs from the exclusivist's belief that there is a single best way to live. Pluralism assumes an absolute reality that includes a higher power, but insists there are a variety of ways to approach it. From this perspective, many religions have something worthwhile to offer. As one writer puts it: "God is one, yet the pathways to God are truly different and they do not always travel in the same or in parallel directions" (Leliaert, 1989, p. 113).

This respect for religious diversity does not limit the pluralist's own ability to commit to a particular set of religious beliefs and practices. Pluralists can be found within (and outside of) many religious traditions. Steinberg (1975) illustrates the pluralist position within modern Judaism: "The Jewish modernist prefers not to put religions in contrast with one another. He is content that each has its share of verity and worth, that all have the right to be, that out of their diversity, God, man, and the truth are better served in the long run. As for himself, he is at peace in Judaism" (p. 104). Within a helping relationship, the pluralist assists the individual in a manner respectful of that person's tradition while remaining true to his or her own religious perspective.

More than the other positions, religious pluralism involves a sharing of orientations. Like the constructivist, the pluralist tries to understand how the client sees the world. The pluralist works within the individual's orienting system, assisting in the search for solutions in that frame of reference. Unlike the constructivist, however, the pluralist assumes an individual's orienting system is not always capable of generating answers to difficult questions; to arrive at solutions, old problems may require new vantage points. The pluralist does not claim to be neutral. He or she offers a different perspective on problems and solutions, one that grows out of a body of psychological theory and research and, as importantly, one that is interwoven with the helper's own particular history, identity, and beliefs about significance. Thus, while the pluralist enters the world of the client, the client also enters the world of the pluralist. As a result, the worlds of both may be enriched.

There is, however, the potential for coercion here, given the power differential between a counselor and client. To protect against this danger, the pluralist strives for a spirit of openness and collaboration—

from the negotiation of goals and choice of therapeutic methods to the evaluation of whether counseling has been successful. The pluralist conveys a deep interest in the individual's approach to life, but does not stop there. Also communicated is an openness about the pluralist's own theoretical framework, methods of helping, and views of significance. This openness extends to an explicit acknowledgment of the helper's religious orientation when religious issues become a part of counseling.

What is not communicated is the sense that the helper is the possessor of all truths or holds the sole key to well-being. The helper's views are offered tentatively, as thoughts worth considering. Listen, for example, how carefully one therapist broaches a religious issue in counseling: "I have a feeling that a part of your problem may stem from some of your concepts about God. It would be interesting for us to talk about this, but you genuinely have a right to close off this discussion in the event you find this is something you don't want to pursue" (Nelson & Wilson, 1984, p. 31). However the individual chooses to respond to comments such as these is acceptable. The pluralist tries to create an atmosphere in which the individual feels free to accept or reject the helper's thoughts and suggestions, partially or totally. Ultimately, it is the individual who shoulders the responsibility for his or her decisions.

As they share their orientations, the similarities and differences that arise between counselor and client come as no surprise. Religious pluralism assumes no two orienting systems are totally alike, not even those of two coreligionists. There are many interpretations of Judaism, Christianity, Buddhism, Hinduism, and other faiths. Variations can be found within the many subgroups of each tradition (e.g., conservative Christianity, Orthodox Judaism) as well. On the other hand, areas of agreement in basic beliefs and practices can often be found between a counselor and client even when they come from different religions. Any helping encounter then is likely to include points of agreement and disagreement. This is not a concern from the pluralist perspective. Change and growth are said to occur by grappling with these areas of convergence and divergence (Tyler, Brome, & Williams, 1991).

Finding points of commonality offers validation to the individual and helps to build a sense of trust in the relationship. That the counselor and client both hold to a basic belief in a higher power may be particularly important to the development of a "helping rapport." Just as important, though, are the differences between counselor and client, for they provide the creative tension necessary for change and the source of creative solutions to problems. This point is nicely illustrated by Genia (1990), who developed interreligious encounter groups to assist spiritually troubled people. The groups, she notes, are not ecumenical—the goal is not religious unification. Instead, diversity is prized: "The greater the diversity of the group membership, the greater the potential for growth as each participant encounters within the group, the heritage, ideas, and wisdom of the great spiritual traditions of our time" (p. 47).

Although pluralism has only begun to be articulated in the literature, my sense is that it is a widely practiced religious orientation to helping. It is easy to understand why. Pluralism is applicable to a wide variety of people in need, including those of diverse as well as similar religious backgrounds. The pluralist's own sense of spirituality enhances an appreciation for the religious expressions of others. Nevertheless, this appreciation is not uncritical. Any approach to living, religious or otherwise, has its strengths and limitations. The pluralist facilitates the search for significance not through religious indifference on the one hand or religious zealotry on the other, but through a sharing of orientations. More than the other religious approaches, this perspective makes explicit the important role of the counselor's orienting system in the helping process. Overall, I believe religious pluralism offers the most compelling orientation for helping.

Of course, pluralism is not without problems. Perhaps the biggest limitation of pluralism is the difficulty in doing it. The religious pluralist must have a rich understanding of the varieties of religious life. Stereotypes will not do. Pluralism requires knowledge of how religion works in ordinary and extraordinary times, how religion is helpful or harmful, and how the helper's own religious beliefs and practices are likely to impact on others. In addition, pluralism calls for skills in religious assessment and intervention. I turn now to some of these practical matters.

ASSESSING RELIGION IN THE COPING PROCESS

Griffith (1986) has noted that a therapist who tries to help people "without locating God" in the system faces the same problem as the 19th-century astronomers who were unable to predict the movement of the planets accurately until they realized there was another unseen planet, Neptune, exerting its own gravitational force. Attention to the religious dimension, he argues, is an essential part of the therapeutic process. Unfortunately, helpers often overlook religious issues in their work with people. In one study of oncology nurses, only 44% could correctly identify the religious affiliation of their patients (Sodestron & Martinson, 1987). When it does occur, assessment of religion is frequently limited to a few brief questions about the individual's religious background. Yet for substantial numbers of people, religion is more a part of the foreground than the background (cf. Koltko, 1990).

How does the helper assess religion? A complete answer to this important question would take us far beyond the scope of this book. Fortunately, some excellent books on religious assessment have been written for pastors (e.g., Fitchett, 1993a; Pruyser, 1976) and mental health professionals (Lovinger, 1984). Here I will highlight the special issues that arise in assessing religion from a coping perspective.

The Standard for Comparison

Assessment, like intervention, grows out of a theoretical framework. Evaluations of religion require a standard for comparison (see Fitchett, 1993b, for a review). The standard may be the definition of mature spirituality offered by a particular religious tradition. Malony (1993), for instance, has developed a method of religious assessment based on explicitly Christian criteria of religious maturity (e.g., belief that the individual has been saved by God's grace from sin). The standard of comparison may be a stage theory of religious development, moving from immature to mature forms of faith, as illustrated by Fowler's (1987) work. In this book, coping theory has been offered as still another standard for comparison. From this perspective, religion is evaluated according to the role it plays in the search for significance in stressful times. Recall that people experience stress when significance is threatened or lost. Through the coping process, people try to hold on to significance or, if necessary, develop new sources of significance. However, as noted earlier, coping does not always go smoothly. In any particular situation, problems can arise in the goals the person is seeking (Problems of Ends), in the appropriateness of the method of coping to the situation and the individual's goals (Problems of Means), or in the tension between the individual and the larger social system (Problems of Fit). The problem may also go beyond the individual's response to a specific situation and reflect limitations in the individual's more general orientation to the world. Resources may go untapped or may be insufficient to the tasks of coping. Burdens may interfere with the ability to generate and implement solutions to the immediate crisis and others that may arise.

To what degree is religion a part of these problems? To what degree is it or could it be a part of the solution? These are the most basic questions when religion is evaluated from a coping perspective.

The Starting Point

In most cases, the problems presented to counselors (including religious counselors) are not explicitly religious (Ball & Goodyear, 1993; Shafranske & Malony, 1990). Later, religion may prove to be a central part of the problem or solution, but it is not typically the starting point of assessment. Instead, the assessment initially focuses on the "presenting problem." How has the problem affected the objects of greatest significance to the individual? How has the individual tried to make sense of the situation and deal with it? What has worked and what has not? How has the individual been helped or hindered by the larger social system?

Religious issues may emerge in response to any of these open-ended questions. According to one survey of clinical psychologists, 60% of clients often express themselves in religious language (Shafranske & Malony, 1990). Following the clients' lead when they raise religious issues can be fairly straightforward.

But what if religion is not mentioned spontaneously? Does that mean it is irrelevant? Not necessarily. Religion may be an important part of the client's life, but the client may not see it as an appropriate topic for counseling. Another possibility is that the individual has simply overlooked religion as a source of potential solutions in this situation. Or religion may be a sore spot, a topic too painful to talk about. The failure to mention religion is not a good reason to discount it automatically. Consider the following case.

> Several years ago I worked with a client who sought psychotherapy for depression. She had been physically assaulted by a stranger a year earlier and was in a great deal of turmoil. Avoidance had been her basic method of coping: She tried to put the experience out of her mind, had not spoken of the attack to family or friends, and did her best to appear "perfectly normal" to the outside world. Inside, however, she was barely holding on. When I asked her how the assault had affected the things that mattered most to her, she talked about how she no longer felt clean, how the experience had left her feeling contaminated. Nothing she had tried had succeeded in eliminating that sense of pollution. In the initial assessment, this woman made no explicit mention of religion. Yet the religious theme of profanity and purification seemed to run throughout her narrative. I asked her whether she saw herself as a religious or spiritual person, and she responded with what seemed to be a disinterested shrug. But when pressed about what she meant by that shrug, she admitted that church attendance, communion, and confession had once been important parts of her life. No longer, though; not since the attack. It had left her with two painful religious feelings: anger that God had abandoned her when she was most vulnerable, and anxiety that perhaps God was punishing her for misdeeds on her part that she could only guess at. Had I ignored the religious dimension or taken her religious disinterest at face value, I would have overlooked a very salient element of her crisis,

one that had to be addressed before she could experience a sense of cleansing and renewal in her life.

Probes about religious matters should become a routine part of assessment even for the client who does not spontaneously raise these issues. General questions about whether the person is religious or spiritual, what denomination the individual belongs to, how often he or she goes to religious services and prays, and whether the person believes in God are logical starting points, but only starting points. By now it should be clear that religion has many meanings, methods, and functions. It is by no means certain that counselor and client, even those from the same tradition, will speak the same religious language. Recall the many meanings of the term "religiousness" among Protestant clergy and among Roman Catholic clergy (Pargament et al., 1995). Similarly, religious beliefs and practices that are seemingly benign to some will have different implications for others, depending on their histories of experience. Barr (1995) describes her encounter with one woman who felt a great deal of anxiety whenever she heard the words "Our Father" in the Lord's Prayer. A prayer so comforting to many people was, for her, a terrible reminder of the sexual abuse by her minister that she had suffered as a child.

It is important to go beyond simple descriptions of religion and shift from macro to microreligious assessment. Those who view themselves as religious should be asked more pointed questions, such as: "In what ways are you religious? What purpose does religion serve in your life? How is religion involved in the way you are coping with your present problems?" Those who belong to a denomination should be asked: "How did you become affiliated with your denomination? What aspects of being a member of your denomination do you find particularly important to you? How has your congregation or clergy been involved in the way you are coping with your present problems?" Those who pray should be asked: "How do you pray? What do you pray for? What role does prayer play in the way you are coping with your difficulties?" Those who believe in God should be asked: "How do you envision God? What type of relationship do you have with God? How has this relationship changed over the years? How has your relationship with God affected the way you are coping with your present problems?"

Of course, religion will not be relevant to all problems. Knowing when and how far to pursue the religious dimension can be a very subjective business. In an effort to assist the counselor in this process, my colleagues and I delineated several religious warning signs of trouble in coping (Pargament et al., in press). These religious "red flags" were developed within each of the three major problem areas in the process of coping (Problems of Ends, Problems of Means, and Problems of Fit) (See Table 12.2 for illustrative red flags). The items hint at the kinds of religious difficulties described in the previous chapter, such as one-sidedness and errors of explanation, control, and moderation. It should be stressed that the red flags were not designed to be definitive indicators of problems; rather, they were meant to alert the counselor to statements that signal the need for further religious exploration.

To test the validity of the warning signs, we worked with members of a Roman Catholic church and college students who had experienced a major negative life event in the past few years (Pargament et al., in press). The participants indicated how they had coped with their stressor on a measure that included the religious red flags. Scores on the red flag items were then correlated with measures of mental health and the outcome of the negative event. In support of our predictions, endorsements of the red flags were, with some exception, associated with poorer mental health and poorer outcomes of the negative life event. In a more recent study, clergy and mental health professionals also identified religious indicators such as these as signs of trouble (Butter, 1997). Remember, however, the religious warning signs are only that—warning signs. They call for a deeper, more contextual assessment of religion.

TABLE 12.2. Religious Red Flags in Coping with Negative Life Events

Problems of ends: Wrong direction

I have decided to turn away from God and live life for myself alone.
I have lost interest in God, other people, myself, and everything else.
I have decided to stop taking care of myself and focus only on what God wants for me.
I realize that the world is not important to me and I have decided to spend all of my energies serving God.

Problems of means: Wrong road

I believe that God is punishing me for my sins.
I know God will make the situation better if I just wait long enough.
I am not bothered at all because the situation is God's will.
I pray that God will punish the real sinners.

Problems of fit: Against the wind

My family or friends speak to me about religion in a way I do not agree with.
I disagree with the church's view about why this event happened to me.
I feel that God is not being fair to me.
I question whether God really exists.

Assessing Religion in Context

Life for the counselor would be easier if religion could be pulled apart from the other elements of coping, as if it were a loose thread on a sweater. We have seen, though, that all of the threads of coping, including the religious thread, are intertwined; to pull on one thread can unravel the whole fabric. The challenge of religious assessment then is to understand religion in the full *context* of coping.

Religious coping has to be assessed in the context of nonreligious coping methods and goals. For example, the client who describes an illness as God's will is not necessarily discounting the role of other important causal factors (see Loewenthal & Cornwall, 1993; Pargament et al., 1982). God may be seen as acting in concert with other personal, social, and biological forces or apart from them. Only by exploring religious and nonreligious *patterns* of attribution can it be determined whether the individual is making an error of explanation. Similarly, the client who says that she is now devoting her life to God may not be describing her own self-debasement, but rather a reprioritization of her goals and values. Indeed, participants in our red flags study who endorsed items such as "I realize the world is not important to me and I have decided to spend all of my energies serving God" reported generally *better* mental health and outcomes in coping. Additional exploration of the character of significance, religious and nonreligious, would be needed to determine whether the client is headed in a wrong direction.

Religious coping must also be assessed within a broader situational, social, and personal context. The merits of a coping method, religious or otherwise, cannot be evaluated apart from the situations confronting the individual. Religious passivity in the face of an uncontrollable event has a very different meaning than religious passivity in a situation that calls for action. An angry religious struggle with God in the midst of a traumatic experience has different implications for the individual than the same struggle 5 years after the crisis has been resolved. Similarly, methods of coping cannot be assessed apart from a larger religious social context. The young man who decides to admit his homosexuality will receive a different reception from a mainline congregation than a fundamentalist congregation. Finally, methods of coping cannot be evaluated apart from the larger personal context. A plea for help from God signals an attempt at fundamental transformation for the independent woman who has taken pride in self-sufficiency throughout her life, while the same plea represents an effort to preserve a way of life for the woman who has consistently found refuge in her faith. In short, the assessment of religion from a coping perspective requires a judicious weighing and balancing of a dynamic array of situational, social, and personal forces.

Multiple methods of assessment are needed to evaluate religion within the context of coping. Listening to the client's own story is a critical part of the process, but it is not sufficient. Some aspects of the coping process may be difficult to put into words, particularly phenomena as elusive as the sacred and significance. Some people may be unaware of what matters most to them or the part the sacred plays in their lives. The general rule for assessment becomes especially important here: look beyond *what* is said to *how* it is said. I recall one woman who spent a good part of our initial session describing how she no longer cared about anything. She was doing a good job of it, talking about her work, her marriage, and her future in a voice so flat and lifeless that I felt myself becoming glassy-eyed. Toward the end of the hour, I asked her offhandedly what her plans were for the upcoming Christmas holiday. Much to her own surprise, she started to cry. These were not the tears of someone who had stopped caring. It turned out that holiday times with her extended family were a painful reminder of what she had tried to forget—her infertility. The focus in counseling shifted from the presenting problem, her inability to find something significant in life, to the more basic problem—her difficulty in coming to terms with a terrible loss of significance. In this case, feelings more than words revealed why this woman had come to counseling.

Narrative accounts can also be supplemented by questionnaires. Few religious measures have established norms for people in counseling. Nevertheless, responses to religious scales can be helpful when the findings are interwoven with other sources of information. I have already reviewed measures of religious coping and their implications for the well-being of the client. Measures of the individual's more general religious orienting system of resources and burdens could also prove useful in assessment. For example, Glock and Stark's (1966) brief multidimensional measure of religiousness could help the counselor identify religious resources of Christian clients (e.g., beliefs, practices, experiences) that could be tapped more fully in stressful situations.

Measures of various religious burdens could help the counselor identify religious issues that interfere with the individual's ability to generate effective solutions to problems not only in the immediate situation but in others likely to arise as well. For instance, high scores on the measure of indiscriminate proreligiousness (Pargament, Brannick, et al., 1987) suggest that the client has an undifferentiated religious system, one that may make it difficult to come to terms with suffering. High scores on the religious introjection scale of Ryan et al. (1993) suggest the client is burdened by a fragmented approach to religion based on guilt, anxiety, and external pressures. Low scores on the Quest scale suggest religious rigidity (Batson & Schoenrade, 1991a). Image of God scales that assess the degree to which the divine is seen in positive or negative terms could point to insecure religious attachments (e.g., Spilka et al., 1964).

Both interviews and questionnaires rely on the individual's own experience of the world. As meaningful as these perceptions are, they cannot serve as the only basis for assessment. Coping must be viewed against the backdrop of other perspectives and broader realities. For example, it is important to consider not only how a religious tradition is perceived, but how well that tradition is actively understood. Toward that end, the counselor would be well advised to learn more about the beliefs and practices of diverse religious groups through firsthand experience, readings, or consultation with knowledgeable religious figures (see Lovinger, 1984, for a good resource). The counselor should also gauge the individual's appraisals of his or her resources, burdens, and life events against the evaluations of others who are a part of the person's world. Friends, family members, and coworkers can provide an invaluable perspective on the coping process.

Unfortunately, there are no simple formulas for the assessment of processes as dynamic and multidimensional as religion and coping. The counselor must gather information about many aspects of a client's life from a variety of sources and then integrate this information into a coherent whole. All of this requires situational, social, and personal wisdom (cf. Oden, 1983). How large religion figures into this process will vary from person to person. Certainly, religion will not be a part of the problem or solution for everyone who comes to counseling. But helpers, particularly mental health professionals, appear to be in little danger of spending too much time on the religious realm. The greater danger seems to be religious neglect. In this section, I have examined how religion can be assessed as something more than a "background variable." By attending more closely to religion in the context of coping, we develop a more complete picture of the person struggling for significance in difficult times. It is this picture that guides the counselor's decisions about how best to help.

APPLICATIONS OF RELIGIOUS COPING TO COUNSELING

Religious solutions to problems are not often proposed in counseling (e.g., Bergin & Jensen, 1990). While this pattern of neglect could reflect the counselor's discomfort about religious matters, even explicitly religious practitioners do not make a great deal of use of the intervention techniques of their own tradition (Jones, Watson, & Wolfram, 1992).

The problem may be a matter of "know-how." Many helpers might be willing to incorporate spiritually sensitive methods in counseling if they knew how to do it. To be useful to helpers, DiBlasio and Benda (1991) suggest, religious concepts must be presented in less abstract ways and their applications to problems must be clearer. Thinking about religion and coping can help bridge religious abstractions and the concrete problems of living. In the following sections some of the practical applications of religious coping to counseling are illustrated.

To organize this discussion, let us consider two of the most basic questions about coping. The question of ends: Is the person heading in a good direction? And the question of means: Is the person taking a good road to get there? If we think about these two questions together, then we can identify four possible clinical responses (see Figure 12.1). Religious coping methods can be incorporated into each of these responses in counseling.

Preservation

Sometimes the answers to both questions—about the person's direction and road—is yes. The individual may be heading in a good direction and taking the right road to get there. Why then enter counseling? In some instances, the individual may be unaware that he or she is doing all that can be done to cope with the problem. The thoughts and feelings

Heading in a Good Direction?

		YES	NO
Taking a Good Road?	YES	Preservation: A Conservation of Means and Ends	Re-valuation: A Conservation of Means and Transformation of Ends
	NO	Reconstruction: A Transformation of Means and Conservation of Ends	Re-creation: A Transformation of Means and Ends

FIGURE 12.1. Questions of pathways and destinations in coping: Four clinical responses.

brought on by the crisis may be new and disturbing. Assessment, however, may reveal that the person is actually coping quite well. Reassurance and support are the appropriate forms of counseling here. The religious client can be encouraged to persevere in his or religious way of life and seek out religious support from God, friends, family, and clergy. In other instances, the crisis may have temporarily disrupted a tried and true way of life.

> A while ago I worked with an older client, Bob, who came to therapy after witnessing a tragic accident. A good Samaritan, he had pulled over to help a motorist whose car was stuck in the middle of the road. Suddenly a motorcyclist came around the bend in the road at high speed and hit the disabled car head on. The motorcyclist was killed immediately, literally blown apart by the impact. Bob was within a few feet of the car when he saw this whole process unfold. Since that time, he had been plagued by nightmares, panic attacks, and flashbacks in which he witnessed the accident again and again in painfully slow motion. These experiences were affecting his performance on the job, and he was becoming moody and irritable at home. Although his physician had prescribed a variety of medications, Bob had not experienced any relief.

As I got to know Bob, I found that he had had no history of psychological trouble prior to the accident. In fact, he took a great deal of pride in his accomplishments: a happy marriage of 35 years, children who were out on their own doing well, and a good job. But he had never encountered anything like this accident before. As he said, "It threw me over the edge."

Clearly, Bob had been taking a good path and heading in a good direction before the accident. The task of therapy, I thought, was to help Bob keep himself together and preserve his way of life. The work itself was not all that difficult, for I was dealing with a competent man; we did not have to start from scratch. Bob already had a network of supportive resources; however, he had stopped using it. Part of therapy focused on helping him return to what had worked so well for him.

God and church were a part of this process. In the course of therapy Bob described himself as a religious man, a regular churchgoer who prayed often and lived by his convictions. However, when I asked him whether he had spoken to his minister, someone he liked a great deal, or prayed to God for help in his ordeal, he said he had not. Religion had become compartmentalized from the specifics of his life. I encouraged him to think about how he might draw on his faith to help him through this tragedy. Bob began reading the Bible before he went to bed and found particular solace in the psalms. Bob also decided to share what he had been going through with the minister of his church, as well as other friends and family members. And in the midst of a panic attack or flashback to the accident, we found that Bob was helped by repeating a simple prayer to himself: "God is with me." By breaking down the barriers to his religious resources, Bob was able to tap more fully into this reservoir, seek out religious support, and keep himself together through the most traumatic period of his life. Fundamental change was not the goal here; survival was. This is the essence of preservation.

Reconstruction

In other instances, people come to counseling not because their goals are inappropriate, but because their methods for attaining these goals are flawed. They are heading in the right direction, but taking the wrong road to get there. Problems in the orienting system are often central here. As a result of internal or external changes, the individual's resources are no longer sufficient to the tasks of coping. Preservation would not be the appropriate coping method in this case because the guiding system for coping is itself in need of repair. Instead, the individual needs help in rebuilding his or her way of reaching significance.

Reconstruction may be literal, not just figurative. At a recent conference on disabilities and rehabilitation, one of the wheelchair bound participants spoke of her frustration in gaining access to her church. Ironically, the congregation had posted a "welcome" sign at the bottom of the steps to the social hall, steps too narrow for her to negotiate with her wheelchair. Even more challenging for her was the effort to gain the support and encouragement of her fellow members. "It's the stares that are the bigger problem," she said, "not the stairs." If this woman were to enter counseling, she might be encouraged to press for a physical reconstruction of the church and an attitudinal reconstruction of its members. If that proved infeasible, the counselor might explore the possibility of religious switching to a more receptive congregation.

Often in counseling, reconstruction focuses on the individual's internal world. Religious coping methods can be used to create changes within the religious orienting system. Claypool (1968, cited in Meigs, 1969), for example, describes the religious reframing a minister offered to a member of his church who had just learned that his son had been killed in battle. The father had engaged in a reframing of his own; the death was seen as an abandonment by God: "I want to know," he asked the minister, "where was God when my son was being killed?" (p. 87). From the minister's perspective the father was making an error of explanation. The minister responded with a different type of religious reframing: "I guess you would say that He was right where He was while His Boy was being killed" (p. 87). This reframing of God as loving but limited had a reportedly "revolutionary impact on the man, for it brought God from afar right into the circle as a grieving companion" (p. 87). Capps (1990) presents a number of other striking and compelling examples of religious reframing for pastoral counselors.

Religious purification methods can also be integrated into counseling. Saucer (1991) describes a therapeutic approach for evangelical Christians and evangelical Catholics who engage in behavior that is inconsistent with their values and principles. This approach begins with an analysis of the individual's moral action and self-defeating behavior. The client is gently admonished for these actions and then encouraged to confess the misbehavior. Confession is followed by prayer for forgiveness, absolution, and healing. Therapy concludes with attempts by the individual to make amends for wrong behavior through symbolic acts (e.g., saying the Rosary) and acts of mercy (e.g., feeding and sheltering the homeless).

Other therapists have integrated aspects of religious purification more selectively in their counseling. Confronting their clients in supportive fashion, they point out the inconsistencies between their behavior and values, and their beliefs and practices. The clients' methods of understanding and dealing with the world are contrasted with the pathways followed by their religious models. The dissonance and tension that grows out of this confrontation is resolved when clients adopt more fully integrated orienting systems that are more closely aligned with their religious traditions. This method of religious confrontation and correction has been used to deal with various errors of religious control and moderation, such as passivity of battered women toward their abusive spouses (Whipple, 1987), beliefs that any expression of anger is sinful (Bassett, Hill, Hart, Mathewson, & Perry, 1992), and religiously based guilt about sexual thoughts and feelings (Aust, 1990).

For example, Miller (1988) describes the case of Jon, a 24-year-old seminary student who came to therapy because of severe depression and anxiety.

Jon was "a bright, energetic, well-intentioned young man" who was going to extremes in his commitment to helping others (p. 48). He came by it honestly. Both of his parents were missionaries. For one of his birthdays they gave him a Bible with the inscription: "Of him to whom much has been given, much will be required" (p. 47).

After Jon dismissed the therapist's plan to treat the anxiety and depression through deep-muscle relaxation and behavioral changes as "self-indulgent," the therapist decided to use Jon's religious frame of reference as an aid in therapy. He confronted the inconsistency between Jon's religious values and his own behavior. The therapist pointed out that even Jesus and his followers took time to rest and reflect. He noted how Jon's belief that "no matter how hard [he] works, it's never good enough" contradicted his own theology, which held that grace is free and unearned (p. 48). He commented how, in spite of his desire to serve others, Jon was actually spending a great deal of time focusing on himself and how others were responding to him.

The therapist went on to "correct" Jon, encouraging him to replace older, dysfunctional messages with religious self-statements more consistent with his religious values: "Even Jesus took time to rest and recharge. If I want to serve, I also need to take care of myself. God, through Jesus Christ, accepts me as I am. Don't worry about how other people are evaluating *me*. Focus on *their* needs instead" (p. 49).

Working within Jon's orienting system to increase its flexibility and differentiation, the therapist was able to help Jon develop a new way of looking at himself and a way to sustain himself in his efforts to serve others. As with all reconstructive approaches, the task here was a change, not of ultimate goals or values, but of the methods to reach these goals. Gradually, Jon became less depressed and anxious. Four years later, the therapist reports, Jon was pursuing his mission in ministry and service to others with "renewed energy" (p. 50).

Re-Valuation

In some cases, people seek counseling because they have lost their direction. Their paths in life are worthwhile, but they have lost sight of where they are heading or the destination is now out of reach. The method of choice for counseling in these cases is re-valuation—helping people discover new sources of significance and sustain themselves in the process.

Rituals of Transition

Before new significance can be found though, lost objects of significance must be relinquished. Many people come to counseling because their grieving is incomplete, they have been unable to let go of a loved one. Religious rituals of transition can facilitate the mourning process in counseling.

Boehnlein (1987) presents the case of a 45-year-old widow with symptoms of posttraumatic stress disorder. She had come to the

United States from Cambodia, where she had witnessed her father kill himself because he feared he was about to be captured by the Khmer Rouge forces. One of her greatest concerns was that her father's body had been buried in a mass grave, rather than cremated. The oldest child in her family, she had felt it was her duty to ensure her father's reincarnation through proper adherence to the Buddhist funeral ceremonies. This, of course, had been impossible. Yet she remained obsessed with the past, haunted by guilt and fear about her father's spiritual condition.

As part of the therapy, the counselor encouraged this woman to participate in local Buddhist ceremonies and Cambodian anniversary festivals. These rituals offered a "corrective emotional experience"; they provided her with an opportunity to venerate the soul of her father, assist his transition to a better life in his next incarnation, protect herself from vengeful spirits, and become a part of her new community (see Eisenbruch, 1991). In the process, she was able to let go of her focus on the past. She experienced a series of dreams in which her father appeared happy in his next life and suggested several ways to alleviate her symptoms. These suggestions proved helpful. Stronger in the knowledge that her father was now content in his next incarnation, her condition improved and she was able to turn her attention to finding new significance for herself in her new community.

Seeking Religious Purpose

Religion can be an important resource in the search for new values in counseling. At the core of most religious traditions is the belief that every human life has value. No matter how limited we are by external circumstances or personal shortcomings, each of us is said to carry a spark of the divine. No matter what our condition may be, everyone is said to have a special purpose or mission in life. This message may carry extraordinary power to those who have lost what was most significant to them.

Some counselors are quite explicit in their efforts to help others find religious purpose. For instance, in his approach to premarital pastoral counseling, Capps (1981) acts as a spiritual mentor, instructing the couple about the moral foundation of marriage and pointing to the religiously based virtues that should guide and nourish their relationship. Similarly, Rupp (1988) presents a number of prayers to assist those who have suffered a loss of significance find new purpose:

> God of Exodus, I am off on an inner road never traveled before. Deep within, where only your eyes see, there is so much mystery, greyness, restlessness. I want so much to have a sense of direction, to know where I am and where I ought to be headed. But the dark and the questions stay. . . .

God of my depths, I cry out to you to be my guide. Help me to have a strong sense of inner direction and grant that I may have the reassurance of knowing that I am on the right path. Take all that is lost in me and bring it home to you. (pp. 139–140)

The search for meaning and purpose also lies at the heart of Frankl's logotherapy, although the religious nature of this search may be more implicit than explicit.

Frankl (1984) cites the case of a mother who tried to kill herself after the suicide of her 11-year-old son. With her youngest child dead and her oldest child crippled through infantile paralysis, life had lost meaning. Frankl encourages her to find a new meaning for herself. In therapy he asks her to imagine herself at age 80, on her deathbed, looking back on her life. What would she conclude had she pursued a career of financial and material success? The woman decides that her life would have been an easy one, full of wealth and excitement, but still a life of failure. What would she conclude had she dedicated herself to caring for her handicapped son? This is what she imagines herself saying in retrospect: "I have made a fuller life possible for him; I have made a better human being out of my son. . . . As for myself, I can look peacefully on my life; for I can say my life was full of meaning, and I have tried hard to fulfill it; I have done my best—I have done the best for my son. My life was no failure!"(p. 140)

To put it in the language of coping, Frankl is facilitating a re-valuation—a shift from emptiness and despair over her son's suicide to a life of new significance despite the loss. He is not asking her to make a radical change in the way she has lived her life up to this point. He is asking her to live with new direction and purpose.

Is Frankl's logotherapy religious? I believe so. Frankl asks people to *discover* new meaning in life. Implicit in his therapy is the assumption that there is a "right" and "true" meaning for every individual and every situation, a meaning that, in some sense exists "out there." In this respect, logotherapy is fundamentally religious; it assists people in a basic method of religious coping—the search for religious purpose, the search for each individual's spiritual vocation in life.

Re-Creation

In re-valuation the emphasis is on finding new destinations of significance while holding on to a way of life. But there are times when people lose their bearing completely—when they head off on a road that leads nowhere, when they have no idea where else to go or how to get there.

These instances call for a more radical change in coping. Religion can be a part of the re-creative process in counseling.

Religious Forgiveness

Forgiveness is one of the coping methods some counselors have used to foster radical change among those who have suffered abuse and injustice (Freedman & Enright, 1995; McCullough & Worthington, 1994a). As noted earlier, mistreatment and its many psychological, social, and physical consequences can become the organizing force for the lives of these individuals, their object of greatest significance, negative as it is, and the pain suffered by victims can be unwittingly passed along to others. Forgiveness, rooted in religious tradition, offers one method for breaking this cycle of pain.

Bergin (1988) describes one religiously based counseling approach to promoting forgiveness among victims of family abuse: "the transitional figure technique." Bergin asks his clients to envision themselves at a fork in the road in the history of their families. Looking back, he points out how each new generation has suffered abuse at the hands of the previous generation, only to pass it on to the next one. "Somebody," he argues, should "stop the process of transmitting pain from generation to generation. Instead of seeking retribution, one learns to absorb the pain, to be forgiving, to try to reconcile with forebears, and then become a generator of positive change in the next generation" (p. 29). Bergin encourages his clients to follow the model of exemplary religious figures, to see themselves as transitional figures capable of shifting their focus from anger and pain to understanding and acceptance. Asking people to forgive those who have hurt and betrayed them is not an easy request. It is a call for radical change, a change in the core of significance and the approach to life built around it.

Religious Conversion

Religious conversion is another method of religious coping that can be drawn on in counseling. Propst (1991) presents a case in point in which she encourages her client to make a profound change, one akin to conversion.

> The client was a 42-year-old single elementary school teacher who came to counseling because of sadness and loneliness. She felt controlled by her parents, who insisted that she spend all of her free time with them, and she felt afraid to initiate new relationships. Her only social activity was participation in the nursery and the Sunday

School at her local church. After she attended a wedding she became suicidal. "What's the use," she felt; she had "lost the chance for happiness and marriage" (p. 4).

What was this woman seeking? She seemed to be trying to avoid pain at all costs, "covering even painful words with nervous smiles." If she felt a tear in her eye, her entire face became beet red, further aggravating her embarrassment. Her stated philosophy was "It is better to avoid people than to be hurt again. Suicide is an option; I am tired of the struggle. I want to be with Jesus, and then I will not have to feel the pain'" (p. 6). Passivity, lethargy, even self-destruction, were a part of the path this woman was taking to the end of a pain-free existence. Religion, too, was a part of this path. To be with Jesus was not an end in itself, but rather a way to "feel no pain."

Propst asked her client to make a dramatic change in means and ends—a shift from an avoidance of pain as an end itself to the experience of pain as a means to the ultimate end of spiritual growth. Propst encouraged her to approach the situations she feared, in other words, to "practice *feeling badly*" (p. 8). Drawing on her client's "latent spirituality," she enlisted Jesus Christ as her ally in this process. When her client resisted changing, Propst confronted her with the gap between her own behavior and her religious model for living. She asked her client to rate her belief in the idea that "Jesus was vulnerable and in pain, but still healthy humanness." Her client said she agreed with that 100%. However, when asked the same question about herself she said she could believe that only 50%. After a moment of silence she then said, "I guess I expect more of myself than I do of Jesus" (p. 13).

The confrontation in this case was more than reconstructive. Propst encouraged her client to consider not only new beliefs and practices, but new goals for her life as well. She confronted her with a choice of ultimate directions. What would it be: a life shaped by her past and her desire to "play it safe," or one shaped by her desire to live more in the image of God? If she were to pursue this latter end, Propst told her, she could not expect a pain-free existence. Rather, she would have to view her own suffering, like the suffering of Jesus, as a necessary part of the path to God and her own resurrection. Like Saint John of the Cross, she would have to undergo her own "dark night of the soul." In this sense, the tables would be turned. Jesus would not be a way to the absence of pain. Instead, pain would be a part of the path to Jesus Christ.

Propst was calling for a re-creation here, a life transformation similar to a religious conversion. She asked her client to give up her avoidant strategies and her goal of a life free of discomfort for a willingness to accept her limitations and vulnerability in the search for closeness with God. How successful she was is not entirely clear, but Propst does note that the client began to free herself from her parents and take more risks in her life.

The Efficacy of Religious Counseling

Earlier, I reviewed the results of research showing that several types of religious coping appear to be generally helpful to people when applied by themselves to difficult situations (see Chapter 10). On the basis of these results, we might expect that religious coping methods would also add to the effectiveness of counseling. What does the research show?

Relatively few systematic studies have examined the effectiveness of religious counseling (see Worthington, Kurusu, McCullough, & Sandage, 1996, for an extensive review). It seems apparent from this research that people do make improvements in religiously oriented counseling. For example, in one study, Mormon college students were treated with a religiously oriented cognitive-behavioral therapy for self-defeating perfectionism (Richards, Owen, & Stein, 1993). Over the course of treatment, the participants made significant gains on several measures: perfectionism, depression, self-esteem, and spiritual well-being. However, the study lacked comparison groups and, as a result, the researchers could not determine whether the religious approach was more effective than a comparable secular treatment or more effective than the changes people would make on their own.

Those studies that have compared religious forms of treatment to nonreligious counseling have yielded mixed results. A few investigations have found religious counseling to be more effective than standard approaches in working with religious clients (Azhar, Varma, & Dharap, 1994; Propst, 1980; Propst, Ostrom, Watkins, Dean, & Mashburn, 1992). Other studies have shown few differences in the efficacy of religious and secular treatments (Johnson, DeVries, Ridley, Pettorini, & Peterson, 1994; Johnson & Ridley, 1992; Pecheur & Edwards, 1984). A few studies suggest that the helpfulness of religious counseling varies from problem to problem (Koss, 1987) and across different measures of outcome (Beutler et al., 1988).

If studies of people naturally coping with stressful life situations are a guide, then these mixed results should not be surprising. As we have seen, the efficacy of religious coping depends on a number of factors: the methods of coping, who is doing the coping, the situations they are struggling with, and their social contexts. These factors have not been teased out in the counseling outcome research. The "religious ingredients" of counseling are often described in vague terms. To say that prayer, scriptural reading, or religious imagery are part of counseling says little about *how* these resources are actually used in the coping process.

Coping theory suggests a different direction for studies of religious counseling—the microanalytic approach that focuses on the helpfulness of particular methods of religious coping thoughtfully and carefully selected to meet the needs of particular groups and the demands raised by particular life stressors and transitions. For instance, theoretically, religious forgiveness should be a method of coping well suited to people who have been mistreated by others. However, as noted earlier, religious forgiveness may not be of value to every victim of abuse. For example, when the injustice is terribly deep or when the perpetrator has shown no remorse, attempts to encourage forgiveness in counseling may prove fruitless or counterproductive (see McCullough & Worthington, 1994a). By focusing more sharply on specific religious coping methods, their appropriateness to some problems and populations and their inappropriateness to others, we may learn much more about the elements of religion that enhance or impede counseling. With that knowledge it may be possible to integrate religion more fully and effectively into the helping process.

THE BROADER PRACTICAL IMPLICATIONS OF RELIGION AND COPING

This discussion has focused on the practical implications of religion and coping for counseling. Counseling is, after all, the major tool of the helping professions. It is not, however, the only tool. As traditionally practiced, counseling is constrained by three assumptions: (1) mental health professionals are the most appropriate deliverers of help for personal problems, (2) individuals are the most appropriate targets of help, and (3) the most appropriate time for help is *after* problems have occurred (Rappaport, 1977). Religion and coping theory suggests three broader working assumptions: (1) there are many capable deliverers of help besides mental health professionals, (2) there are many important targets for help besides individuals, and (3) there are other times to help besides after the problem has occurred. In the following sections, I consider the broader implications of religion and coping for helping.

Expanding the Pool of Helpers

No group has a monopoly on helping. Assistance in coping can come from many sources.

Health Care Professionals

Health care professionals are in a particularly strategic position to assist people in their most critical moments. In one study of terminally ill patients in a major nonsectarian medical center, 76% indicated that they wanted to be able to talk to their nurses about God, 55% wanted their nurses to assist them with prayer, and 46% wanted their nurses to acknowledge and respect their religious beliefs (Sodestron & Martinson, 1987). Health care professionals are, in turn, showing a growing interest in the spiritual needs of their patients. For example, in a survey of hospice caregivers, a majority stated that they listened to their patients talk about God, shared their own spirituality, used prayer, and read scriptures with their patients (Millison & Dudley, 1992). Many of these activities were performed as frequently by the caregivers as they were by the clergy. Nevertheless, health care professionals appear to be treading gingerly around religious issues. Surveys indicate that they, like their mental health counterparts, are uncertain about how best to respond to their patients' spiritual needs (Taylor & Amanta, 1994b).

Even if health and mental health professionals were more willing and able to address religious issues in their work, many people would still be left without help. Epidemiological surveys indicate that the numbers of people with significant personal problems in the United States far exceeds the capacity of health professionals to serve them (Regier et al., 1988). Mental health services are being further restricted by cutbacks in insurance reimbursement that have followed the growth in managed health care. There are, however, other places to go for help.

Clergy

The most obvious sources of professional religious assistance in coping are the clergy. Clergy have several advantages as helpers that go beyond their spiritual orientation. First, they are accessible. There are far more clergy in the United States (over 545,000) than mental health professionals (approximately 40,000) (Jacquet & Jones, 1991). Clergy can be found in virtually every community in the United States, including those rural and urban areas that receive little service by other professionals. Second, clergy have traditionally shared the most critical life transitions with their members—birth, coming of age, marriage, illness, death— those times when people may be in greatest need of support. Third, unlike mental health professionals, who wait for their cases to come to them, clergy have the right to reach out to their members in times of trouble. Thus, they can intervene more quickly and directly than other helping professionals. Finally, many people may feel less stigma in seeking help from their clergy than from other professionals. As noted earlier, large numbers of people prefer to take their problems to religious leaders. Studies show that ministers see many of the same types of problems as those seen by psychologists, psychiatrists, and social workers (Hohmann & Larson, 1993).

Concerns, however, have been raised about the ability of clergy to provide counseling for significant personal problems. A small but significant number of clergy have received extensive clinical training and supervision by accrediting bodies. For example, the American Association of Pastoral Counselors (AAPC) has certified more than 3,200 pastoral counselors and 100 pastoral counseling centers in the United States (Wyrtzen, 1996). However, these clergy may be among the exceptions to the rule. Although interest in counseling is growing within seminaries, most graduates still receive relatively little training in this area (e.g., Linebaugh & Devivo, 1981). The lack of preparation for counseling, a source of dissatisfaction among clergy themselves (e.g., Kaseman & Anderson, 1977), may help explain why clergy are less knowledgeable than other groups about mental health issues. For example, in one study of religious leaders from a variety of traditions, clergy demonstrated less expertise about psychopathology than doctoral clinical psychologists, graduate students in clinical and counseling psychology, and undergraduates in abnormal and introductory psychology courses (Domino, 1990).

Whether the lack of training and formal knowledge about psychopathology means that clergy are ineffective as counselors is unclear. Few studies have directly examined the efficacy of clergy as counselors. People report quite positively on the counseling they receive from their ministers (Veroff et al., 1981), but these reports are difficult to interpret without comparison groups of those who have not had counseling or have gone into counseling with other professionals. Propst et al. (1992) did find that a pastoral form of counseling was more effective in the treatment of clinical depression than a standard cognitive-behavioral treatment. However, the "pastoral" counseling was delivered by religiously sensitive students, not clergy.

Some in the religious community have screamed "foul" at the attempt to evaluate clergy by the standards of mental health. After all, how well would mental health professionals do on a test of *religious* knowledge? The role of the clergy, it has been argued, should not be confused with the role of the mental health professional. In this vein, theologian Thomas Oden (1983) has criticized the loss of religious identity among pastors who have tried to emulate other professions in their work. He writes:

> It is true that the good pastor functions as philosophical guide and psychological counselor and social change agent and moral mentor at various times. . . . But when these are disconnected from their historical identity and tradition and from the history of revelation and the capacity of God to address the heart, they easily become too cheaply accommodative to the present culture and lose the finely balanced judgment that the tradition has called wisdom. (p. 55)

Oden makes a compelling argument. Clergy are not mental health professionals in religious garb. As "shepherds of the soul," clergy are distinctly concerned about the embodiment of the spiritual as well as the biological, social, and psychological in the life of the whole person. It follows that evaluations of pastoral counseling that reduce the clergy to simply another group of mental health workers are likely to underestimate the power of this unique role. Spiritual criteria of success in the search for significance should be integrated in future studies of counseling if we are to develop a more complete understanding of the efficacy of clergy (and other professionals) as helpers.

Self-Help, Lay Persons, and Mutual Support

For most people, the telephone call to the helping professional is more likely to be the last resort than the initial reaction when problems arise. Most people try to solve their problems themselves or with the help of family and friends. Only when these methods fail are they likely to look for professional assistance. These methods, however, do not necessarily fail. Nonprofessional help may be quite effective, and this help can be sensitive to matters of religion.

One potentially valuable source of help is religious self-help materials. Many people try to solve their problems through scriptural study or religious television. A quick visit to any bookstore, drugstore, or supermarket checkout line also reveals an abundant supply of religious self-help books, pamphlets, and articles. They cover the gamut of life's crises: the death of a child, divorce, imprisonment, life-threatening illness, suicide, and so on. Many of these readings contain recommendations about religious coping. For example, one pamphlet entitled "Walking with God through Grief and Loss" encourages the reader to express his or her religious discontent ("As we grieve our loss, it helps to deliberately pray our pain, to cry out to God, to express our anger"), seek out spiritual support ("We can picture God sitting by our side, looking upon us with much love, or walking with us and listening to our story of sorrow"), and reframe the relationship with God ("We may think God is absent, yet God is there in ways we may not have noticed") (Rupp, 1990). Although the effectiveness of religious self-help materials has not been examined directly, studies of other self-administered treatments indicate that they may be as helpful as therapist-administered treatments, at least for problems that are well suited to educational interventions (see Christensen & Jacobson, 1994).

Lay members of churches, mosques, temples, and synagogues represent another pool of potential support and help. Like clergy, they are able to access many of the hardest to reach people in our communities and, like clergy, they are able to draw on a tradition of caring and support for one another in stressful times. Several lay counseling programs have been developed to train and organize congregation members as lay ministers to others in need (see Tan, 1990). For example, the Stephen Series teaches church members to assist fellow members who are typically identified and referred by the minister (Haugk, 1985). This program is explicitly rooted in the Christian belief in the "priesthood of all believers" (1 Peter 2:5–9). Stephen ministers receive extensive training in crisis intervention, listening skills, dealing with feelings, community resources, and the distinctive nature of Christian caring. Over 30,000 lay ministers have been trained from 1,100 congregations and 40 different denominations. One church reported that, over an 18-month period, its ministers made 736 direct contacts and 648 phone contacts with members experiencing a wide range of problems, including divorce, grief, unemployment, depression, and chronic illness. Researchers are only just beginning to assess the effectiveness of lay counselors (Tan, 1990). The results are, however, promising (see Toh & Tan, in press).

Mutual support groups have also become increasingly popular forms of help. It has been estimated that there are approximately 500,000 self-help groups in the United States, attended by over 15 million people (see Atkins, 1991). A sizable portion of these groups are 12-Step programs, modeled after Alcoholics Anonymous (AA). These groups have been described as modern religious movements that encourage fundamental changes in relationships, worldviews, and lifestyles. Indeed, a close look at the 12 steps themselves reveals some strong parallels between these methods and the methods of religious coping, especially religious conversion and rituals of purification (see Table 12.3). In the first three steps, the individual is encouraged to make a radical change, to recognize the powerlessness of the self and to incorporate the sacred into the self. In the next six steps, the person is asked to identify his or her shortcomings, to seek out God's help in removing these limitations, and to make amends to those who have been hurt. In the final two steps, the individual looks to God for religious direction and strength, and commits him- or herself to helping others.

Evaluations of AA members suggest that they achieve as high or higher rates of abstinence than professionally treated alcoholics (Emrick, 1987). Evaluation of other mutual support groups, while limited in number and design, have also yielded promising results (Christensen & Jacobson, 1994).

Mental health professionals are not the only deliverers of help. There are many sources of assistance in coping, and each source has something distinctive to offer people in times of trouble. There is no need for rivalry among helpers, particularly at a time when changes in the health and human service system may leave increasing numbers of people without assistance. Personal problems are numerous enough, serious enough, and diverse enough to require help from many quarters.

Expanding the Targets of Help

Typically, people in western culture think about problems and solutions in individual terms. Mental health professionals are no exception to this

---

Table 12.3. The 12 Steps of Alcoholics Anonymous

---

1. We admitted we were powerless over alcohol—that our lives had become unmanageable.
2. Came to believe that a Power greater than ourselves could restore us to sanity.
3. Made a decision to turn our will and our lives over to the care of God *as we understand Him.*
4. Made a searching and fearless moral inventory of ourselves.
5. Admitted to God, to ourselves, and to another human being the exact nature of our wrongs.
6. Were entirely ready to have God remove all these defects of character.
7. Humbly asked Him to remove our shortcomings.
8. Made a list of all persons we had harmed, and became willing to make amends to them all.
9. Made direct amends to such people wherever possible, except when to do so would injure them or others.
10. Continued to take personal inventory and when we were wrong promptly admitted it.
11. Sought through prayer and meditation to improve our conscious contact with God *as we understand Him,* praying only for knowledge of His will for us and the power to carry that out.
12. Having had a spiritual awakening as the result of these steps, we tried to carry this message to alcoholics, and to practice these principles in all our affairs.

Note. From *Alcoholics Anonymous* (1977, pp. 59–60). The Twelve Steps are reprinted with permission of Alcoholics Anonymous World Services, Inc. Permission to reprint the Twelve Steps does not mean that AA has reviewed or approved the contents of this publication, nor that AA agrees with the views expressed herein. AA is a program of recovery for alcoholism *only*—use of the Twelve Steps in connection with programs and activities which are patterned after AA, but which address other problems, or in any other non-AA context, does not imply otherwise.

rule. The American Psychiatric Association's *Diagnostic and Statistical Manual of Mental Disorders* catalogues the variety of individual psychological problems in living. The most widely practiced and accepted forms of treatment are also targeted to the individual. One reflection of this individualistic bias is the traditional refusal of many insurance companies to reimburse costs for marital or family therapy.

From a coping perspective, individuals represent an important target for change, but not the only target. Stressful situations affect systems as well as individuals. When an individual gets cancer, the saying goes, the whole family gets cancer (Schafer, 1984). The same point holds true for religious systems. For example, cases of sexual misconduct by religious leaders create powerful waves that wash over not only those directly involved, but the congregation as a whole. Like the individual, the system must cope with the negative event and, like the individual, the system can encounter troubles in coping.

Religious resources may be helpful to social systems in times of trouble. Families, for example, are accorded sacred status from the perspective of most religious traditions. Religions prescribe norms and values that encourage family closeness and stability and discourage attitudes and behaviors that pose threats to the well-being of the family (D'Antonio, Newman, & Wright, 1982). Research studies have shown positive relationships between measures of religiousness and marital and family adjustment (Hansen, 1992; Stinnett, 1979). Counselors have begun to draw on religious resources and coping methods to help families struggling through change and transition (see Prest & Keller, 1993; Worthington, 1989).

Griffith (1986), for example, describes the case of Byron, a 20-year-old evangelical Christian who was having difficulty in the transition to college. An honors student in high school, he was experiencing problems concentrating on his studies and was almost failing. Griffith learned that Byron was preoccupied with concerns about his mother, who had been lonely and isolated since the death of her own mother several years earlier. Byron's mother was, in turn, preoccupied with her son: "Byron and I are so close," she said, "that when he takes a bath, I feel clean" (p. 610). To reduce the degree of enmeshment between mother and son, Griffith decided to work with the family. He challenged mother and son from their own religious frame of reference. "For many years," he said to Byron in the presence of his mother, "you have been more a husband to your mother than her own husband; now, by acting as her protector against every natural disaster, you are trying to be her God" (p. 610). By relabeling Byron's obsessive focus on his mother as a sin, a usurpation of God's powers, Griffith encouraged his client to engage in a re-valuation—a shift of significance from a one-sided focus on his mother to a commitment to his religious faith. Ultimately, Byron chose to become more involved in his religious life and, in the process, he developed greater emotional independence from his mother.

Religious forms of help could be applied to other increasingly common family problems, such as the difficulties that arise in coping with interfaith marriages or interfaith blended families (e.g., Weidman, 1989) and family conflicts about abortion, euthanasia, and life-sustaining measures for the terminally ill (e.g., Sonnenblick, Friedlander, & Steinberg, 1993). Religious help is also applicable to other social systems, including churches and synagogues coping with internal and external changes (Pargament et al., 1991), and communities facing problems of poverty, crime, and deteriorating neighborhoods.

For example, Cohen and his colleagues (Cohen et al., 1992) have documented the extensive involvement of religious denominations and local congregations in efforts to deal with homelessness. These efforts go well beyond financial assistance or temporary shelter offered to individual families. Religious institutions have advocated for affordable housing at state and federal levels. They have targeted specific neighborhoods for housing development, crime prevention, and demolition of deteriorating buildings. Some congregations have joined forces to construct and manage their own affordable housing for low- and moderate-income families. Cohen et al. note that religious organizations offer "strength, personnel, vision, stability, continuity, and intellect" to the daunting problem of homelessness (p. 324).

In short, even though helping professionals are used to thinking about problems and solutions in individual terms, there are other relevant targets for religiously based change. Life stressors affect families, organizations, and communities as well as individuals. Problems in coping can be conceptualized and addressed at any of these social or individual levels of analysis. Helping social systems is relatively new and challenging work, yet it offers opportunities to enhance the quality and to extend the range of help to other important problems and populations.

Expanding the Time to Help

Students of community psychology are often presented with the following hypothetical dilemma. A young woman hiking alongside a river hears the cries of several people trying to stay afloat in the middle of the river. She jumps into the river and helps the people ashore, only to hear the calls of several others in the same distress. Confused, she looks up and notices that the bridge upriver has been swept away. Drivers, unaware the bridge is out, are plunging into the waters. Should she continue to rescue people as they come downriver, one by one? Or should she race upstream and warn the other drivers before they fall into the river? Most students try to find a way to do both: save those who are drowning and prevent others from falling in. Helping people after a crisis has occurred and helping people steer clear of the crisis both make sense.

In the real world, however, most helping takes place after the fact. Professional helpers are generally socialized into a "waiting mode" (cf. Rappaport, 1977), remaining in their offices to treat people who come to them for help after a problem has occurred. This pattern has been perpetuated by the traditional reluctance of health insurance companies to provide reimbursement for preventive services. Yet many lives, considerable anguish, and a great deal of expense could be spared by preventing serious problems, such as AIDS or alcohol/drug abuse, from developing in the first place. Preventive programs have proven successful in reducing the incidence of a variety of disorders and problems (Price, Cowen, Lorion, & Ramos-McKay, 1988).

Religion is not usually thought of as a resource for prevention. Religious helpers themselves do not typically speak the language of prevention (Anderson, Maton, & Ensor, 1992). In fact, as Spilka and Bridges (1992) have noted, according to some traditions, prevention is a "theological impossibility." The fundamental problem of sin is basic to the human condition. It can be transcended through the grace of God; it cannot be prevented through human action. From this point of view, prayer for salvation in the world-to-come rather than prevention in this world is the proper response to the human plight. Religious groups that hold strictly to this position may discourage "sinful" acts (e.g., homosexuality), but they may also be less than willing to support efforts that prevent the potential consequences of these acts (e.g., AIDS education), consequences that could be viewed as deserved punishments from God.

Many other religious traditions see the human condition differently. Personal and social suffering can be defined as the result of human ignorance and "social sin" (Spilka & Bridges, 1992). To remake the world along the lines of greater understanding, compassion, and social justice are, from this perspective, central religious tasks. Prevention is quite consistent with the religious mission defined in this manner. In some but not all of its forms, then, religion can serve important preventive roles (see Pargament, Maton, et al., 1992). How does religion contribute to prevention? In two ways. First, religious involvement can be inherently preventive. Second, religious groups and institutions have begun to offer formal prevention programs of their own.

Regular involvement in a system of religious beliefs and practices can have naturally preventive consequences. Many religions teach their members to avoid high-risk behaviors. For example, Seventh-Day Adventists, a group that discourages the consumption of coffee and meat, have lower than average mortality rates from bowel, prostate, and breast cancer. The Amish, who have strong sanctions against extramarital sex, have lower rates of cervical cancer (see Jenkins, 1992, for a review). Involvement in religious systems that proscribe the destruction of life, substance use, and extramarital relationships has been associated with lower risks of suicide, drug and alcohol abuse, and family breakup (see Payne, Bergin, Bielema, & Jenkins, 1992, for a review).

Involvement in day-to-day religious life can also strengthen the orienting system and increase the individual's resilience to crisis. On the social side, long-term participation in a religious congregation offers the individual a source of support and access to rites of passage that facilitate the transition through important junctures of the lifespan. On the personal side, religion can contribute to a well-differentiated, well-organized, and comprehensive framework for understanding and dealing with the world. With this framework, the individual is more capable of generating religious coping methods that buffer the effects of stress and prevent the development of serious life problems (see Chapter 10).

Religious institutions have begun to develop formal programs for people before they encounter problems. For example, one survey in a large Western city in the United States revealed that half the congregations had conducted drug or alcohol education programs within the last 3 years (Lorch, 1987). Many churches and synagogues are also sponsoring marital enrichment programs to help couples view their relationship in a spiritual light, anticipate problems that may arise, build communication skills, and identify religious resources to strengthen their marriage (e.g., Worthington, 1990).

It is important to note that religious institutions are particularly well positioned to help some of the most disenfranchised, at-risk groups in society. The black church, for example, is a central institution in the lives of African-Americans, many of whom have only limited access to mainstream health and human services. Its ethos of commitment to serving the full range of social, psychological, physical, and spiritual needs is quite compatible with the ethos of prevention (Levin, 1984). Black churches and many other congregations are involved in outreach programs to high-risk groups. In 1991, 9 out of 10 congregations were reportedly supporting or operating human service, health, or welfare programs (Goodstein, 1993). These programs span a broad spectrum, from church-based crisis counseling, health education, and jobs skills training for the hard-core unemployed to school-based tutoring and

Family Life Centers (see Eng & Hatch, 1992; Maton & Pargament, 1987; Maton & Wells, 1995).

Although its involvement in formal preventive programming is a recent phenomenon, religion may be a particularly potent resource for prevention. This point is illustrated by an evaluation of Project RAISE (Raising Ambition Instills Self Esteem), a Baltimore City project aimed at providing inner-city youth with academic and social support over a 7-year period (Maton & Seibert, 1991). Six churches and seven community organizations recruited mentors to help the students with schooling, provide attention and caring, and serve as role models for success and responsibility. Three years into the program, Maton and Seibert found that the students served by the church were more likely to have established a stable long-term relationship with the sponsor than students served by other community organizations. Furthermore, students with congregational sponsors made more consistent academic gains than a non-RAISE comparison sample.

Maton and Seibert (1991) offer several reasons for the distinctive impact of the church-based sponsors. The church may have provided more support to sustain the mentors over the course of the 7-year project. The parents of the students and students themselves may have been more likely to trust and respond to outreach from church-based individuals, given the central role of the church in the community and the similarity of religious and cultural background. The church provided mentors and students with a variety of congregational activities in which they could meet and form a deeper, on-going relationship. Finally, the deeper commitment of the church-based mentors to this program may have been motivated by their belief in the special religious calling to their work.

Prevention is not as popular a form of helping as counseling to those already in distress. Mother Teresa and Albert Schweitzer are far better known than John Snow and Ignatz Semmelweiss, public health figures who discovered how to prevent cholera and child-bed fever, respectively. Yet, in terms of lives saved and suffering spared, the impact of Snow and Semmelweiss was arguably equal to or greater than that of Mother Teresa and Albert Schweitzer. Traditionally, religious ministry has been more closely associated with healing the sick and suffering than with prevention. But there is nothing about religion per se that restricts it to helping after the fact. On the contrary, religious resources and preventive methods of coping represent a potentially powerful form of assistance to people before they encounter trouble or before small problems become big problems.

There are many exciting opportunities for work in the area of religion and prevention. One possibility would be to design a religious

educational curriculum that promotes comprehensive, well-differentiated, flexible religious orienting systems relevant to a broad range of
life's existential questions and crises. For example, one religious musical
series devoted one album to teaching problem-solving skills from a
religious perspective (Rettino & Rettino, 1985). A second possibility
would be to target other disenfranchised groups whose only institutional
link may be the congregation. Following their survey of almost 50,000
street injection-drug users across the United States, McBride, McCoy,
Chitwood, Hernandez, and Mutch (1994) concluded that "churches,
temples, and other religious organizations could be perceived by high
risk groups, to whom the government often has very little credible access,
as a believable, valid source of AIDS prevention information" (p. 332).
A third possibility would be to develop specialized programs to facilitate
religious coping among particular groups of people vulnerable to serious
problems. Congregations could develop outreach programs to elderly
widows who have begun to isolate themselves from their communities
and run a greater risk of depression (see Siegel & Kuykendall, 1990).
The opportunities for religious involvement in prevention have only
begun to be explored.

BRIDGING THE WORLDS
OF PSYCHOLOGY AND RELIGION
THROUGH RESOURCE COLLABORATION

As I have gotten to know psychologists and other mental health professionals, I have been struck by the number who once aspired to go into
the ministry or received training in seminary. Many clergy, I have also
found, seriously considered careers in the mental health profession earlier
in their lives. The affinity between the two kinds of professionals makes
sense; both are interested in understanding and improving the human
condition. What makes less sense is the fact that, once the career choice
is made, the two groups so often head down very separate paths. In spite
of their shared interests and concerns, helpers from psychological and
religious communities have traditionally had relatively little to do with
each other.

In the first chapter, I noted how stereotypes, rivalry, and suspicion
are partly responsible for this schism. In other chapters of this book, I
have tried to challenge some of these misconceptions: the notion that
religion is merely a defense against anxiety on the one hand, and the
notion that there is no room in psychology for anything but self-centered
concerns on the other. We have seen that religion can contribute to the
search for significance in stressful times in a rich variety of ways. We

have also seen that psychology is capable of stretching itself as a science and profession to explore and grapple with the most profound human longings and dilemmas. To be sure, there are important differences between psychological and religious disciplines in worldviews, practices, and methods of study. But these differences could be a source of dialogue rather than division.

Even though writers have long called for closer ties between religious and mental health disciplines, until recently these calls have gone largely ignored. Members of the two communities have had little actual contact with one another, and are often poorly informed about the resources the other has to offer. Those interactions that have taken place have typically been one-sided. A subset of clergy has been quite receptive to the theories and methods of psychotherapy, integrating this body of knowledge into pastoral counseling. A subset of clergy has also been willing to refer cases for counseling to mental health professionals. Although mental health professionals have been happy to accept these referrals and to provide educational programs to congregations, they have not drawn on the resources and wisdom of religious communities to enhance their own work and professional development in return. Surveys indicate that clergy refer far greater numbers of cases to mental health professionals than they receive (e.g., Carson, 1976; Meylink & Gorsuch, 1986).

Some leaders of religious communities have voiced dissatisfaction with the one-sidedness of the relationship between religion and mental health (Kloos, Horneffer, & Moore, 1995). Bickel (1978), for one, put it this way: "For decades there have been calls on all sides for a 'dialogue between religion and mental health.' What has resulted has been to a large extent a monologue in which the clerical and lay members of the religious community have sat at the feet of the mental health professional" (p. 1).

Fortunately, there are signs of change. The publication of several important basic texts in the psychology of religion underscores the growing audience of psychologists interested in learning more about religious phenomena (Batson et al., 1993; Hood, Spilka, Hunsberger, & Gorsuch, 1996; Paloutzian, 1996; Wulff, 1997). Books and papers by psychologists on religion and counseling reflect a heightened awareness of the need to understand and deal with the client's religious world (Lovinger, 1984; Propst, 1988; Shafranske, 1996). Graduate programs in psychology have formed that explicitly attempt to integrate psychological theories and methods within particular religious traditions (e.g., Biola University, Fuller Theological Seminary, George Fox College, Wheaton College).

Researchers and practitioners within the mainstream of psychology and other helping professions have also begun to apply methods of coping rooted in the religious world to a broader population. These methods include the use of forgiveness to help people give up old resentments and move on to new goals and interests (e.g., McCullough & Worthington, 1994b), the use of rituals to facilitate important transitions in life (e.g., Imber-Black & Roberts, 1993), and the use of meditation to reduce anxiety and stress (e.g., Benson, 1984). Interventions such as these provide a measure of correction to the more traditional control-oriented interventions of psychology. But it is important to add that in many instances these coping methods have been divested of their original religious association and meaning: Forgiveness has been promoted on purely secular grounds; rituals have been suggested that have little, if any, spiritual connection; and meditation has centered around nonreligious matters and mantras. It remains to be seen whether these methods of coping retain their potency when separated from their religious roots.

Overall, there appears to be an increasing willingness among many members of psychological and religious communities to learn about and learn from the other. But there is further to go (e.g., Weaver, Koenig, & Larson, 1997). For the relationship between these groups to evolve, more direct contact and interaction must replace the one-sided relationships of the past. Neither psychology nor religion holds all of the answers to life's most difficult questions, but each has a method and a message of importance to those they serve and to each other. What is needed is a shift from monologue to dialogue, from isolation to collaboration.

Tyler, Gatz, and I (Tyler, Pargament, & Gatz, 1983) proposed the resource collaborator role as an appropriate model for interactions between psychologists, clients, and other disciplines, including religious helpers. The resource collaborator model rejects the notion that one partner in a helping relationship is superior to another by virtue of education or occupation. Instead, it assumes that the participants are equal in their basic worth. This is not to say that they bring identical qualities to the relationship. Both partners are assumed to have distinctive resources and deficits. But these differences do not have to result in estrangement. On the contrary, the process of sharing distinctive resources creates opportunities for mutual growth. Resource collaboration rests on a deep respect for our unique identities, strengths, and weaknesses, and the belief that we can enhance the well-being of ourselves and each other by sharing our resources.

Resource collaboration is well suited to the relationship between religious and psychological helping communities. It underscores the uniqueness of the two disciplines. Congregations and clergy are not to be confused with quasimental health centers and mental health professionals (Rappaport, 1981). Psychologists and other health professionals are not to be dismissed as modern-day clergy. The missions of the two overlap, both are concerned with the search for significance, but they are not identical. Each community may articulate a destination of significance and a pathway to reach it that is, in some ways, distinctive.

The resource collaborator model also alerts us to the strengths and limitations of both psychological and religious helpers, and the exciting possibilities for exchange. Limited in its own access to the most underserved populations and limited in its understanding of culturally diverse religious expressions, psychology could expand its reach by working more closely with religious institutions that have a history of trusted relationship with many disenfranchised and diverse groups. With its difficulty in facing and resolving difficult value-related issues, psychology could draw on the wealth of religious literature on morality, ethics, and matters of deepest significance. Less than adequate in its own ways of understanding and dealing with the limits of human control, psychology could learn a great deal from the theologies of the religious world and its methods of coming to terms with human finitude.

Religion, in turn, could address its own shortcoming by drawing on psychological resources. Struggling at times with its own ways to enhance personal power, religion could learn more about psychological theories and methods of change. Unequipped to evaluate its own efforts to bring people closer to the sacred, religion could call upon the methods of science for assistance. In these respects, psychology and religion complement each other very nicely; both disciplines have something to gain through exchange. For their part, many religious leaders have expressed an openness to genuine collaboration between psychology and religion (Kloos et al., 1995).

Collaboration will not be possible in all instances. Fundamental differences in values may be, in some cases, too great to support any hopes of collaboration (e.g., abortion, homosexuality, deference to religious authority). More often than not, however, I believe psychology and religion can find enough common ground for exchange.

Examples of resource collaboration are already available. Mental health professionals and clergy have joined forces to counsel people who are encountering a mixture of psychological and religious problems (e.g., York, 1987). Of particular note are the relationships with "cultural brokers," leaders from new or nontraditional religious groups, that are forming to assist mental health professionals in their work with increasing numbers of culturally diverse religious clients (e.g., Waldfogel & Wolpe, 1993). Holistic health centers have developed that are staffed by clergy, medical, and mental health professionals who work together to address the well-being of the whole person—physical, mental, and spiritual (McSherry, 1983). Psychologists and religious leaders have created successful partnerships to implement and evaluate alcohol abuse prevention programs in local congregations (Roberts & Thorsheim, 1987). Religious institutions and other community organizations have established effective alliances to develop a variety of community revitalization programs (Scheie, Markham, Mayer, Slettom, & Williams, 1991). In my research with my colleagues (Pargament et al., 1991), we have provided churches and synagogues with a data-based consultation program to help them evaluate themselves and plan for the future in exchange for the opportunity they give us to learn about the roles of religion in coping in the lives of their members.

In the future, helpers from psychological and religious communities could collaborate in the development and evaluation of psychospiritual interventions for groups coping with major life crises. Joint educational forums could also be established in which leaders of religious and psychological communities teach each other about their worldviews, practices, and methods of study. These are just a few of the intriguing possibilities that emerge when we are willing to reach beyond the boundaries of our own disciplines and work with others who share a commitment to bettering the world.

The search for significance in stressful times is not a simple or straightforward process. The individual must grapple with powerful and, at times, opposing forces: the controllable and the uncontrollable, the intellectual and the emotional, the good and the bad, the possible and the impossible, the personal and the interpersonal, the immediate and the ultimate. Committed and caring as we may be, no single helper or helping profession can succeed in unraveling all of these complexities. Collectively, however, we are likely to be more successful, and the beneficiaries of this collaboration are not restricted to those we serve.

Helpers from every discipline have their limitations. The failure to take these limitations and needs for renewal seriously has exacted a toll in burnout and frustration among helpers in religious and mental health communities. We have become "wounded healers" (Lerner, 1994). Resource collaboration offers a partial remedy, an opportunity for helpers to replenish themselves and grow personally as well as professionally. By working together, we bridge two worlds that have been isolated for too long, opening each up to new resources and possibilities. Through this process, we may discover that we are better able to help others and ourselves in the search for significance.

APPENDICES

APPENDIX A. Proportion of People Who Involve Religion in Coping

Study	Sample	Method	Results
Baider & Sarell (1983)	33 Jewish Israeli women with breast cancer	Structured interview of who/what is to blame for their illness	60.6% report God is to blame for the cancer.
Balk (1983)	33 white teenagers who experienced death of a sibling	Structured interview on response to death of sibling	69.7% report religion was important or very important after the loss.
Bowker (1988)	1,000 battered wives	Interviews and surveys regarding where help was sought for their situation	One-third sought help from clergy.
Bulman & Wortman (1977)	28 victims of severe accidents	Spontaneous responses to question "Why me?"	35% indicate that God had a reason for the accident.
Cain (1988)	30 middle-class white women divorced after age 60	Interviews and questionnaires of how coped with divorce	Two-thirds report turned to religion in coping (e.g., congregation affiliation, clergy, rituals).
Carlson & Cervara (1991)	37 wives of prison inmates	Self-reports of use of religion in coping with husband's incarceration	27% indicate religion was used to cope.
Compas, Forsythe, & Wagner (1988)	65 undergraduates	Checklist over 4 weeks on whether sought or found spiritual comfort and support for a negative academic and negative interpersonal event	29.2% involve religion in dealing with academic event; 21.5% involve religion in dealing with interpersonal event.
Conway (1985–1986)	65 older women reporting medical problems	Checklist of prayer as a coping mechanism for medical problem	91% report prayer as coping mechanism.

(continued)

407

Study	Sample	Method	Results
Croog & Levine (1972)	324 men who had heart attack; Catholic, Protestant, and Jewish	Survey of whether they had seen or planned to see clergy for aid; survey of causes of heart attack	11% obtained or planned to seek aid from clergy; 40% rate Will of God as influential factor; 13% rate Payment for Sins and Punishment for Doing Wrong in Life as influential.
Dalal & Pande (1988)	41 patients from India with major injuries due to an accident	Questionnaire and interview on causal attributions using 1 to 5 scale	God's wishes received highest rating as cause of the accident (4.42).
Ellison & Taylor (1996)	1,299 African-American adults	Interviews of whether person prayed or had someone pray for them in response to major life crisis and/or personal problem too great to handle alone	80% reported use of prayer to cope.
Gilbert (1989)	54 parents who lost fetus or child	Minimally structured interview of how coped with loss of fetus or child	78% report religious involvement in coping, positive or negative.
Greil, Porter, Leitko, & Riscilli (1989)	29 parents with infertility	Spontaneous mention of supernatural entity in response to "Why me?"	86% address "Why me?" in religious sense.
Gurin, Veroff, & Feld (1960)	National sample of 2,460 adults	First spontaneous mention of how one handles worries	16% mention prayer as first response; 4% mention clergy as first response.
Hayden & Przybysz (1995)	42 metastatic cancer patients; Protestant and Catholic	Interviews about "Why me?"	29% indicate religious explanations in attempt to resolve the question.
Hughes et al. (1994)	56 parents of infants in a neonatal intensive care unit	Self-report of reliance on religious faith in coping	33% report rely on religious faith to cope.

Study	Sample	Method	Results
Kesselring et al. (1986)	45 Swiss and 40 Egyptian cancer patients	Interviews on expectations of what will help with illness	37% Swiss say God will help; 92% Egyptian say God will help.
Koenig (1988)	263 elderly; mostly Protestant	Report of use of prayer and religious beliefs to cope with a recent stressor	95% report use of prayer and 81% report use of religious beliefs to cope.
Koenig, George, & Siegler (1988)	100 older adults; mostly Protestant	Spontaneous mention of religious coping in response to 1 of 3 stressful events	45% indicate religion involved in coping.
Koenig et al. (1992)	850 hospitalized, ill, elderly men; largely conservative Protestant	Spontaneous mention of religion as most helpful way of coping with illness	20% mention religion as primary coping method.
Kubacka-Jasiecka, Dorczak, & Opozzynska (1990)	30 college students in Poland reporting stressful situations	Spontaneous mention of religion as a coping mechanism in a stressful situation	Two-thirds mention some form of religion or religious values in coping.
LaGrand (1985)	901 college students reporting death of loved one	Survey of coping through religious beliefs in response to the loss	35% report used religious beliefs in coping.
Leyser (1994)	82 Israeli Orthodox Jewish parents of disabled children	Checklist and open-ended questions about ways of coping with disabled child	46% indicate prayers as way of coping; 35% spontaneously mention faith in God as way of coping.
Lindenthal et al. (1970)	938 adult residents of New Haven	Survey of whether prayed for help after a life crisis over the past year	44% reportedly prayed for help.
Manfredi & Pickett (1987)	51 older adults mostly in senior housing	Survey of ways of coping with stressful event experienced in last month	Prayer most frequently used strategy; $M = 2.35$ on 4-point scale.

(continued)

Study	Sample	Method	Results
Mattlin, Wethington, & Kessler (1990)	977 married nonblack adults in Detroit	Report of religious coping with most recent stressor	73% report religion was used to cope from a little to a lot.
McCrae (1984)	255 community adults with recent life event of loss, threat, or challenge	Survey of whether coped by putting faith in God	60% report coped through faith in God.
Pargament, Ensing, et al. (1990)	586 members of 10 mainline Christian churches	Survey of whether religion was involved in understanding and/or dealing with serious life event in past year	78% indicate religion involved from slightly to great deal in coping.
Segall & Wykle (1988–1989)	59 black family caregivers to dementia relatives	Spontaneous mention of religious coping; surveys of faith and prayer as way of coping on 1 to 5 scale	65% say prayer, faith in God were ways of coping; prayer and faith rated 4.34 and 4.00.
Thompson et al. (1993)	71 cancer patients; mostly white, married	Open-ended question about how tried to control emotions	22% reportedly tried to control emotions through faith.
Wicks (1990)	Random sample of 400 residents of Toledo	Survey of whether religion was involved in understanding and/or dealing with serious life event in past year	58% indicate religion involved from slightly to great deal in coping.

APPENDIX B. Predictors of Religious Coping

Study	Sample	Predictor	Religious coping	Results
Personal predictors of religious coping				
Bearon & Koenig (1990)	36 elderly reporting physical symptoms; Protestant	Gender, race, Baptist versus other denominations	Reports of prayer over symptoms	Less educated were more likely to pray. Blacks (60%) more likely to pray than whites (44%). Baptists more likely to pray than others.
Berman (1974)	198 people who had a life-threatening experience; Jewish, Protestant, and Catholic	Religious activity	Frequency of prayer after life-threatening experience	Prayer was reported more frequently by more religiously active people.
Bjorck & Cohen (1993)	293 college students; Protestant and Catholic	Gender and intrinsic religiousness	Scale of religious coping with hypothetical life stressors	Religious coping was tied to female status and intrinsicness.
Carver, Scheier, & Weintraub (1993)	59 women with breast cancer at presurgery, and four times postsurgery	Optimistic personality	Scale of religious coping with breast cancer	No relationship of religious coping to optimism at any point in time.
Courtenay et al. (1992)	16 older adults (60 to 100+ years old)	Measures of religiousness	Reports of reliance on prayer, religious beliefs, and church attendance in coping with health and family problems	Reliance on prayer and religious beliefs were associated with ideological, experiential, and consequential religiousness, not intellectual religiousness. No relation to church attendance.

(continued)

411

Study	Sample	Predictor	Religious coping	Results
Croog & Levine (1972)	324 who had had a heart attack; Catholic, Protestant, and Jewish	Denomination, social status	Survey of whether they had seen or planned to see clergy for aid; survey of whether heart attack was God's Will	Catholics and Protestants were more likely to seek aid from clergy than Jews; less educated were more likely to seek help from clergy; Catholics, Protestants, and Jews see God's Will successively less influential; there was no relation of social status to God's Will ratings.
DeVellis, DeVellis, & Spilsbury (1988)	72 parents responding to vignettes of hypothetical illness in their children	Belief in divine influence in child's recovery from illness	Reports of spiritual action in response to illness	Spiritual action was associated with belief in divine influence over child's recovery from illness.
Dufton & Perlman (1986)	232 college students from Canada completing measure of loneliness	Nonbelievers versus nonconservative believers versus conservative believers	Frequency of supernatural attributions of cause and cure of loneliness; frequency of coping with loneliness through prayer, reading Bible, talking to fellow believers	Supernatural attributions of cause and cure of loneliness and religious coping responses to loneliness increase from nonbelievers to nonconservative believers to conservative believers.
Ellison & Taylor (1996)	1,299 African-American adults	Age, gender, education, personal mastery, subjective religiousness, nonorganizational religiousness	Interview question on whether person prayed or had someone pray for him or her in response to a problem	Praying to cope was more common among women, more subjectively religious, more nonorganizationally religious, and those with less personal mastery. There was no relation to age and education.

Study	Sample	Predictor	Religious coping	Results
Ferraro & Koch (1994)	National sample of 3,417 adults	SES, gender, age, marital status, race	Frequency seek spiritual comfort and support in response to problems	Religious coping was more frequent among females, older, black, married people. There was no relation to SES.
Gorsuch & Smith (1983)	164 college students at evangelical college	Fundamentalism and nearness to God measures	Attributions to God as responsible for the outcomes of four hypothetical vignettes	Attributions to God were associated with fundamentalism and nearness to God.
Gurin, Veroff, & Feld (1960)	National sample of 2,460 adults	Gender, age, education, income place of residence, Protestant versus Catholic	First spontaneous mention of prayer as way of handling worries	Prayer was noted more frequently by females, elderly, less educated, lower income, and Protestant. There was no relation to place of residence.
Hathaway (1992)	Five intrinsic and five extrinsic	Intrinsic versus extrinsic people	Scale of religious coping with daily hassles over a 90-day period	Intrinsics reported more religious coping than extrinsics.
Johnson & Spilka (1991)	103 women with breast cancer; mostly Protestant and Catholic	Intrinsic and extrinsic religious orientations	Varied religious approaches to coping with cancer	Intrinsicness was associated with more clergy involvement, beliefs of God's involvement in cancer, and satisfaction with religion in coping. Extrinsicness was not generally related to religious coping.
Koenig, George, & Siegler (1988)	100 older adults; mostly Protestant	Gender	Spontaneous mention of religious coping in response to 1 of 3 stressful events	58% females versus 32% males mention religion.

(continued)

Study	Sample	Predictor	Religious coping	Results
Koenig et al. (1990)	100 older Protestant, adults from South U.S.	Cattell 16PF	Nonreligious copers, occasional religious copers, and consistent religious copers with three stressors	Few differences in personality, but religious copers were less hostile and more humble and submissive than nonreligious copers.
Koenig et al. (1992)	850 hospitalized, ill, elderly men; largely conservative Protestant	Demographic variables, functional status, medical diagnosis	Three-item religious coping index	Religious coping was greater among older, black, retired, and those with history of psychiatric problems and poorer cognitive status. There was no relation to living situation, marital status, income, functional status, and medical diagnosis.
Kunst, Tan, & Bjorck (1994)	329 college students responding to vignettes of uncontrollable negative events; Protestant and Catholic	Religious salience and church attendance	Degree religious attributions made for the negative events	Greater religious salience and church attendance were tied to attributions to God's will, God's love, and evil spiritual forces. There was no relation to God's punishment.
Lilliston & Klein (1990)	50 college students	Self-discrepancy measure	Measure of behavioral, affective, and cognitive religious coping in response to worst personal crisis imagined	"Actual–ought" self-discrepancy was related to more behavioral and affective religious coping.
Lindenthal et al. (1970)	753 adult residents of New Haven who experienced crisis in past year	Degree of psychological impairment	Survey of whether prayed for help after life crises	Frequency of prayer increased with psychological impairment; more impaired people prayed more frequently in more controllable situations.

Study	Sample	Predictor	Religious coping	Results
McCrae & Costa (1986)	Two adult community samples of 255 and 151	NEO inventory of personality	Rating of extent faith used to cope with recent stressors	Religious coping was related to greater neuroticism in second sample only and to less openness in both samples. There was no relation to extraversion.
Pargament, Olsen, et al. (1992a)	586 members of 10 mainline Christian churches	Gender, age, education, marital status, income, religiousness measures	Survey of whether religion was involved in understanding and/or dealing with serious life event in past year	Religious coping was associated with female status, intrinsicness, orthodoxy, religious experience, loving God image, prayer, and collaborative and deferring religious coping styles. Religious coping was negatively related to self-directed coping and extrinsicness. There was no relation to quest orientation, age, education, marital status, or income.
Pargament & Sullivan (1981)	209 college students	Self-rated religiousness and general frequency of church attendance	Attributions to God control over six hypothetical situational domains	More religious students attributed more control to God than less religious.
Park & Cohen (1993)	96 college students who had experienced death of a close friend in past year; Protestant and Catholic	Measures of religiousness and gender	Scale of religious coping with death of a friend	Religious coping was tied to female status, intrinsic and extrinsic religiousness, and fundamentalism.

(continued)

Study	Sample	Predictor	Religious coping	Results
Ritzema (1979)	32 college students	Measures of religiousness	Attributions to God over four hypothetical situational domains	Religious attributions were associated with devotionalism, creedal assent, and salience of religious cognition. There was no relation to salience of religious behavior.
Sattler et al. (1994)	322 survivors of Hurricane Iniki	Demographic variables	Self-report of degree turned to religion in coping with hurricane	Religious coping was tied to female status. No relation to age, marital status, income, or education.

Situational predictors of religious coping

Study	Sample	Predictor	Religious coping	Results
Bjorck & Cohen (1993)	293 college students responding to hypothetical life stressors; Protestant and Catholic	Threat, loss, and challenge stressor vignettes	Scale of anticipated religious coping	Religious coping was greater in response to threat and loss than challenge, and in response to threat than loss.
Brown (1966)	1,111 children 12–17 from United States, New Zealand, and Australia	Seven hypothetical situations when prayer might occur	Ratings of efficacy of and appropriateness of prayer in these situations	Prayer seen as less effective and suitable for immoral, natural, and trivial situations than for situations of personal danger.
Ellison & Taylor (1996)	1,299 African-American adults	Different types of crises and problems	Interview question on whether person prayed or had someone pray for him or her in response to a problem	Praying to cope was more common in response to bereavement, personal health, and others' health problem than other stressors.

Study	Sample	Predictor	Religious coping	Results
Fry (1990)	278 elderly, homebound, with death concerns	Seven fears about death and dying	Scale of religious coping with death concerns	Religious coping was associated with concerns about physical suffering, sensory loss, personal safety, and rejection by God. It was not related to self-esteem concerns or vacuum beyond death.
Gorsuch & Smith (1983)	164 college students at evangelical college	Four hypothetical vignettes varying in extremity and probability of outcome	Attributions to God as responsible for the outcomes of the hypothetical vignettes	Attributions to God were associated with more unlikely event outcomes, and with more extreme outcomes for those who report being nearer to God.
Harris et al. (1995)	40 adult heart recipients; mostly Protestant and Catholic	Two months, 7 months, and 12 months post-transplant	Close-ended question on whether prayer was used to cope with health problems	51% used prayer to cope at 2 months posttransplant. There was no significant change over time.
Hathaway (1992)	Five intrinsic and five extrinsic mainline church members	Days of the week	Scale of religious coping with daily hassles over a 90-day period	Extrinsics reported more religious coping on Sundays than on other days of the week; intrinsics did not vary in religious coping by days of the week.

(continued)

Study	Sample	Predictor	Religious coping	Results
Hood (1977)	23 male high school seniors involved in week-long nature experience	Anticipatory stress; high stress situations versus low stress situations; congruity of anticipations of stress and stress of situation	Reports of religious mystical experience during nature experience	Lower anticipatory stress related to higher mysticism in several situations; low-stress situation related to lower mysticism; anticipations of low stress in high-stress situations were associated with high mysticism.
Hood (1978)	93 male high school seniors involved in solo overnight nature experience	Anticipatory stress; high stress (rain) versus low (dry) night; congruity of anticipation of stress and stress of situation	Reports of religious mystical experience during overnight solo	Lower anticipatory stress marginally related to higher mysticism; stress of situation unrelated to mysticism; mysticism was greater in incongruent conditions (high anticipation–low stress and low anticipation–high stress) than in congruent conditions.
Lindenthal et al. (1970)	753 adult residents of New Haven who experienced life crisis in past year	Event types	Survey of whether prayed for help after the life crisis	Prayer was more common after health and catastrophic events than legal, financial, job, marriage, interpersonal, family, education, or relocation events.
Mattlin, Wethington, & Kessler (1990)	1,556 married nonblack adults in Detroit coping with major life events and chronic difficulties	Seven types of stressful events	Report of religious coping with stressor	Religious coping was more common in dealing with illness and death than in dealing with practical and interpersonal problems.

Study	Sample	Predictor	Religious coping	Results
McCrae (1984)	255 community adults who had reported a recent life event	Events objectively sorted into categories of loss, threat, and challenge	Rating of whether faith was involved in coping with the event	People used faith more in loss (75%) and threat (72%) than challenge (43%).
Pargament, Olsen, et al. (1992a)	586 members of 10 mainline Christian churches	Number of life events in past year; appraisals of negative event experienced in past year; kind of negative event experienced in past year	Survey of whether religion was involved in understanding and/or dealing with negative event in past year	Religious coping was associated with greater number of life events; with appraisals of event as a threat, loss, challenge, God's will, and inability to cope with it; with deaths, mental health concerns, health problems, religious conflicts, and less with work concerns, financial problems, and accidents.
Pargament & Hahn (1986)	124 college students	Hypothetical health-related scenarios of responsible or irresponsible behavior followed by positive or negative outcome	Degree turn to God for help in coping	People turned to God for help in coping more in negative outcome than in positive outcomes, regardless of whether behavior was responsible.
Poggie, Pollnac, & Gersuny (1976)	108 fishermen from three ports in New England	Length of time spent at sea—1 day versus longer trip	Recall of number of ritual taboos practiced on fishing trip	More taboos were recalled during longer trips than 1-day trips.
Ritzema (1979)	32 college students	Eight hypothetical vignettes varying in positive versus negative outcomes and event domain	Attributions to God for causality of the outcomes	Attributions to God were associated with positive outcomes and interpersonal, emotional, and financial situations more so than medical situations.

(continued)

Study	Sample	Predictor	Religious coping	Results
Spilka & Schmidt (1983)	(1) 135 Christian youth from college and church; (2) 85 Christian religious youth from college and church	Hypothetical vignettes varying in event characteristics	Degree explanation for the event involves God	Attributions to God were greater for more important events, medical more than economic or social events, and more positive outcome events; mixed results for personal versus impersonal event.
Welford (1947)	63 male, Protestant, college and seminary students	Hypothetical scenarios rated for degree of arousal and frustration	Likelihood of prayer in the hypothetical scenario	Prayer was related to frustration and arousal.

Contextual predictors of religious coping

Study	Sample	Predictor	Religious coping	Results
Ellison & Taylor (1996)	1,299 African-American adults	Subjective family organizational religiousness	Interview question on whether person prayed or had someone pray for him or her in response to a problem	Praying to cope was associated with organizational religiousness. There was no relation to subjective family closeness.
Ferraro & Koch (1994)	National sample of 3,417 adults	Geographical location	Frequency seek spiritual comfort and support in response to problems	Religious coping was more frequent among people living in the South.
Gurin, Veroff, & Feld (1960)	National sample of 2,460 adults	Frequency of church attendance	First spontaneous mention of prayer as way of handling worries	More frequent church attendance was associated with more frequent mention of prayer.
Jenkins (1995)	422 HIV-positive military personnel	Membership in spiritual groups; affiliation with organized religion	Overall use of religious coping activities	Greater religious coping among members of spiritual groups and those identified with organized religion.

Study	Sample	Predictor	Religious coping	Results
Koenig (1995)	96 male inmates over 50 years	Security level of prison; location of prison	Three-item religious coping index	There were no relations.
Kunst, Tan, & Bjorck (1994)	329 college students responding to vignettes of uncontrollable negative events; Protestant and Catholic	Frequency of church attendance	Degree religious attributions made for the negative events	Church attendance was tied to attributions to God's will, God's love, and evil spiritual forces. There was no relation to God's punishment.
Pargament, Olsen, et al. (1992a)	586 members of 10 mainline Christian churches	General frequency of church attendance; congregational affiliation; measures of church mission, climate, and satisfaction	Survey of whether religion was involved in understanding and/or dealing with serious life event in past year	Religious coping was associated with more frequent church attendance; levels of religious coping varied across the 10 congregations; religious coping was related to perceptions of active church mission, greater sense of community, and greater satisfaction with services, programs, and facilities of church.
Pargament & Sullivan (1981)	209 college students	General frequency of church attendance	Attributions to God control over six hypothetical situational domains	More frequent church attenders attributed more control to God than less frequent attenders.
Spilka & Schmidt (1983)	85 Christian youth from college and church	Response to hypothetical vignettes in a church versus nonchurch context	Degree explanation for the event involves God	Attributions to God were no different in church and nonchurch contexts.

(continued)

Study	Sample	Predictor	Religious coping	Results
Wood & Parham (1990)	85 black and white, rural and urban caretakers of relatives with Alzheimer's disease	Race and residence	Reports of thinking about religion and prayer to cope with caregiving	Rural whites made less use of religion in coping than urban whites and rural and urban blacks.

Study	Sample and stressor	Measure of religious orientation	Measure of adjustment	Results (pos./neg./nonsig.)
Personal religious expressions (religious belief, faith, salience, prayer)				
Bahr & Harvey (1979b)	44 widows of miners who had died in a fire; M age = 37	Item on self-rated religiousness	Self-rated stability of quality of life over past 5 years	Higher proportion of people who rated themselves as more religious reported a more stable quality of life. (1/0/0)
Bivens et al. (1994–1995)	167 gay men with AIDS, HIV-positive, and uninvolved	Rating of strength of belief in God; scales of religious orthodoxy	Fear of death scale and death threat scales	Belief in God tied to less death threat ($r = -.29$) only; Christian orthodoxy tied only to less death threat ($r = -.20$). (1/0/5)
Brant & Pargament (1995)	179 African-Americans coping with racist and other negative life events	Self-rated religiousness and frequency of prayer items	Positive and negative affect, event-specific outcome, and religious outcome scales	Self-rated religiousness tied to better event-specific ($r = .19$) and religious ($r = .37$) outcomes. There was no relationship to frequency of prayer. (2/0/6)
Carey (1974)	74 terminally ill patients	Six religious belief items	Emotional adjustment scale rated by clergy	Only religious belief in Jesus Christ related to adjustment (gamma = .66). (1/0/5)
Franks et al. (1990–1991)	51 gay men with AIDS and 64 gay men without AIDS	Rating of strength of religious attachment	Death anxiety scale	There was no relationship. (0/0/1)

(continued)

423

Study	Sample and stressor	Measure of religious orientation	Measure of adjustment	Results (pos./neg./nonsig.)
Gass (1987)	100 women widowed in past year; mostly white and Catholic; M age = 71	Strength of religious beliefs (measure not described)	Measures of physical and psychosocial dysfunction	Religious beliefs tied to less psychosocial dysfunction (r = –.28), but not to physical dysfunction. (1/0/1)
Gibbs & Achterberg-Lawlis (1978)	16 terminally ill cancer patients; white and African-American; mostly fundamentalist and lower SES	Item on strength religious beliefs	Items on fear of death and discomfort	Strength of religious beliefs tied to less fear of death (r = .77).
Gray (1987)	50 adolescents who had a parent die within last 5 years	Item on whether had religious beliefs	Depression scale and diagnosis of depression	Religious beliefs related to lower depression and to less frequent diagnosis of major depression. (2/0/0)
Harris et al. (1995)	40 heart transplant recipients 2 months and 12 months postsurgery; mostly Protestant and Catholic	Items on degree religious beliefs influence life and frequency of prayer	Seven physical health, mental, health, and health concern scales and 12 months postsurgery	Degree religious beliefs influence life was related to better physical functioning (r = –.36), less anxiety (r = –.28), better self-esteem (r = –.29), fewer health worries (r = –.39), and less difficulty with regime (r = –.37). Frequency of prayer and Catholic was related to less difficulty with regime (r = –.33) only. (6/0/8)

Study	Sample and stressor	Measure of religious orientation	Measure of adjustment	Results (pos./neg./nonsig.)
Kass et al. (1991)	83 adult outpatients with serious medical disorders participating in 10-week relaxation program; M age = 46; Protestant, Catholic, and Jewish	Scale of spiritual experiences and beliefs	Scales of frequency of medical symptoms, degree of discomfort and interference of symptoms with daily life. Scales of life purpose and self-confidence in stressful situations. Measures taken before and after 10-week treatment	Spiritual experience tied to improved life satisfaction and reduced number of medical symptoms. It was not related to other scales. (2/0/3)
Koenig (1995)	96 male inmates over 50; mostly Protestant	Items of belief in God, frequency of prayer or Bible reading	Number of physical symptoms, severity of illness, and depression	There was no relationship. (0/0/3)
Koenig, Kvale, & Ferrel (1988)	836 elderly from community and a geriatric clinic; M age = 73; 61% Protestant and 36% Catholic	Three-item scale on personal religious practices	Item on efficacy of coping with tension in life	Personal religious practices tied to greater perceived coping efficacy (r = .12). (1/0/0)
Lasker, Lohmann, & Toedter (1989)	138 women who had an abortion, or fetal or neonatal death; mostly white; M age = 28	Scale of importance of religious belief, prayer, and God in person's life; item on self-rated religiousness	Three perinatal grief subscales and total grief score assessed at 2 months and 2 years postloss	Importance of religion related to less grief on two of four scales 2 months after loss (r's = −.16 and −.21) and to one of four scales 2 years postloss (r = −.23). There was no relationship with self-rated religiousness. (3/0/13)

(continued)

Study	Sample and stressor	Measure of religious orientation	Measure of adjustment	Results (pos./neg./nonsig.)
Long & Miller (1991)	147 people with multiple sclerosis; white	Items on self-rated religiousness, belief in supreme being, and scale of religious orthodoxy	Measure of suicidal ideation	Suicidal ideation was related to lower self-rated religiousness ($r = -.39$), less orthodoxy ($r = -.24$), and less belief in supreme being ($r = -.40$). (3/0/0)
McIntosh, Silver, & Wortman (1993)	124 parents of infants who died of SIDS; white and African-American	Item on self-rated importance of religion	Measures of well-being and psychological distress 3 weeks and 18 months after the loss	Importance of religion related only to greater well-being 3 weeks after loss ($r = .18$). (1/0/3)
Mercer, Lorden, & Falkenberg (1995)	107 victims of drunk driving	Items on importance of daily religious beliefs	Eight scales of well-being, psychological symptoms, PTSD, and event impact	Importance of religious beliefs tied to greater well-being only ($r = .14$). (1/0/7)
Oxman, Freeman, & Manheimer (1995)	232 patients undergoing elective open heart surgery	Self-rated religiousness	Mortality within 6 months of surgery	Lower self-rated religiousness was tied to greater risk of mortality. (1/0/0)
Pargament, Ensing, et al. (1990)	586 members of mainline Christian churches coping with a major negative life event; M age = 46; mostly white	Doctrinal orthodoxy scale and item on frequency of prayer	Measures of current psychological status, event-specific outcome, and religious outcome of the event	Orthodoxy related to better outcomes on two of three measures (r's = .18 and .31). Prayer related to better outcomes on two of three measures (r's = .14 and .30). (4/0/2)

Study	Sample and stressor	Measure of religious orientation	Measure of adjustment	Results (pos./neg./nonsig.)
Pargament et al. (1995)	225 people coping with 1993 floods in Midwest; mostly Protestant and Catholic	Items of frequency of prayer and self-rated religiousness	Measures of positive and negative affect, physical health, mental status, and religious outcome	Religious measures tied to better mental status (r's = .14 and .27) and better religious outcomes (r's = .26 and .46); self-rated religiousness tied to less negative affect (r = −.20). (5/0/5)
Park & Cohen (1993)	96 undergraduates coping with recent death of a close friend	Scale of religious orthodoxy	Measures of depression, event-related outcome, and personal growth	There was no relationship. (0/0/3)
Plante & Manuel (1992)	86 college students coping with Persian Gulf war	Item of strength of religious faith	Four symptom checklist subscales	Strength of religious faith was unrelated to symptom subscales. (0/0/4)
Rabins et al. (1990)	62 caregivers of people with Alzheimer's or cancer	Item of strength of religious beliefs	Measures of negative and positive affect 2 years later	Stronger religious beliefs related to less negative affect (r = .46) and more positive affect (r = .36). (2/0/0)
Reynolds & Nelson (1981)	154 chronically ill male veteran patients	Single item of religious commitment	Mortality 1 year after interview	Religious commitment tied to lower risk of mortality. (1/0/0)
Sherkat & Reed (1992)	156 family members of accident victims and suicides; Protestant and Catholic	Item on frequency of prayer	Measures of depression and self-esteem	There were no relationships. (0/0/2)
Smith, Nehemkis, & Charter (1983–1984)	20 terminally ill patients	Importance of religion	Three fear of death scales	There was no relationship. (0/0/3)

(continued)

Study	Sample and stressor	Measure of religious orientation	Measure of adjustment	Results (pos./neg./nonsig.)
VandeCreek et al. (1995)	150 family members and friends in hospital waiting for loved one going through major heart surgery	Items of frequency of prayer and self-rated religiousness	Event-specific outcome, religious outcome, anxiety and depression scales	Frequency of prayer and self-rated religiousness tied to better event-specific outcome (r's = .32 and 29) and better religious outcome (r's = .53 and .52); frequency of prayer related to more depression (r = .26). (4/1/5)
Yates et al. (1981)	71 advanced cancer patients; M age = 59	Scale of religious beliefs; item on importance of church and religion	Measures of well-being, presence and level of pain; duration of survival	Religious beliefs tied to one of four well-being measures (r = .41), to lower pain level (r = –.29), but not to presence of pain or to duration of survival. Importance of church and religion tied to two of four well-being measures (r's = .31 and .24), less pain (r = –.33), but not to presence of pain or duration of survival. (5/0/9)

Organizational religious expressions

Acklin, Brown, & Mauger (1983)	26 cancer patients with M age = 48	Frequency of church attendance	Six subscales from Grief Experience Inventory	Church attendance tied only to less anger/hostility (r = –.39) and less social isolation (r = –.32). (2/0/4)

Study	Sample and stressor	Measure of religious orientation	Measure of adjustment	Results (pos./neg./nonsig.)
Acklin, Brown, & Mauger (1983)	18 patients receiving treatment for nonthreatening condition; *M* age = 42	Frequency of church attendance	Six subscales from Grief Experience Inventory	Church attendance related only to less anger/hostility (*r* = −.50) and less social isolation (*r* = −.40). (2/0/4)
Bahr & Harvey (1979b)	44 widows of miners who had died in a fire; *M* age = 37	Items on belonging to church, frequency of church attendance, and participation in church social events	Self-rated stability of quality of life over past 5 years	Membership, attendance at church and participation in social events tied to more stable quality of life. (3/0/0)
Bivens et al. (1994–1995)	167 gay men with AIDS, HIV-positive, and uninvolved	Frequency of church attendance	Fear of death scale and death threat scales	Frequency of church attendance tied to less death threat (*r* = −.26). (1/0/1)
Bohannon (1991)	143 bereaved mothers and 129 bereaved fathers; white; respective *M* ages = 38 and 40; mostly Protestant	Frequent church attenders (more than twice a month) and infrequent attenders (less than twice a month)	Multiscale Grief Experience Inventory	Men and women frequent attenders reported less grief than infrequent attenders. Frequent women attenders reported fewer grief-related problems on 8 of 12 scales. Frequent men attenders reported fewer grief-related problems on 3 of 12 scales. (13/0/13)
Brant & Pargament (1995)	179 African-Americans coping with racist and other negative life events	Item of frequency of church attendance	Positive and negative affect, event-specific outcome, and religious outcome scales	Frequency of church attendance related only to better religious outcome (*r* = .38). (1/0/3)

(continued)

Study	Sample and stressor	Measure of religious orientation	Measure of adjustment	Results (pos./neg./nonsig.)
Franks et al. (1990–1991)	51 gay men with AIDS and 64 gay men without AIDS	Item on frequency of church attendance	Death anxiety scale	Church attendance tied to greater death anxiety. (0/1/0)
Harris et al. (1995)	40 heart transplant recipients 2 months and 12 months postsurgery; mostly Protestant and Catholic	Items on frequency attend religious services, how active in congregation, and financial contributions to congregation at 2 months postsurgery	Nine physical health, mental, health, and health concern scales at 12 months postsurgery	More frequent church attendance was related to less anxiety ($r = -.36$) and fewer health worries ($r = -.30$). Activity in congregation was related to better self-esteem ($r = -.30$) and less difficulty with regime ($r = -.30$). There was no relationship to financial contributions. (4/0/17)
Koenig (1988)	708 elderly men and women; mostly Protestant	Item on involvement in religious community activities	Item on feelings about death	There was no relationship. (0/0/1)
Koenig (1995)	96 male inmates over 50; mostly Protestant	Frequency of church attendance	Number of physical symptoms, severity of medical illness, and depression	Frequency of church attendance tied to less depression. (1/0/2)
Koenig, Kvale, & Ferrel (1988)	836 elderly from community and a geriatric clinic; M age = 73; 61% Protestant and 36% Catholic	Two-item scale on frequency of church attendance and religious group activities	Item on efficacy of coping with tension in life	Religious activity tied to greater perceived coping efficacy ($r = .14$). (1/0/0)

Study	Sample and stressor	Measure of religious orientation	Measure of adjustment	Results (pos./neg./nonsig.)
Lasker, Lohmann, & Toedter (1989)	138 women who had an abortion, or fetal or neonatal death; mostly white M age = 28	Item of frequency of church attendance	Three perinatal grief subscales and total grief score assessed at 2 months and 2 years postloss	There was no relationship. (0/0/8)
McGloshen & O'Bryant (1988)	226 recent widows	Items on frequency of church attendance and other religious activities	Measures of positive and negative affect	Frequency of church attendance was related to more positive affect (partial r = .19). There were no other relationships. (1/0/3)
McIntosh, Silver, & Wortman (1993)	124 parents of infants who died of SIDS; white and African-American	Item of frequency of attendance at religious services	Measures of well-being and psychological distress 3 weeks and 18 months after the loss	More frequent attendance related only to greater well-being at 3 weeks postloss (r = .18) (1/0/2)
Mercer, Lorden, & Falkenberg (1995)	1,423 victims of drunk drivers	Items on precrash religious attendance	Eight scales of well-being, psychological symptoms, PTSD, and event impact	Precrash attendance tied to well-being (r = .09), less anxiety (r = −.05), less depression (r = −.06), and less PTSD (r = −.07). (4/0/3)
O'Brien (1982)	126 chronic dialysis patients; majority African-American and Protestant	Item on frequency of participation in church services in past year	Measures of interactional behavior, quality of interaction, alienation, and treatment compliance	Church attendance tied to more interactional behavior, better quality of interaction, less alienation, and more compliance with treatment. (4/0/0)

(continued)

Study	Sample and stressor	Measure of religious orientation	Measure of adjustment	Results (pos./neg./nonsig.)
Oxman, Freeman, & Manheimer (1995)	232 patients undergoing elective open heart surgery	Frequency of church attendance and number of people known in congregation	Mortality within 6 months of surgery	There were no relationships to mortality. (0/0/2)
Pargament, Ensing, et al. (1990)	586 members of mainline Christian churches coping with a major negative life event; M age = 46; mostly white	Single item of frequency of church attendance	Measures of current psychological status, event-specific outcome, and religious outcome of the event	More frequent attendance tied to better outcomes on two of three measures (r's = .14 to .30). (2/0/1)
Pargament et al. (1995)	225 people coping with 1993 floods in Midwest; mostly Protestant and Catholic	Item on frequency of church attendance	Measures of positive and negative affect, physical health, mental status, and religious outcome	Frequency of church attendance related to less negative affect (r = −.23), better physical health (r = −.20), better mental status (r = .19), and better religious outcomes (r = .36). (4/0/1)
Sanders (1979–1980)	102 adults who experienced death of spouse, parent, or child; M age = 52	Item of frequency of church attendance	14 grief experience scales	More frequent church attenders reported more optimism and less appetite loss than less frequent attenders. There were no differences on other scales. (2/0/12)
Sherkat & Reed (1992)	156 family members of accident victims and suicides; Protestant and Catholic	Items on frequency of church attendance	Measures of depression and self-esteem	Frequency of church attendance was related to less depression (beta = −.13) but not self-esteem. (1/0/1)

Study	Sample and stressor	Measure of religious orientation	Measure of adjustment	Results (pos./neg./nonsig.)
Smith, Nehemkis, & Charter (1983–1984)	20 terminally ill patients	Frequency of church attendance	Three fear of death scales	Frequency of church attendance related to less positive images of death ($r = -.41$). (0/1/2)
VandeCreek et al. (1995)	150 family members and friends in hospital waiting for loved one going through major heart surgery	Item of frequency of church attendance	Event-specific outcome, religious outcome, anxiety, and depression scales	Frequency of church attendance tied to better event-specific outcome ($r = .21$) and better religious outcome ($r = .33$) only. (2/0/2)
Yates et al. (1981)	71 advanced cancer patients; M age = 59	Frequency of attendance at church services in past month	Measures of well-being, presence and level of pain; duration of survival	Attendance tied to three of four well-being measures (r's = .32 to .35), to less pain ($r = -.24$), but not to presence of pain or to duration of survival. (3/0/3)

Traditional measures of religious orientation (intrinsic, extrinsic, quest, and indiscriminate proreligiousness)

Acklin, Brown, & Mauger (1983)	26 cancer patients; M age = 48	Intrinsic and extrinsic	Six subscales from Grief Experience Inventory	Intrinsic tied only to less anger/hostility ($r = -.34$). There were no relationships with extrinsic orientation. (1/0/5)
Acklin, Brown, & Mauger (1983)	18 patients receiving treatment for nonlife threatening conditions	Intrinsic and extrinsic	Six subscales from Grief Experience Inventory	Intrinsic tied only to greater denial ($r = .52$); extrinsic tied only to less depersonalization ($r = -.48$). (1/1/10)

(continued)

Study	Sample and stressor	Measure of religious orientation	Measure of adjustment	Results (pos./neg./nonsig.)
Astin, Lawrence, & Foy (1993)	53 battered women	Single item of intrinsic religiousness	Measures of PTSD symptoms and intrusion	Intrinsic religiousness was related to more PTSD symptoms ($r = .21$) and less intrusion ($r = -.21$). (1/1/0)
Bivens et al. (1994–1995)	167 gay men with AIDS, HIV-positive, and uninvolved	Intrinsic and extrinsic religiousness scales	Fear of death scale and death threat scales	There were no relationships. (0/0/4)
Carey (1974)	74 terminally ill hospital patients	Intrinsic and extrinsic	Emotional adjustment scale rated by clergy	Intrinsic related to better adjustment (no correlation reported). Extrinsic tied to poorer adjustment (r=.30). (1/0/1)
Carey (1977)	119 widows and widowers; *Mdn* age = 57; Protestant and Catholic	Intrinsic	Adjustment scale	There was no relationship. (0/0/1)
Gibbs & Achterberg-Lawlis (1978)	16 terminally ill cancer patients; white and African-American; mostly fundamentalist and lower SES	Intrinsic and extrinsic	Items on fear of death and discomfort	There was no relationship of intrinsic and extrinsic.
Harris & Spilka (1990)	136 alcohol abusers; *M* age = 43; mostly male and white	Intrinsic and extrinsic	Success in abstaining from drinking	There was no relationship. (0/0/2)
Johnson & Spilka (1991)	103 women with breast cancer; *M* age = 53; mostly Protestant and Catholic	Intrinsic and extrinsic	Single item of helpfulness of religion in coping with breast cancer	Intrinsic related to more helpfulness of religion ($r = .70$). There was no relationship with extrinsic. (1/0/1)

Study	Sample and stressor	Measure of religious orientation	Measure of adjustment	Results (pos./neg./nonsig.)
Koenig (1995)	96 male inmates over 50; mostly Protestant	Intrinsic and extrinsic religiousness scales	Number of physical symptoms, severity of medical illness, and depression	Intrinsic tied to less depression ($r = -.24$). There was no relationship to extrinsic. (1/0/5)
Koenig, Kvale, & Ferrel (1988)	836 elderly from community and a geriatric clinic; M age = 73; 61% Protestant and 36% Catholic	Intrinsic	Item on efficacy of coping with tension in life	Intrinsic tied to greater perceived coping efficacy ($r = .12$). (1/0/0)
McIntosh, Inglehart, & Pacini (1990)	117 Christian students adjusting to transition to college	Combined index centrality and flexibility of religious beliefs. High values obtained by high intrinsic, low extrinsic, high seeking, and low doubt orientation scores	Measure of esteem, subjective well-being, happiness at college, and grade-point average	Central-flexible beliefs tied to greater well-being ($r = .20$), esteem ($r = .19$), happiness ($r = .19$) and GPA ($r = .22$). (4/0/0)
Mickley & Soeken (1993)	50 Anglo and Hispanic women with breast cancer; mostly Catholic and Protestant	Intrinsic and extrinsic religiousness scales	Measures of spiritual, religious, and existential well-being	Intrinsic religion tied to greater spiritual, religious, and existential well-being (r's = .63 to .77). There was no relationship to extrinsic. (3/0/3)

(continued)

Study	Sample and stressor	Measure of religious orientation	Measure of adjustment	Results (pos./neg./nonsig.)
Newman & Pargament (1990)	327 college students coping with most important problem in past 3 years	Intrinsic	Scales of degree religion helpful in comforting, redefining, generation solutions, decision making, and implementing solutions in coping.	Intrinsic orientation tied to greater helpfulness of religion in each aspect of problem solving (r's = .27 to .62). (5/0/0)
Pargament, Ensing, et al. (1990)	586 members of mainline Christian churches coping with a major negative life event; M age = 46; mostly white	Intrinsic, extrinsic, and quest	Measures of current psychological status, event-specific outcome, and religious outcome of the event	Intrinsic tied to better outcomes on all measures (r's = .11 to .41). Extrinsic tied to better outcomes on two of three measures (r's = .15 and .18). Quest was not related. (5/0/4)
Pargament et al. (1994)	271 college students coping with stresses of Persian Gulf war	Intrinsic	Measures of positive and negative affect, and recent mental health status 2 days before assault of Kuwait and 1 week after suspension of hostilities	There were no relationships. (0/0/6)
Pargament et al. (1995)	225 people coping with 1993 floods in Midwest; mostly Protestant and Catholic	Intrinsic religious scale	Measures of positive and negative affect, physical health, mental status, and religious outcome	Intrinsic religiousness tied to better mental status (r = .14), better religious outcome (r = .39), and less negative affect (r = −.19). (3/0/2)
Park & Cohen (1993)	96 undergraduates coping with recent death of a close friend	Intrinsic and extrinsic	Measures of depression, event-related outcome, and personal growth	Intrinsic related only to personal growth (r = .20). Extrinsic was not related to measures. (1/0/5)

Study	Sample and stressor	Measure of religious orientation	Measure of adjustment	Results (pos./neg./nonsig.)
Rosik (1989)	159 elderly white widows and widowers	Intrinsic, extrinsic, and indiscriminate proreligious- ness	Measures of grief and depression	Extrinsic tied to greater grief (r = .41) and depression (r = .23) for widows, greater grief (r = .29) and depression (r = .15) for widowers. Indiscriminate proreligious tied to greater grief (r = .12) and depression (r = .21) for widowers but not for widows. Intrinsic was not related to grief or depression. (0/6/6)
Rutledge & Spilka (1993)	174 single men and women; ages 41–50	Intrinsic and extrinsic	Depression scale	Extrinsic related to depression (r = .17). There was no relation to intrinsic. (0/1/1)

Mixed personal and organizational religious expressions

Folkman et al. (1994)	82 HIV-positive caregivers and 162 HIV-negative caregivers to partners with AIDS	10-item measure of religious and spiritual beliefs and activities	Scale of caregiver burden	Religious/spirituality was uncorrelated with caregiver burden for HIV-positive and HIV-negative caregivers. Regression analyses showed religious/spirituality tied to lower caregiver burden for HIV-positive caregivers only (beta = −.16). (0/0/2)

(continued)

Study	Sample and stressor	Measure of religious orientation	Measure of adjustment	Results (pos./neg./nonsig.)
Pressman et al. (1990)	20 female patients recovering from surgery for broken hips; over 65 years	Mixed index of self-rated religiousness, frequency of church attendance, and comfort from God items	Depression scale and ambulatory status assessed by physical therapist within 48 hours of surgery and before discharge	Greater religiousness related to less depression at discharge ($r = -.61$) and better ambulatory status at discharge ($r = .45$) after controlling for severity of illness. (2/0/0)
Videka-Sherman (1982)	194 bereaved parents; 70% women; M age = 41	Three-item scale of frequency of attendance at religious services, change in attendance since death, belief that religion offers security in life measured at two times after death	Measures of depressive symptoms, negative affect, and personal growth assessed at two times after death	Religiousness measured at Time 2 related to depressive symptoms (beta = .05), less negative affect (beta = −.05), and more growth (beta = .05). Religiousness at Time 1 was unrelated to adjustment. (2/1/3)

APPENDIX D. Summary of Research on the Relationship between Religious Coping Methods and the Outcomes of Negative Events

Study	Sample and stressor	Measure of religious coping	Measure of outcome	Results (pos./neg./nonsig.)
Spiritual forms of coping (e.g., spiritual support, spiritual discontent)				
Barbarin & Chesler (1986)	74 parents of children living with cancer; white	Coding of open-ended coping responses that reflect reliance on religion for comfort and explanation	Scales of medically related stress, quality of relations with medical staff, and items on number of hospitalizations, and coping effectiveness	There were no relationships. (0/0/4)
Belavich & Pargament (1995)	222 college students coping with hassles	Spiritually based coping scales	Measures of depression, and positive and negative affect	Spiritually based coping tied to more negative affect. ($r = .17$)
Brant & Pargament (1995)	179 African-Americans coping with racist and other negative life events	Spiritually based coping scale	Positive and negative affect, event-specific outcome, and religious outcome scales	Spiritually based coping tied to better outcomes on three of measures (r's = .31 to .61). (3/0/1)
Cook & Wimberly (1993)	114 bereaved parents; mostly white and Protestant	Item on perceived change in strength of religious beliefs after loss of child	Items on self-assessed adjustment, physiological adjustment, and perceived helpfulness of religion	Perceptions of strengthened religious beliefs tied to better emotive ($r = .19$) and physiological ($r = .18$) adjustment, and perceived helpfulness of religion ($r = .54$). (3/0/1)
Harris et al. (1995)	40 heart transplant recipients 2 months and 12 months postsurgery; mostly Protestant and Catholic	Items on degree consult God to make important decisions at 2 months postsurgery	Seven physical health, mental, health, and health concern scales at 12 months postsurgery	Consult God tied to better physical functioning and less difficuty with regime ($r = .44$). (2/0/5)

(continued)

439

Study	Sample and stressor	Measure of religious coping	Measure of outcome	Results (pos./neg./nonsig.)
Jenkins (1995)	422 HIV-positive military personnel	Spiritually based coping scale	Four measures of affect and four measures of evaluation of social support	Spiritually based coping tied to more positive evaluations of social support (r's = 08 to .14), but is not related to affect. (1/0/1)
Mercer, Lorden, & Falkenberg (1995)	107 victims of drunk driving	Items on degree seek spiritual comfort in life and degree ask what God wants in decision making	Eight scales of well-being, psychological symptoms, PTSD, and event impact	Seeking spiritual comfort and God's guidance in decision making tied to greater well-being (r's = .12 and .10) only. (2/0/14)
O'Brien (1982)	126 chronic dialysis patients; majority African-American and Protestant	Item on importance of faith in coping with dialysis	Measures of interactional behavior, quality of interaction, alienation, and treatment compliance	Importance of faith tied to more interactional behavior, better quality of interaction, less alienation, and more compliance. No effect sizes reported. (4/0/0)
Oxman, Freeman, & Manheimer (1995)	232 patients undergoing elective open heart surgery	Degree of strength and comfort from religion	Mortality within 6 months of surgery	Absence of strength and comfort from religion tied to three times the risk for mortality. (1/0/0)

Study	Sample and stressor	Measure of religious coping	Measure of outcome	Results (pos./neg./nonsig.)
Pargament, Ensing, et al. (1990)	586 members of mainline Christian churches coping with a major negative life event; *M* age = 46; mostly white	Loving image of God; religious experiences of closeness with God; spiritually based coping activities	Measures of current psychological status, event-specific outcome, and religious outcome of the event	Loving images of God tied to better outcomes on all measures (*r*'s = .10 to .13). Experiences of closeness with God tied to better outcomes on all measures (*r*'s = .18 to .43). Spiritually based coping activities tied to better outcomes on all measures (*r*'s = −.12 to .22). (12/0/0)
Pargament et al. (1994)	271 college students coping with stresses of Persian Gulf war	Spiritually based coping scale	Measures of positive and negative affect, and recent mental health status 2 days before assault of Kuwait and 1 week after suspension of hostilities	Spiritually based coping related to more positive affect at Time 1 (*r* = .18) and Time 2 (*r* = .25), more negative affect at Time 1 only (*r* = .15), and better mental health status at Time 2 only (*r* = −.14). (3/1/2))
Pargament et al. (in press)	49 Roman Catholic church members coping with a major negative event in past few years	Anger at God scale; doubts about God and faith scale	Measures of negative mood, event-related outcome, and religious outcome	Anger at God tied to more negative mood (*r* = .46) and poorer event-outcome (*r* = −.46), not to religious outcome. (0/2/1)
Pargament et al. (in press)	98 college students coping with death of friend or loved one in past few years	Anger at God scale; doubts about God and faith scale	Measures of negative mood, event-related outcome, and religious outcome	Anger at God tied to more negative mood (*r* = .57), poorer event-outcome, (*r* = −.40), and poorer religious outcome (*r* = −.32). (0/3/0)

(continued)

Study	Sample and stressor	Measure of religious coping	Measure of outcome	Results (pos./neg./nonsig.)
Pargament et al. (in press)	98 college students coping with unjust life event in past few years	Anger at God scale; doubts about God and faith scale	Measures of negative mood, event-related outcome, and religious outcome	There were no relationships. (0/0/3)
Pargament et al. (1995)	225 people coping with 1993 floods in Midwest, mostly Protestant and Catholic	Spiritually based coping scale	Measures of positive and negative affect, physical health, mental status, and religious outcome	Spiritually based coping tied to positive affect (r = .15), better mental status (r = .30), and better religious outcome (r = .63). (3/0/2)
Park & Cohen (1993)	96 undergraduates coping with recent death	Spiritually based coping scale	Measures of depression, event-related outcome, and personal growth	Spiritually based coping related to personal growth (r – .29), not to other two measures. (1/0/5))
Thompson & Vardaman (in press)	150 family members of homicide victims; mostly female, African-American, and Protestant	Spiritually based coping scale	Four scales of psychological distress and posttraumatic stress (PTS)	There were no relationships. (0/0/5)
Wright, Pratt, & Schmall (1985)	240 Alzheimer's caregivers	Item on use of spiritual support	Caregiver burden scale	Spiritual support tied to less caregiver burden (r = –.25). (1/0/0)
Yates et al. (1981)	71 advanced cancer patients; M age = 59	Item of felt closeness to God or nature in past few weeks	Measures of well-being, presence and level of pain; duration of survival	Closeness to God or nature tied to two of four well-being measures (r's = .33 and .43), to less of a presence of pain (r = –.29), a lower pain level (r = –.25), but not to duration of survival. (4/0/3)

Study	Sample and stressor	Measure of religious coping	Measure of outcome	Results (pos./neg./nonsig.)
Congregational forms of coping (e.g., congregational support and discontent)				
Belavich & Pargament (1995)	222 college students coping with hassles	Scale of support from clergy and church members in coping; discontent with church and God	Measures of depression and positive and negative affect	Religious support related to more positive affect (r = .24). There was no relationship to discontent. (1/0/5)
Brant & Pargament (1995)	179 African-Americans coping with racist and other negative life events	Scale of support from clergy and church members in coping; religious discontent with church and God	Positive and negative affect, event-specific outcome, and religious outcome scales	Religious support tied to two of four outcomes (r's = .22 and .38); discontent related to more negative affect (r = .35). (2/1/5)
Carey (1974)	74 terminally ill hospital patients	Perceived concern by local clergy	Emotional adjustment scale rated by clergy	Clergy concern related to better adjustment (r = .25).
Gibbs & Achterberg-Lawlis (1978)	16 terminally ill cancer patients; white and African-American; mostly fundamentalist and lower SES	Report of emotional support from church	Items on fear of death and discomfort	Emotional support from church related to less difficulty sleeping (r = −.72).
Jenkins (1995)	422 HIV-positive military personnel	Scale of support from clergy and congregation in coping; religious discontent with church and God	Four measures of affect and four measures of evaluation of social support	Religious support tied to more positive evaluations of social support (r's = .09 to .12) but not related to affect. Discontent related to poorer affect (r's = .31 to .39) and more negative evaluations of social support (r's = −.14 to −.27). (4/8/4)

(continued)

Study	Sample and stressor	Measure of religious coping	Measure of outcome	Results (pos./neg./nonsig.)
Lasker, Lohmann, & Toedter (1989)	138 women who had an abortion, or fetal or neonatal death; mostly white; *M* age = 28	Scale of strength and support from church, members, or clergy after loss	Three perinatal grief subscales and total grief score at 2 months and 2 years postloss	There was no relationship. (0/0/8)
Pargament, Ensing, et al. (1990)	586 members of mainline Christian churches coping with a major negative life event; *M* age = 46; mostly white	Scale of support from clergy and church members in coping; religious discontent with church and God	Measures of current psychological status, event-specific outcome, and religious outcome of the event	Religious support tied to better outcomes on all measures (*r*'s = .10 to .51). Religious discontent tied to poorer outcomes on all measures (*r*'s = −.12 to .22). (3/3/0)
Pargament et al. (1994)	271 college students coping with stresses of 1991 Persian Gulf war	Scale of support from clergy and church members in coping; religious discontent with church and God	Measures of positive and negative affect, and recent mental health status	Religious support tied to more positive affect at Time 1 (*r* = .21) and Time 2 (*r* = .27), more negative affect at Time 1 only (*r* = .16), and better mental health status at Time 2 only (*r* = −.20). Religious discontent related to more negative affect at Time 1 (*r* = .37) and Time 2 (*r* = .24) and poorer mental health status at Time 1 only (*r* = .24). (3/4/5)
Pargament et al. (in press)	49 Roman Catholic church members coping with major negative event in past few years	Conflict with members and clergy scale; conflict with church dogma scale	Measures of negative mood, event-related outcome, and religious outcome	Conflict with church dogma tied to poorer religious outcomes (*r* = −.34). There were no other relationships. (0/1/5)

Study	Sample and stressor	Measure of religious coping	Measure of outcome	Results (pos./neg./nonsig.)
Pargament et al. (in press)	98 college students coping with death of friend or loved one in past few years	Conflict with members and clergy scale; conflict with church dogma scale	Measures of negative mood, event-related outcome, and religious outcome	Conflict with members and clergy, and conflict with church dogma tied to more negative mood (r's = .51 and .42) and poorer religious outcomes (r's = −.33 and −.37). (0/4/2)
Pargament et al. (in press)	98 college students coping with unjust life event in past few years	Conflict with members and clergy scale; conflict with church dogma scale	Measures of negative mood, event-related outcome, and religious outcome	Conflict with members and clergy tied to more negative mood (r = .27). There were no other relationships. (0/1/5)
Pargament et al. (1995)	225 people coping with 1993 floods in Midwest; mostly Protestant and Catholic	Scale of support from clergy and church members in coping; religious discontent with church and God	Measures of positive and negative affect, physical health, mental status, and religious outcome	Religious discontent tied to poorer status on all measures but positive affect (r's = −.18 to 40); religious support tied to better religious outcomes only (r = .44). (1/4/5)
Thompson & Vardaman (in press)	150 family members of homicide victims; mostly female, African-American, and Protestant	Scale of support from clergy and church members in coping; religious discontent with church and God	Four scales of psychological distress and PTS	Religious support tied to less hostility (r = −.21) only; discontent related to greater distress on all measures (r's = .19 to .31) and PTS (r = .27). (1/5/4)

(continued)

Study	Sample and stressor	Measure of religious coping	Measure of outcome	Results (pos./neg./nonsig.)
Religious reframing (God's will; God's love; God's punishment)				
Dalal & Pande (1988)	44 hospitalized patients from India with major injuries due to an accident; mostly male, lower middle-class, Hindu	Causal attributions of accident to Karma and to God's wishes	Scale of psychological recovery	Attributions to Karma related to psychological recovery ($r = .37$). There was no relationship with attributions to God's wishes. (1/0/0)
Grevengoed (1985)	149 university students who had experienced death of family member or close friend in past 4 years; mostly Protestant and Catholic	Attributions of death to God's anger, God's will, and God's love	Scales of death anxiety, depression, and mental health. Items on how much learned from event, how well handled feelings, and how well handled the death	Attributions to God's will and God's love related to better event-specific outcomes (r's = .16 to .38). Attributions to God's anger related to poorer event-specific outcomes (r's = −.22 to −.25). There was no relationship to death anxiety, depression, or mental health. (6/3/9)
Jenkins & Pargament (1988)	62 cancer patients; M age = 56; mostly white	Item of perceived control by God over the cancer	Scales of self-esteem, life threat, adjustment to illness, and nurses' ratings of adjustment	Perceptions of control by God tied to higher self-esteem ($r = .25$), better adjustment ratings by nurses ($r = −.23$). There was no relationship to life threat and self-rated adjustment. (2/0/2)

Study	Sample and stressor	Measure of religious coping	Measure of outcome	Results (pos./neg./nonsig.)
Pargament, Ensing, et al. (1990)	586 members of mainline Christian churches coping with a major negative life; *M* age = 46; mostly white	Appraisals of negative event to God's will, God's punishment, and threat to spiritual well-being	Measures of current psychological status, event-specific outcome, and religious outcome of the event	Appraisals to God's will tied to better outcome on two of three measures (r's = .16 and .19). Appraisals to God's punishment tied to poorer outcomes on two of three measures (r's = −.17). Appraisals of event as a spiritual threat tied to poorer outcomes on all measures (r's = −.09 to −.17). (2/5/2)
Pargament et al. (in press)	49 Roman Catholic church members coping with major negative event in past few years	God's punishment scale; positive religious reappraisal scale	Measures of negative mood, event-related outcome, and religious outcome	Appraisal of negative event as God's punishment tied to more negative mood (r = .28) and poorer event-specific outcome (r = −.35). Positive religious reappraisal tied to better outcomes on all measures (r's = −.39 to .40). (3/2/1)
Pargament et al. (in press)	98 college students coping with death of friend or loved one in past few years	God's punishment scale; positive religious reappraisal scale	Measures of negative mood, event-related outcome, and religious outcome	Appraisal of death as God's punishment tied to more negative mood (r = .28) only. Positive religious reappraisals tied to better event-specific outcome (r = .28) and better religious outcome (r = .33). (2/1/3)

(continued)

Study	Sample and stressor	Measure of religious coping	Measure of outcome	Results (pos./neg./nonsig.)
Pargament et al. (in press)	98 college students coping with unjust life event in past few years	God's punishment scale; positive religious reappraisal scale	Measures of negative mood, event-related outcome, and religious outcome	There was no relationship with God's punishment. Positive religious reappraisals tied to better event-specific outcome ($r = .21$) and better religious outcome ($r = .47$). (2/0/4)
Park & Cohen (1993)	96 undergraduates coping with recent death of a close friend	Single items of attribution of event to loving God and to purposeful God	Measures of depression, event-related outcome, and personal growth	Attributions to purposeful God related to personal growth ($r = .25$) only. (1/0/5)

Religious approaches to agency and control (self-directing, deferring, collaborative, pleading)

Study	Sample and stressor	Measure of religious coping	Measure of outcome	Results (pos./neg./nonsig.)
Belavich & Pargament (1995)	222 college students coping with hassles	Scale of pleading to God and bargaining for a miracle	Measures of depression, and positive and negative affect	Pleading tied to more depression ($r = .26$) and more negative affect ($r = .35$). (0/2/1)
Brant & Pargament (1995)	179 African-Americans coping with racist and other negative life events	Scale of pleading to God and bargaining for a miracle	Positive and negative affect, event-specific outcome, and religious outcome scales	Pleading tied to more positive affect ($r = .24$), more negative affect ($r = .40$), more positive event-specific ($r = .20$) and religious outcomes ($r = .46$). (3/1/0)
Friedel & Pargament (1995)	105 emergency health care workers coping with most stressful work event in past 6 months	Self-directing, collaborative, and deferring religious coping with stressful event	Measures of mental health status, event-specific outcomes, job satisfaction, and turnover intention	Collaborative related to better mental health status ($r = .28$). There were no other relationships. (1/0/11)

Study	Sample and stressor	Measure of religious coping	Measure of outcome	Results (pos./neg./nonsig.)
Harris & Spilka (1990)	136 alcohol abusers; M age = 43; mostly male and white	Self-directing, collaborative, and deferring coping styles	Success in abstaining from drinking	Self-directing tied to success in abstaining from drinking (r = −.32). There was no relationship to deferring and collaborative. (1/0/2)
Jenkins (1995)	422 HIV-positive military personnel	Scale of pleading to God and bargaining for a miracle	Four measures of affect and four measures of evaluation of social support	Pleading tied to more negative affect (r's = .15 to .22) and less positive evaluations of support on one scale (r = −.08). (0/5/3)
Pargament, Ensing, et al. (1990)	586 members of mainline Christian churches coping with a major negative life event; M age = 46; mostly white	Scale of pleading to God and bargaining for a miracle. Self-directing, collaborative, and deferring coping styles	Measures of current psychological status, event-specific outcome, and religious outcome of the event	Pleading and bargaining tied to poorer psychological status (r = −.11) and better religious outcome (r = 17). Deferring tied to better outcomes on all measures (r's = .12 to .42). Collaborative tied to better outcomes on all measures (r's = .14 to .46). Self-directing coping tied to poorer outcomes on all measures (r's = −.10 to −.30). (7/4/1)

(continued)

Study	Sample and stressor	Measure of religious coping	Measure of outcome	Results (pos./neg./nonsig.)
Pargament et al. (1994)	271 college students coping with stresses of 1991 Persian Gulf war	Scale of pleading to God and bargaining for a miracle; self-directing, deferring, and collaborative styles	Measures of positive and negative affect, and recent mental health status 2 days prior to assault of Kuwait and 1 week after suspension of hostilities	Pleading tied to more negative affect ($r = .25$) and poorer mental health status ($r = .21$) before assault, more negative affect ($r = .31$) and more positive affect ($r = .24$) after the assault. Collaborative tied to more positive affect ($r = .14$) before and after assault ($r = .18$). Self-directing tied to less positive affect after assault ($r = -.13$). Deferring tied to better mental health status before assault ($r = -.17$). (4/4/16)
Pargament et al. (in press)	49 Roman Catholic church members coping with major negative event in past few years	Scale of passivity and deferral to God	Measures of negative mood, event-related outcome, and religious outcome	Passivity tied to better religious outcome ($r = .34$) only. (1/0/2)
Pargament et al. (in press)	98 college students coping with death of friend or loved one in past few years	Scale of passivity and deferral to God	Measures of negative mood, event-related outcome, and religious outcome	Passivity tied to better religious outcome ($r = .53$) and poorer event-specific outcome ($r = -.20$). (1/1/1)
Pargament et al. (in press)	98 college students coping with unjust life event in past few years	Scale of passivity and deferral to God	Measures of negative mood, event-related outcome, and religious outcome	Passivity tied to better religious outcome ($r = .59$) only. (1/0/2)

Study	Sample and stressor	Measure of religious coping	Measure of outcome	Results (pos./neg./nonsig.)
Pargament et al. (1995)	225 people coping with 1993 floods in Midwest; mostly Protestant and Catholic	Self-directing, collaborative, deferring religious coping with flood	Measures of positive and negative affect, mental status, and religious, outcome	Collaborative and deferring tied to better mental status (r's = .20 and .25) and better religious outcome (r's = .51 and .47); self-directing related to poorer mental status (r = −.17) and poorer religious outcome (r = −.41). There were no other relationships. (4/2/6)
Park & Cohen (1993)	96 undergraduates coping with recent death of a close friend	Scale of pleading to God and bargaining for a miracle	Measures of depression, event-related outcome and personal growth	Pleading and bargaining tied to greater depression (r = .19) and event-related distress (r = .49), but were not related to personal growth. (0/2/1)
Rutledge & Spilka (1993)	174 single men and women; ages 41 to 50	Self-directing, collaborative, and deferring coping styles	Depression scale	Self-directing related to more depression (r = .23). Collaborative related to less depression (r = −.22). There was no relationship to deferring. (1/1/1)
Thompson & Vardaman (in press)	150 family members of homicide victims; mostly female, African-American, and Protestant	Scale of pleading to God and bargaining for a miracle	Four scales of psychological distress and PTS	Pleading tied to greater distress on all measures (r's = .20 to .27). (0/5/0)

(continued)

Study	Sample and stressor	Measure of religious coping	Measure of outcome	Results (pos./neg./nonsig.)
VandeCreek et al. (1995)	150 family members and friends in hospital waiting for loved one going through major heart surgery	Self-directing, collaborative, deferring, and pleading religious coping with the wait	Event-specific outcome, religious outcome, anxiety, and depression scales	Collaborative, pleading, and deferring tied to better event-specific outcome (r's = .33 to .49), better religious outcome (r's = .54 to .76), more anxiety (r's = .22 to .46), and more depression (r's = .30 to .52); self-directing related to poorer religious outcome only ($r = -.25$). (6/7/3)
Yelsma & Montambo (1990)	55 patient after heart attack; mostly male	Self-directing, collaborative, and deferring coping styles	Physiological measure of recovery	There were no relationships. (0/0/3)

Religious rituals

Bahr & Harvey (1979b)	44 widows of miners who had died in a fire; M age = 37	Change in church attendance since fire	Self-rated stability of quality of life over past 5 years	There was no relationship. (0/0/1)
Belavich & Pargament (1995)	222 college students coping with hassles	Scale of participation in rituals and good deeds as a way of coping with hassles	Measures of depression, and positive and negative affect	Religious good deeds and rituals tied to more positive affect (r = .20). (1/0/2)

Study	Sample and stressor	Measure of religious coping	Measure of outcome	Results (pos./neg./nonsig.)
Brant & Pargament (1995)	179 African-Americans coping with racist and other negative life events	Scale of participation in rituals and religious good deeds as a way of coping with negative event	Positive and negative affect, event-specific outcome, and religious outcome scales	Religious good deeds and rituals tied to more positive affect (r = .30), more negative affect (r = .15), and better event-specific (r = .31) and religious outcomes (r = .62). (3/1/0)
Gass (1987)	100 women widowed in past year; mostly white and Catholic; M age = 71	Practice of death and mourning rituals	Measures of physical and psychosocial dysfunction	Ritual practice related to less physical dysfunction (r = −.28), but not to psychosocial dysfunction. (1/0/1)
Griffith, Mahy, & Young (1986)	16 members of West Indian Spiritual Baptist sect; some seeking physical health and spiritual strength	Participation in 7-day "mourning" ritual	Psychological symptomatology scales assessed pre- and postritual	Improvements in symptomatology on 11 of 12 scales pre- and postritual. (11/0/1)
Jenkins (1995)	422 HIV-positive military personnel	Scale of participation in rituals and religious good deeds as way of coping with negative event	Four measures of affect and four measures of evaluation of social support	Religious good deeds and rituals tied to more positive evaluations of social support on two scales (r's = .09 and .12). There was no relationship to affect. (2/0/6)
Lasker, Lohmann, & Toedter (1989)	138 women who had an abortion, or fetal or neonatal death; mostly white; M age = 28	Scale of loss-related rituals	Three perinatal grief subscales and total grief score at 2 months and 2 years postloss	There was no relationship. (0/0/8)

(continued)

Study	Sample and stressor	Measure of religious coping	Measure of outcome	Results (pos./neg./nonsig.)
Morris (1982)	24 physically ill in England; mostly Catholic; M age = 60	Pilgrimage to Lourdes	Changes in measures of anxiety and depression before pilgrimage, 1 month after, and 10 months after	Pilgrimage associated with decrease in anxiety and depression 1 month after and 10 months after. No effect size reported. (2/0/0)
Pargament, Ensing, et al. (1990)	586 members of mainline Christian churches coping with a major negative life event; M age = 46; mostly white	Scale of participation in rituals and religious good deeds as way of coping with negative event	Measures of current psychological status, event-specific outcome, and religious outcome of the event	Religious good deeds and rituals tied to better outcomes on all measures (r's = .13 to .55). (3/0/0)
Pargament et al. (1994)	271 college students coping with stresses of 1991 Persian Gulf war	Scale of religious participation in rituals and religious good deeds as way of coping	Measures of positive and negative affect, and recent mental health status 2 days before assault of Kuwait and 1 week after suspension of hostilities	Religious good deeds and rituals tied to more positive affect and more negative affect at Times 1 and 2 (r's .16 to .24), and better mental health status at Time 2 only (r = −.16). (3/2/1)
Pargament et al. (1995)	225 people coping with 1993 floods in Midwest; mostly Protestant and Catholic	Scale of participation in rituals and religious good deeds as way of coping with flood	Measures of positive and negative affect, physical health, mental status, and religious outcome	Religious good deeds and rituals related to less negative affect (r = −.16), better mental status (r = .27), and better religious outcomes (r = .52). (3/0/2)

Study	Sample and stressor	Measure of religious coping	Measure of outcome	Results (pos./neg./nonsig.)
Park & Cohen (1993)	96 undergraduates coping with recent death of a close friend	Scale of religious participation in rituals and religious good deeds as way of coping with the death	Measures of depression, event-related distress, and personal growth	Religious good deeds and rituals tied to greater event-related distress ($r = .21$) and more personal growth ($r = .22$). There was no relationship to depression. (1/1/1)
Rothbaum & Jackson (1990)	18 Orthodox Jewish Mikvah (ritual bath attenders), 23 Orthodox Jewish non-Mikvah attenders, 35 Protestant and 45 Catholic women	Attendance at Mikvah and religious affiliation	Menstrual symptoms	No differences among four groups in menstrual symptoms. (0/0/1)
Rutledge & Spilka (1993)	174 single men and women; ages 41–50	Attending singles socials at church	Depression scale	Attendance at singles socials related to more depression ($r = .15$). (0/1/0)
Thompson & Vardaman (in press)	150 family members of homicide victims; mostly female, African-American, and Protestant	Scale of participation in rituals and good deeds as a way of coping with homicide	Four scales of psychological distress and PTS	Religious good deeds tied to greater anxiety ($r = .16$) and somatization ($r = .19$) only. (0/2/3)
Zeidner & Hammer (1992)	261 Jewish Israelis threatened by missiles in Persian Gulf war	Items about engagement in religious activities to deal with stressor	Measures of anxiety, symptoms and cognitive function	Increase in religious activities tied to greater anxiety ($r = .33$) and symptoms ($r = .29$), but not cognition. (0/2/1)

(continued)

Study	Sample and stressor	Measure of religious coping	Measure of outcome	Results (pos./neg./nonsig.)
		Patterns of religious coping		
Frazier, Krasnoff, & Port (1995)	239 renal transplant patients 3 months posttransplant; 170 12 months posttransplant	10-item religious coping index	Brief symptom inventory and life satisfaction	Religious coping related to greater life satisfaction 3 months posttransplant (r = .19) and 12 months posttransplant (r = .23). There was no relationship to psychological symptoms. (2/0/2)
Koenig (1988)	708 elderly men and women; mostly Protestant	Use of prayer and religious beliefs in coping generally and in coping with a major life stressor	Item about feelings related to death	Prayer and religious beliefs in coping tied to less death anxiety. (1/0/0)
Koenig (1995)	96 male inmates over 50 years; mostly Protestant	Three-item index of religious coping	Number of physical symptoms, severity of medical illness, and depression scales	There were no relationships. (0/0/3)
Koenig et al. (1992)	850 hospitalized, ill, elderly men; largely conservative Protestant	Three-item religious coping index	Social support, alcohol use, cognitive status, self- and observer-rated depression, self-rated depression for 202 men 6 months later	Religious coping related to more social support (beta = .12), less alcohol use (beta = −.14), better cognitive status (beta = .10), less self-rated (beta = −.14) and observer-rated depression (beta = −.19), and less self-rated depression (beta = −.18) 6 months later. (6/0/0)

Study	Sample and stressor	Measure of religious coping	Measure of outcome	Results (pos./neg./nonsig.)
Koenig et al. (1995)	832 older medical inpatients	Three-item religious coping index	Self- and observer-rated cognitive and somatic scales of depression	Religious coping related to lower levels of cognitive symptoms according to self-rated scale (r = −.16) and other rated scales (r = −.15 and −.14). There was no relationship with somatic symptoms. (3/0/3)
Pargament, Smith, & Koenig (1996)	310 members of two churches located near Oklahoma City bombing, 6 weeks after the blast	Scales of positive and negative religious coping	Measures of stress-related growth, religious outcome, and PTSD	Positive religious coping related to stress-related growth (r = .62), religious outcome (r = .59), and PTSD (r = .25); negative religious coping tied to stress-related growth (r = .21), and PTSD (r = .48). (3/2/1)
Sattler et al. (1994)	322 survivors of Hurricane Iniki 7 weeks after hurricane	4-item religious coping index	Measure of psychological symptoms	Religious coping associated with more psychological symptoms (r = .22). (0/1/0)

APPENDIX E. Summary of Studies of Religion as a Moderator and/or Deterrent of the Relationship between Stressors and Adjustment

Study	Sample and stressor	Measure of religiousness	Measure of adjustment	Results
Anson et al. (1990)	225 members of religious and nonreligious kibbutz in Israel respond to list of recent life events	Two kibbutz types; self-related religiousness item; religious practice scale; frequency of private prayer item; item on extent of comfort from God in times of distress	Subjective evaluation of health; frequency of symptoms; reported disability; reported chronic conditions	Partial support for religion as stress moderator, and partial support for religion as stress deterrent
Bahr & Harvey (1979a)	96 widows and survivors of miners in fire, and 128 wives of other miners	Items on church affiliation, frequency of church attendance, religious salience, change in importance of religion since disaster, participation in church social events	Item on loneliness in past week	Partial support for religion as stress moderator, no test of religion as stress deterrent
Bickel et al. (in press)	245 adult members of Presbyterian churches	Collaborative and self-directing religious coping scales	Scale of depression	Support for religion as stress moderator, and support for religion as deterrent
Brown & Gary (1988)	245 African-American women either employed or unemployed	Measure of degree of involvement in religious activities and application of religious beliefs to life	Depression scale	Partial support for religion as stress moderator, and partial support for religion as stress deterrent

Study	Sample and stressor	Measure of religiousness	Measure of adjustment	Results
Ellison (1991)	National sample respond to checklist of three traumatic events	Frequency of attendance; closeness to God and frequency of prayer; items about existential certainty; denomination	Overall life satisfaction and personal happiness	Partial support for religion as stress moderator, and partial support for religion as deterrent
Ellison, Gay, & Glass (1989)	National sample indicating total number of traumatic events in past year	Affiliation; frequency of church attendance; devotionalism (frequency of prayer and closeness to God)	Life satisfaction scale	No support for religion as stress moderator, and partial support for religion as stress deterrent
Ellison & Gay (1990)	2,107 African-Americans noting whether had one or more disruptive health conditions or one or more interpersonal or institutional encounters which bothered them a great deal	Denomination; attendance at religious services; self-rated religiousness; frequency of personal prayer	Single item of life satisfaction	No support for religion as stress moderator, and partial support for religion as stress deterrent
Ellison (1993)	1,933 Black Americans; mostly Protestant and Catholic completed measures of negative life events, chronic illnesses, and physical attractiveness	Measures of public and private religiousness	Measures of self-esteem and personal mastery	Partial support for religion as stress moderator, and partial support for religion as stress moderator

(continued)

Study	Sample and stressor	Measure of religiousness	Measure of adjustment	Results
Ensing (1991)	483 church members who completed checklist of negative life events over past year	Religious practice scale (prayer, Bible reading, church attendance); intrinsic, extrinsic, and quest orientations; self-directing, collaborative, and deferring religious coping measured at 2-year intervals	Adjustment scale of self-esteem, loneliness, and psychological health measured at 2-year intervals	No support for religion as stress moderator, and partial support for religion as stress deterrent
Friedel & Pargament (1995)	105 emergency health care workers coping with most stressful work event in past 6 months varying in controllability	Self-directing, collaborative, and deferring religious coping with event	Measures of mental health status, event-specific outcomes, job satisfaction, turnover intention	Partial support for religion as stress moderator, and no test of religion as stress deterrent
Friedrich, Cohen, & Wilturner (1988)	158 parents of retarded children complete scales of child behavior problems and degree of child's physical incapacitation	Religiousness scale assessing religious practices, belief in God, and frequency of church attendance	Depression scale; index of positive and negative well-being	Partial support for religion as stress moderator, no test of religion as stress deterrent
Harvey, Barnes, & Greenwood (1987)	Canadian sample of 11,071 men and women who were widowed and nonwidowed	Single item on religious salience	Global measure of happiness; measure of positive affect	No support for religion as stress moderator, and support for religion as stress deterrent

Study	Sample and stressor	Measure of religiousness	Measure of adjustment	Results
Idler (1987)	2,756 elderly from New Haven with stressors of chronic medical conditions and functional disability	Measure of church attendance and number of members known in congregation (public); measure of religious salience and degree of comfort and strength from religion (private)	Depression and functional disability scales	Partial support for religion as stress moderator, and partial support for religion as stress deterrent
Idler & Kasl (1992)	603 elderly males experiencing more functional disability over 3 years; Protestant, Jewish, and Catholic	Measures of public and private religiousness	Measures of depression over 3 years	Partial support for religion as stress moderator, no support for religion as stress deterrent
Jamal & Badawi (1993)	325 Muslims in North America coping with job stress	Self-rated religiousness item	Measures of job-related outcomes (e.g., satisfaction, motivation, commitment), psychosomatic symptoms, and happiness	Partial support for religion as stress deterrent, and partial support for religion as stress moderator
Krause & Van Tran (1989)	51 elderly African-Americans responding to checklist of negative life events in past month	Measure of organized religious involvement; measure of personal religious involvement (frequency of prayer, self-rated religiousness, importance of sending children to services)	Measures of self-esteem and mastery	No support for religion as stress moderator, and partial support for religion as stress deterrent

(continued)

Study	Sample and stressor	Measure of religiousness	Measure of adjustment	Results
Maton (1989b), Study 1	81 members of bereaved parents support group divided into high stress and low stress based on recency of death	Scale of spiritual support	Measures of depression and self-esteem	Partial support for religion as stress moderator, and partial support for religion as stress deterrent
Maton (1989b), Study 2	68 high school seniors in transition to college divided into high and low stress based on number of negative life events in past 6 months	Scale of spiritual support; frequency of church attendance assessed precollege	Scales of social adjustment and personal–emotional adjustment; depression scale assessed post-high school	Partial support for religion as stress moderator, no support for religion as stress deterrent
Maton (1989a)	162 members of 3 churches (M age = 31) completed scale of economic stress	Whether part of a high support or low support church as measured by number of material support transactions in the church	Life satisfaction	Partial support for religion as stress moderator, no support for religion as stress deterrent
Pargament et al. (1994)	215 college students completing measure of concerns about 1990–1991 Persian Gulf war prior to invasion of Kuwait	Religious coping activity scales (spiritually based, good deeds, pleading, interpersonal religious support, religious avoidance, religious discontent)	Psychological health, positive and negative affect scales	Partial support for religion as stress moderator, and support for religion as stress deterrent
Park, Cohen, & Herb (1990), Study 1	College undergraduates completed measure of life events	Intrinsic and extrinsic scales; item on degree religion used in coping for each event	Scale of depression and trait anxiety at pretesting and 8 weeks later	Partial support for religion as stress moderator, and partial support for religion as stress deterrent

Study	Sample and stressor	Measure of religiousness	Measure of adjustment	Results
Park, Cohen, & Herb (1990), Study 2	College undergraduates completed measure of life events	Intrinsic and extrinsic scales; item on degree religion used in coping for each event	Scale of depression and trait anxiety at pretesting and 8 weeks later	Partial support for religion as stress moderator, and partial support for religion as stress deterrent
Pollner (1989)	National sample of 1,500 to 3,000 adults	Measure of closeness to God and frequency of prayer (divine relations); 3 subscales of images of God; God as friend or God as hierarchical; frequency of church attendance	General happiness item; marital happiness; life excitement; and life satisfaction scale	No support for religion as stress moderator, and support for religion as stress deterrent
Shams & Jackson (1993)	140 male British Asian employed and unemployed Muslims	Scale of religious values	Measure of mental health	Support for religion as stress deterrent, and support for religion as stress moderator
Siegel & Kuykendall (1990)	825 married or widowed who note whether a close family member had died in past 6 months	Whether belong to a church/temple	Depression scale	Partial support for religion as stress moderator, no support for religion stress deterrent
Sijuwade (1994)	115 elderly Nigerians completed measure of life events	Scale of religious commitment, prayer, and experience presence of God	Self-rated scale of illness	No support for religion as stress moderator or religion as stress deterrent
Simons & West (1984–1985)	299 elderly adults in Midwest noting major life experiences in past year	Scale of frequency prayer, reading religious materials, felt presence of God, and degree of religious commitment	Seriousness of illness rating scale	No support for religion as stress moderator, no support for religion as stress deterrent

(continued)

Study	Sample and stressor	Measure of religiousness	Measure of adjustment	Results
Stouffer et al. (1965)	Soldiers involved in different theaters of operation in World War II	Item on whether prayer helped them when the going was tough	Embedded in religious measure	Partial support for religion as stress moderator, no test of religion as stress deterrent
Williams et al. (1991)	720 adults from New Haven completed scale of number of undesirable life events, and measure of physical health problems	Frequency of church attendance and religious affiliation	Psychological symptom checklist measured over a 2-year period	Partial support for religion as stress moderator, no support for religion as stress deterrent
Zuckerman, Kasl, & Ostfeld (1984)	398 men and women, 62 and older, poor, completed index of health status and symptoms	Scale of church attendance, self-rated religiousness, and strength from religion	Mortality over next 2 years	Support for religion as stress moderator, no support for religion as stress deterrent

NOTES

Chapter Two

1. A similar criticism could be made of definitions of spirituality that exclude some reference to the sacred (see Copp & Copp, 1993). What is it, for example, that makes the values of meaning in life, personal growth, or interconnectedness spiritual unless they are somehow sacralized? How are practices such as guided imagery or meditation more spiritual than other cognitive and behavioral approaches to change unless they are connected to the sacred? Invoking the label "spiritual" adds luster and legitimacy to any number of values and practices, but the label may ultimately lose meaning and power when it is separated from its sacred core.

2. The picture is not always clear when we try to demarcate the boundaries of the concept of God. Do sorcery, witchcraft, or homage to one's ancestors qualify as forms of divine worship? What about astrology, or a belief in the power of a lucky rabbit's foot? Is Nirvana, the highest state of the human spirit in Buddhism, one in which all human desires have been extinguished, godly? There is no easy answer to these questions. Each must be considered separately. Take, for instance, the concept of Nirvana. There has been considerable debate about whether Nirvana is God, and, more generally, whether Buddhism is a religion (Conze, 1951). Buddha explicitly rejected the kind of god defined as a personal creator. Yet the concept of Nirvana embodies many qualities of the divine. It is "permanent, stable, imperishable, immovable, ageless, deathless, unborn, and unbecome . . . it is power, bliss and happiness, the secure refuge, the shelter, and the place of unassailable safety" (Conze, 1951, p. 40). Defined in this fashion, Nirvana seems to fall well within the umbrella of the divine. To be more certain, though, it is important to see how concepts such as Nirvana are actually experienced by individuals and collectives. In this vein, Spiro (1978) has found that, in contrast to their religious leaders and traditional teachings, common

465

Buddhists from Burma hold beliefs in superhuman beings. The weight of the evidence suggests that Nirvana, and at least some expressions of Buddhism, incorporate a sense of higher powers. Delineating the boundaries of the divine is no simple task, but it is a necessary one, for God and that which becomes sanctified represent a critical point of reference for religion.

Chapter Three

1. Important questions can be raised about studies of motivation. In response to the Braden (cited in Clark, 1958, p. 79) study, we can ask how well people are truly able to identify and report the reasons why they do what they do. In studies documenting a connection between religious involvement and meaning, we can ask whether people who derive meaning necessarily seek meaning from religion. Perhaps meaning is a by-product of the search for some other significant end. In response to the popularity of books of the "Why me?" variety, we can wonder how well the reading habits of a population reflect their underlying motivations. Because any single study will have its limitations, the best we can do is approximate a conclusion when it comes to motivations. We can have the greatest confidence in conclusions when our theory coincides with the results of studies of what people have to say about their motives, whether they act consistently with their stated motives, and what they derive from their experiences.

2. The quest orientation may seem to be no different from religion as it has been defined here—the search for significance in ways related to the sacred. But they differ in an important respect. Quest for Batson is a variable; people vary in the degree to which they question themselves and their world on the path to growth and meaning. In contrast, I assume that everyone is involved in a search of one form or another. The search is constant; what varies is the kind of search. From my perspective, Batson's quest is simply one orientation to the religious odyssey, an orientation that involves continual questioning and doubt. While answers, resolutions, and goals achieved are not a part of the quest orientation, they can be a part of the religious search. The search for significance, religious or otherwise, can be successful. This does not mean that people stop striving. Those who find satisfying answers to difficult questions may no longer search for answers but they still struggle to preserve, protect, or enhance their new understanding. This is a very different struggle than the one we hear in the religious quest. In short, the questioning orientation is only one of many religious directions people can take in their search for significance.

3. A similar argument could be made about the relationship of quest to the other orientations. The lack of correlation among these orientations

indicates that some people find room for both questions and answers in their religious experience. In fact, Tillich (1951) defines the theologian in just this way: "Every theologian is committed and alienated; he is always in faith and in doubt; he is inside and outside the theological circle" (p. 10).

Chapter Five

1. That significance can take undesirable as well as desirable forms distinguishes this concept from other terms such as "meaning" or "purpose in life." These latter terms have a distinctly positive connotation. Frankl (1984), for example, notes: "Once an individual's search for a meaning is successful, it not only renders him happy but also gives him the capability to cope with suffering" (p. 163). From my point of view, meaning represents one of many possible objects of significance, constructive and destructive. The attainment of significance does not necessarily bring happiness or well-being.

2. I prefer the more inclusive term "significance" to "personal well-being" here. Admittedly, personal well-being is a central concern for most people when they encounter stress. But stressful events can also threaten, challenge, or harm objects of significance that are not limited to the self, such as friends, families, or communities. These objects may have only indirect implications for the individual's *personal* well-being, and yet we still care about them.

3. A number of researchers have examined the qualities that make events so problematic. Although we cannot review or resolve this debate here, some of the positions can be noted. Some researchers have emphasized the stressfulness associated with the cumulation of major life changes or transitions, be they positive or negative (Holmes & Rahe, 1967). Others have focused on the accumulation of more minor "daily hassles" of life, those irritations and annoyances we feel with the day-to-day problems of family, friends, housework, or financial matters (DeLongis, Coyne, Dakof, Folkman, & Lazarus, 1982). Some have preferred to define the stressfulness of events in terms of particular content areas, such as interpersonal events (e.g., divorce, trouble with children), work-related events (e.g., loss of job), health-related events (e.g., illness, injury), intrapersonal events (e.g., conflict), major calamities (e.g., war, natural disasters), or events affecting significant others (e.g., death, victimization) (Hobfoll, 1988). Still others have attempted to identify the psychologically salient elements of problematic situations; ambiguity, unpredictability, uncontrollability, chronicity, severity, novelty, timing, and the degree to which the event triggers earlier unresolved negative experiences have been tied to stressfulness (Baider & Sarell, 1984; Lazarus & Folkman, 1984). Finally, some theorists have defined crises in terms of

a lack of synchronization among biological, psychological, sociological, and cultural developments (Riegel, 1975).

4. Secondary appraisals in Lazarus and Folkman's (1984) framework include both assessments of resource availability and assessments of the most efficacious coping strategy. These appraisals, they write, refer to "what might and can be done . . . which coping options are available, the likelihood that a given coping option will accomplish what it is supposed to, and the likelihood that one can apply a particular strategy or set of strategies successfully" (p. 35). Because the selection of the most compelling coping strategy for the particular situation has such important implications, I believe it is helpful to assign this process its own label and reserve "secondary appraisals" for assessments of resource availability.

5. Trade-offs between individual and system are not the best we can hope for in coping. Synergistic outcomes are also possible. "Individual–system spirals" can also occur in which the person and his or her system enhance the well-being of each other and themselves (see Pargament & Myers, 1982).

Chapter Seven

1. Our research offers one explanation for a seemingly counterintuitive finding in the psychology of religion literature. People who report that they rely more on God in life do not invariably report greater powerlessness (see Pargament & Park, 1995). In fact, some studies have shown a positive relationship between the sense of control by God and the sense of personal control (e.g., DeVellis, DeVellis, & Spilsbury, 1988; Jackson & Coursey, 1988; Kahoe, 1974). If we think about reliance on God as a synonym for helplessness, then these results are difficult to explain. However, reliance may be used in a different sense. People may be relying on God more as a partner than as a substitute for their own efforts. Knowing that they can call on God for help and knowing that God is on their side would not diminish their sense of efficacy and mastery. It would enhance it. The relationship between reliance on God and personal control may reflect the fact that people view God more as a partner in coping than as a paternal figure who will solve their problems for them. Research using the three styles of religious coping reveals that scores on the collaborative scale are quite a bit higher than scores on the deferring scale. Recall that the collaborative style relates to a greater sense of personal control, unlike its deferring counterpart. Thus, people who report that they rely on God may be endorsing the collaborative approach, one that empowers them in their lives (see also Pargament, Sullivan, Tyler, & Steele, 1982).

2. The three styles of religious coping are moderately intercorrelated. To

assess the independent effects of each style, the effects of the other two styles should be statistically controlled. The intercorrelations among the three styles are interesting in themselves. People who adopt a self-directing approach are less likely to use collaborative or deferring religious problem solving. Collaborative and deferring coping styles, on the other hand, are positively related to each other. Perhaps those who score higher on both measures have a more comprehensive religious coping system, collaborating with God in some situations and deferring to God in others. Or perhaps collaboration is often mixed with some deference in coping. God may be a partner in coping, but a senior partner. We hear this mixture of the two styles in this letter from Bonhoeffer (1971) during his imprisonment in World War II: "I believe that God can and will bring good out of evil, even out of the greatest evil. For that purpose he needs men who make the best use of everything. I believe that God will give us the strength we need to help us resist in all times of distress. But he never gives it in advance, lest we should rely on ourselves and not on him alone" (p. 11). In spite of their connections, it makes an important difference for religion and mental health whether the partnership *with* God or the deference *to* God is emphasized in coping.

Chapter Eight

1. Although most researchers, including several of those cited earlier, use the term "convert" to describe people who change denominations, I have reserved this term for later use when we consider more radical changes in the coping process. I have taken the liberty here of relabeling "converts" as "switchers." There is a critical distinction here. In contrast to the convert, the religious switcher does not seek a wholesale change in values; instead, he or she looks for another way to realize them. My sense is that most people who change denominations, even under stress, are not searching for a new destination in living, but rather a new group to help them reach their old goals. Travisano (1970) has made a similar point. He distinguishes between alternation and conversion as qualitatively different transformations, and argues that the former is much more common than the latter.

2. A willingness to credit God for the good things that happen goes hand in hand with the disinclination to blame God for the bad. Empirical studies have consistently shown that religious attributions are greater for positive than for negative events (Pargament & Sullivan, 1981; Ritzema, 1979; Spilka & Schmidt, 1983). Mark Twain (1974) once wrote facetiously on this tendency: "If science exterminates a disease which has been working for God, it is God that gets the credit, and all the pulpits break into grateful advertising-raptures and call attention to how good he is!" (p. 36). What seems to be at work here is a strong desire to sustain

the image of a benevolent deity involved in the world. Both the willingness to credit God for good occurrences and the reluctance to blame God for bad ones are mechanisms designed to protect the holy itself.

Chapter Nine

1. Beliefs about an afterlife are not restricted to rites of passage. Neither are they necessarily transformational. In the face of death, beliefs in the hereafter may conserve a number of ends: emotional comfort, the sense of intimacy with the deceased, the sense of personal identity, the desire for a better world, and the desire for a sacred connection. To determine the conservational or transformational role of any belief or practice, we have to go beyond a description of the content of that method of coping to a functional analysis of the purposes it serves.

Chapter Ten

1. Although a number of other studies are at least indirectly relevant to this topic, studies were excluded in which (1) the relationship between religiousness and mental health or psychopathology was examined among groups that were not dealing with an explicitly defined stressor; (2) the measure of religiousness was severely confounded by other factors, such as education or socioeconomic status (e.g., Purisman & Maoz, 1977); (3) the measures of religiousness and outcome were highly confounded with each other, as is the case when religiousness is assessed by outcome-like items (e.g., "How much help have you received from your religion?") (Hunter et al., 1974); and (4) there were too few studies of that particular form of religiousness. For example, although there have been a number of studies of the relationship between beliefs in an afterlife and death anxiety (see Spilka et al., 1985), only a few studies have looked at these relationships among those in crisis, with mixed results (Bivens, Neumeyer, Kirchberg, & Moore, 1994–1995; Franks, Templer, Cappelletty, & Kauffman, 1990–1991; Smith, Nehemkis, & Charter, 1983–1984). Several studies examine more than one type of religious orientation variable. In these cases, the various results are separated and presented in the appropriate subsections of the table. Thus, some studies appear several times in the table.

2. The positive results here may have been confounded by the relationship of church attendance to physical health status. Those who participated more regularly in church services may have been in better physical shape, and their physical condition rather than church participation may have been responsible for their better social adjustment. A few other researchers, however, have found that the positive relationship between

church participation and adjustment remains even after controlling for the health status of the sample (e.g., Koenig, Kvale, & Ferrel, 1988).

3. A few studies using more elaborate statistical methods have tested the mediating model of religious coping more directly and yielded some support. Hathaway and Pargament (1990) found that the deferring and collaborative religious problem solving styles mediated the relationship between an intrinsic religious orientation and measures of psychosocial competence. Using path analytic methods, Park and Cohen (1993) found that measures of religious coping activities mediated some, but not all, of the relationships between measures of religious orientation and psychological distress and growth.

4. While these dimensions correspond roughly to some of the religious coping mechanisms described in the last two chapters, they are not an exact match. Several types of religious coping, particularly transformational ones, have gone unstudied (e.g., rites of passage, seeking religious direction, religious forgiveness).

   Studies that examine more than one type of religious coping appear more than once in Table 10.2. The results of these studies are separated and presented in the appropriate subsections. In some published studies, only significant results were presented. The results of these studies are not entered into the tallies of positive, negative, and nonsignificant findings.

5. In some instances, data more extensive than those in the published papers were available from the authors of these studies. These data have been included in Appendix D.

6. It could be argued that the most straightforward way to evaluate the efficacy of pleading would be to see whether the miracle actually occurred. In fact, a few studies have examined the effects of prayers for divine intercession on behalf of those with a physical illness, with mixed results (Byrd, 1988; Collipp, 1969; Joyce & Welldon, 1965). This is a controversial area of research. Perhaps the most difficult question is how to determine what constitutes a divine intercession. The Allied victory in the Persian Gulf war could be seen as a miraculous event to those on the Allied side. Those on the other side who suffered such terrible losses might view the same event as an instance of divine abandonment or retribution. If only God knows what is ultimately best for humankind, then the attempt to "test for miracles" falls outside the province of science.

7. Although religious conversion and religious switching have been conceptualized as ways of coping with negative life events, empirical studies have not tied these approaches to negative life situations and their resolution. For this reason, the religious conversion and religious switching research could not be placed in Table 10.2 and Appendix D.

8. To put it in more scientific terms, the relationship between age, gender, race, income, marital status, and the outcomes of coping may be mediated by the degree of involvement of religion in the individual's

orienting system. Krause (1991) provides some support for this model in a path analysis of drinking behavior. Both gender (female status) and race (minority status) were indirectly associated with alcohol abstinence through their relationship with greater subjective religiousness.

9. This discussion has focused on differences in the *degree* of situational stressfulness rather than differences in the *types* of stressful situations. Unfortunately, few studies have compared the relative efficacy of religious coping in particular types of situations, such as chronic versus acute conditions or major life events versus daily hassles. However, there is some evidence that religion may be especially helpful in coping with death (Mattlin et al., 1990; Neighbors et al., 1983) and in coping with life-threatening illness (Lilliston, Brown, & Schliebe, 1982). Of course, deaths and life-threatening illnesses are also among the most stressful of situations, so these results could simply be another way of saying that religion is most helpful in times of greatest trouble (i.e., the religious stress moderator model).

Chapter Eleven

1. Some researcher have suggested that moderately positive illusions about oneself and the world may facilitate positive mental health. Taylor and Brown (1988), for instance, reviewed a body of research that led them to question whether accuracy in self-perception is a necessary ingredient of psychological adjustment. Others, however, have taken issue with their reading of the research, and the matter is still being hotly debated (see Colvin & Block, 1994; Taylor & Brown, 1994). Certainly, many situations allow for some range of interpretation, and within that range, realistically benign appraisals may be more helpful to the individual than realistically negative ones. But to go beyond that interpretative range, I believe, is likely to lead to serious problems in coping.

2. Some cases of religiously based abuse might also fall under the rubric of religious deception. Spiritual justification may cloak the more basic motivation underlying the abuse: the desire for control, dominance, and mastery over the child.

3. Hunsberger (1996) has suggested a related culprit in all of this—right-wing authoritarianism. There is a strong tendency for fundamentalists to have more authoritarian personalities. Perhaps authoritarian personalities are drawn to religious fundamentalism, or perhaps fundamentalism fosters the development of this type of personality. In either case, Altemeyer and Hunsberger (1993) offer evidence from one study that right-wing authoritarianism is more directly related to prejudice than fundamentalism (whether left-wing authoritarianism is related to other forms of religiousness and prejudice is another interesting but unexplored question).

REFERENCES

Abbott, D. A., & Meredith, W. H. (1986). Strengths of parents with retarded children. *Journal of Applied Family and Child Studies, 35,* 371–375.

Achterberg, J. (1985). *Imagery in healing: Shamanism and modern medicine.* Boston: New Science Library.

Acklin, M. W., Brown, E. C., & Mauger, P. A. (1983). The role of religious values in coping with cancer. *Journal of Religion and Health, 22,* 322–333.

Adams, J. E., & Lindemann, E. (1974). Coping with long-term disability. In G. V. Coelho, D. A. Hamburg, & J. E. Adams (Eds.), *Coping and adaptation* (pp. 127–138). New York: Basic Books.

Ajami, F. (1990/1991). The summer of Arab discontent. *Foreign Affairs, 69,* 1–20.

Alcoholics Anonymous: The twelve steps and twelve traditions (3rd ed.). (1977). New York: Alcoholics Anonymous World Services.

Aldwin, C. M. (1994). *Stress, coping, and development: An integrative perspective.* New York: Guilford Press.

Aldwin, C. M., Levenson, M. R., & Spiro, A. (1994). Vulnerability and resilience to combat exposure: Can stress have lifelong effects? *Psychology and Aging, 9,* 34–44.

Allport, G. W. (1950). *The individual and his religion: A psychological interpretation.* New York: Macmillan.

Allport, G. W. (1954). *The nature of prejudice.* Cambridge, MA: Addison-Wesley.

Allport, G. W. (1960). *Personality and social encounter.* Boston: Beacon Press.

Allport, G. W. (1966). The religious context of prejudice. *Journal for the Scientific Study of Religion, 5,* 447–457.

Allport, G. W. (1968). The fruits of eclecticism: Bitter or sweet? In G. W. Allport (Ed.), *The person in psychology* (pp. 3–27). Boston: Beacon Press.

Allport, G. W., Bruner, J. S., & Jandorf, E. M. (1956). Personality under social catastrophe: Ninety life-histories of the Nazi revolution. In C. Kluckhohn & H. A. Murray (Eds.), *Personality in nature, society, and culture* (2nd ed., pp. 436–455). New York: Knopf.

Allport, G. W., Gillespie, J. M., & Young, J. (1948). The religion of the post-war college student. *Journal of Psychology, 25,* 3–33.

Allport, G. W., & Ross, J. M. (1967). Personal religious orientation and prejudice. *Journal of Personality and Social Psychology, 5,* 432–443.

Altemeyer, B., & Hunsberger, B. (1992). Authoritarianism, religious fundamentalism, quest, and prejudice. *International Journal for the Psychology of Religion, 2,* 113–133.

Altemeyer, B., & Hunsberger, B. (1993). Reply to Gorsuch. *International Journal for the Psychology of Religion, 3,* 33–37.

American Psychiatric Association. (1990). Guidelines regarding possible conflict between psychiatrists' religious commitments and psychiatric practice (official actions). *American Journal of Psychiatry, 147,* 542.

Anderson, R. W., Jr., Maton, K. I., & Ensor, B. E. (1992). Prevention theory and action from the religious perspective. In K. I. Pargament, K. I. Maton, & R. E. Hess (Eds.), *Religion and prevention in mental health: Research, vision, and action* (pp. 195–214). New York: Haworth Press.

Anniversary of Oklahoma City bomb blast. (1996, April 29). *Newsweek,* p. 19.

Anson, O., Carmel, S., Bonneh, D. Y., Levenson, A., & Maoz, B. (1990). Recent life events, religiosity, and health: An individual or collective effect. *Human Relations, 43,* 1051–1066.

Anthony, E. J. (1987). Risk, vulnerability, and resilience: An overview. In E. J. Anthony & B. J. Cohler (Eds.), *The invulnerable child* (pp. 3–48). New York: Guilford Press.

Antonovsky, A. (1987). *Unraveling the mystery of health: How people manage stress and stay well.* San Francisco: Jossey-Bass.

Argyle, M., & Beit-Hallahmi, B. (1975). *The social psychology of religion.* London: Routledge & Kegan Paul.

Astin, M. C., Lawrence, K. J., & Foy, D. W. (1993). Posttraumatic stress disorder among battered women: Risk and resiliency factors. *Violence and Victims, 8,* 17–28.

Atkins, R. G., Jr. (1991). *Twelve-step groups as modern forms of religious life.* Paper presented at the meeting of the Society for the Scientific Study of Religion, Pittsburgh, PA.

Augsberger, D. (1981). *Caring enough to forgive: Caring enough not to forgive.* Scottsdale, PA: Herald Press.

Augustine, Saint. (1950). *The city of God* (M. Dods, Trans.). New York: Modern Library.

Aust, C. F. (1990). Using the client's religious values to aid in therapy. *Counseling and Values, 34,* 125–129.

Azhar, M. Z., Varma, S. L., & Dharap, A. S. (1994). Religious psychotherapy in anxiety disorder patients. *Acta Psychiatrica Scandinavica, 90,* 1–3.

Bahr, H. M., & Harvey, C. D. (1979a). Correlates of loneliness among widows bereaved in a mining disaster. *Psychological Reports, 44,* 367–385.

Bahr, H. M., & Harvey, C. D. (1979b). Widowhood and perceptions of change in quality of life: Evidence from the Sunshine Mine Widows. *Journal of Comparative Family Studies, 10,* 411–428.

Baider, L., & De-Nour, A. K. (1987). The meaning of a disease: An exploratory study of Moslem Arab women after a mastectomy. *Journal of Psychosocial Oncology, 4,* 1–13.

Baider, L., & Sarell, M. (1983). Perceptions and causal attributions of Israeli women with breast cancer concerning their illness: The effects of ethnicity and religiosity. *Psychology and Psychosomatics, 39,* 136–143.

Baider, L., & Sarell, M. (1984). Coping with cancer among Holocaust survivors in Israel: An exploratory study. *Journal of Human Stress, 10,* 121–127.

Bakan, D. (1966). *The duality of human existence: An essay on psychology and religion.* Chicago: Rand McNally.

Bakan, D. (1968). *Disease, pain, and sacrifice: Toward a psychology of suffering.* Chicago: University of Chicago Press.

Baker, M., & Gorsuch, R. (1982). Trait anxiety and intrinsic–extrinsic religiousness. *Journal for the Scientific Study of Religion, 21,* 119–122.

Balch, R. W. (1980). Looking behind the scenes in a religious cult: Implications for the study of conversion. *Sociological Analysis, 41,* 137–143.

Balch, R. W., & Gilliam, M. (1991). Devil worship in western Montana: A case study in rumor construction. In J. T. Richardson, J. Best, & D. G. Bromley (Eds.), *The satanism scare* (pp. 249–262). New York: Aldine de Gruyter.

Baldree, K. S., Murphy, S. P., & Powers, M. J. (1982). Stress identification and coping patterns in patients on hemodialysis. *Nursing Research, 31,* 107–112.

Balk, D. (1983). Adolescents' grief reactions and self-concept perceptions following sibling death: A study of 33 teenagers. *Journal of Youth and Adolescence, 12,* 137–161.

Ball, R. A., & Goodyear, R. K. (1993). Self-reported professional practices of Christian therapists. In E. L. Worthington (Ed.), *Psychotherapy and religious values* (pp. 171–182). Grand Rapids, MI: Baker Book House.

Bandura, A. (1978). The self-system in reciprocal determinism. *American Psychologist, 37,* 122–147.

Bandura, A. (1989). Human agency in social cognitive theory. *American Psychologist, 44,* 1175–1184.

Barbarin, O. A., & Chesler, M. (1986). The medical context of parental coping with childhood cancer. *American Journal of Community Psychology, 14,* 221–235.

Barbour, J. G. (1974). *Myths, models and paradigms: A comparative study in science and religion.* New York: Harper & Row.

Barr, M. (1995). *Sticks and stones: The impact of liturgical language on victims of abuse.* Paper presented at the meeting of the Society for the Scientific Study of Religion, St. Louis, MO.

Barsch, R. H. (1968). *The parent of the handicapped child: The study of child-rearing practices.* Springfield, IL: Charles C Thomas.

Bartkowski, J. P. (1995). Spare the rod . . . or spare the child? Divergent perspectives on Conservative Protestant child discipline. *Review of Religious Research, 37,* 97–116.

Barton, A. H. (1971). Selected problems in the study of religious development. In M. Strommen (Ed.), *Research on religious development: A comprehensive handbook* (pp. 836–855). New York: Hawthorn Books.

Bassett, R. L., Hill, P. C., Hart, C., Mathewson, K., & Perry, K. (1992). Helping Christians reclaim some abandoned emotions: The ACE model of emotions. *Journal of Psychology and Theology, 21,* 165–173.

Batson, C. D. (1975). Rational processing or rationalization? The effect of disconfirming evidence on a stated religious belief. *Journal of Personality and Social Psychology, 32,* 176–184.

Batson, C. D. (1990). How social an animal? The human capacity for caring. *American Psychologist, 45,* 336–346.

Batson, C. D., & Flory, J. D. (1990). Goal-relevant cognitions associated with helping by individuals high on intrinsic, end religion. *Journal for the Scientific Study of Religion, 29,* 346–360.

Batson, C. D., Oleson, K. C., Weeks, J. L., Healy, S., Reeves, P. J., Jennings, P., & Brown, T. (1989). Religious prosocial motivation: Is it altruistic or egoistic? *Journal of Personality and Social Psychology, 57,* 873–884.

Batson, C. D., & Raynor-Prince, L. (1983). Religious orientation and complexity of thought about existential concerns. *Journal for the Scientific Study of Religion, 22,* 38–50.

Batson, C. D., & Schoenrade, P. A. (1991a). Measuring religion as quest: (1) Validity concerns. *Journal for the Scientific Study of Religion, 30,* 416–429.

Batson, C. D., & Schoenrade, P. A. (1991b). Measuring religion as quest: (2) Reliability concerns. *Journal for the Scientific Study of Religion, 30,* 430–447.

Batson, C. D., Schoenrade, P., & Ventis, W. L. (1993). *Religion and the individual: A social-psychological perspective.* New York: Oxford University Press.

Baugher, R. J., Burger, C., Smith, R., & Wallston, K. (1989–1990). A comparison of terminally ill persons at various time periods to death. *Omega, 20,* 103–115.

Baures, M. M. (1996). Letting go of bitterness and hate. *Journal of Humanistic Psychology, 36,* 75–90.

Bearon, L. B., & Koenig, H. G. (1990). Religious cognitions and use of prayer in health and illness. *Gerontologist, 30,* 249–253.

Beck, J. R. (1986). Christian reflections on stress management. *Journal of Psychology and Theology, 14,* 22–28.

Beit-Hallahmi, B. (1992). *Despair and deliverance: Private salvation in contemporary Israel.* Albany: State University of New York Press.

Belavich, T. G., & Pargament, K. I. (1995). *The role of religion in coping with daily hassles.* Paper presented at the meeting of the American Psychological Association, New York, NY.

Bellah, R. N. (1970). *Beyond belief. Essays on religion in a post-traditional world.* New York: Harper & Row.

Bellah, R. N., Madsen, R., Sullivan, W. M., Swidler, A., & Tipton, S. M. (1985). *Habits of the heart: Individualism and commitment in American life.* New York: Harper & Row.

Bem, D. J. (1972). Self-perception theory. In L. Berkowitz (Ed.), *Advances in experimental social psychology* (Vol. 6, pp. 2–62). New York: Academic Press.

Bendann, E. (1930). *Death customs: An analytical study of burial rites.* London: Kegan Paul, Trench, Trubner.

Benner, P., Roskies, E., & Lazarus, R. S. (1980). Stress and coping under extreme conditions. In J. E. Dimsdale (Ed.), *Survivors, victims and perpetrators: Essays on the Nazi Holocaust* (pp. 219–258). Washington, DC: Hemisphere.

Bennis, W. (1989). *Why leaders can't lead: The unconscious conspiracy continues.* San Francisco: Jossey-Bass.

Benson, H. (1984). *Beyond the relaxation response.* New York: Berkley Books.

Benson, P. L., & Spilka, B. (1973). God image as a function of self-esteem and locus of control. *Journal for the Scientific Study of Religion, 13,* 297–310.

Berger, P. L. (1961). *The precarious vision.* Garden City, NY: Doubleday.

Berger, P. L. (1967). *The sacred canopy: Elements of a sociological theory of religion.* New York: Doubleday.

Berger, P. L. (1974). Some second thoughts on substantive versus functional definitions of religion. *Journal for the Scientific Study of Religion, 13,* 125–134.

Bergin, A. E. (1980). Psychotherapy and religious values. *Journal of Consulting and Clinical Psychology, 48,* 95–105.

Bergin, A. E. (1988). Three contributions of a spiritual perspective to counseling, psychotherapy, and behavior change. *Counseling and Values, 33,* 21–31.

Bergin, A. E., & Jensen, J. P. (1990). Religiosity of psychotherapists: A national survey. *Psychotherapy, 27,* 3–7.

Bergin, A. E., Masters, K. S., & Richards, P. S. (1987). Religiousness and mental health reconsidered: A study of an intrinsically religious sample. *Journal of Counseling Psychology, 34,* 197–204.

Bergin, A. E., Stinchfield, R. D., Gaskin, T. A., Masters, K. S., & Sullivan, C. E. (1988). Religious life styles and mental health: An exploratory study. *Journal of Counseling Psychology, 35,* 197–204.

Berkovits, E. (1979). *With God in hell: Judaism in the ghettos and death camps.* New York: Sanhedrin Press.

Berkowitz, W. (1989, April). The ten plagues of our time. *Toledo Jewish News,* p. 14.

Berman, A. L. (1974). Belief in afterlife, religion, religiosity and life-threatening experiences. *Omega, 5,* 127–135.

Bernt, F. M. (1989). Being religious and being altruistic: A study of college service volunteers. *Personality and Individual Differences, 10,* 663–669.

Bertocci, P. A. (1972). Psychological interpretations of religious experience. In M. Strommen (Ed.), *Research on religious development: A comprehensive handbook* (pp. 3–41). New York: Hawthorn.

Beutler, J. J., Attevelt, J. T. M., Schouten, S. A., Faber, J. A. J., Mees, E. J. D., & Geijskes, G. G. (1988). Paranormal healing and hypertension. *British Medical Journal, 296,* 1491–1494.

Bibby, R. W. (1987). *Fragmented gods: The poverty and potential of religion in Canada.* Toronto: Irwin.

Bickel, C. O. (1978). *The uniqueness of pastoral counseling.* Paper presented at the meeting of the Seventh Annual Clinical–Community Psychology Conference, University of Maryland, Silver Spring, MD.

Bickel, C. O., Ciarrocchi, J. W., Scheers, N. J., Estadt, B. K., Powell, D. A., & Pargament, K. I. (in press). Perceived stress, religious coping styles and depressive affect. *Journal of Psychology and Christianity.*

Biegert, J. E. (1985). *Staying in.* New York: Pilgrim Press.

Bijur, P. E., Wallston, K. A., Smith, C. A., Lifrak, S., & Friedman, S. B. (1993). *Gender differences in turning to religion for coping.* Paper presented at the meeting of the American Psychological Association, Toronto, Ontario.

Binger, C. M., Ablin, A. R., Feuerstein, R. C., Kushner, J. H., Zoger, S., & Mikkelsen, C. (1969). Childhood leukemia: Emotional impact on patient and family. *New England Journal of Medicine, 280,* 414–418.

Bivens, A. J., Neumeyer, R. A., Kirchberg, T. M., & Moore, M. K. (1994–1995). Death concern and religious beliefs among gays and bisexuals of variable proximity to AIDS. *Omega, 30,* 105–120.

Bjorck, J. P., & Cohen, L. H. (1993). Coping with threats, losses, and challenges. *Journal of Social and Clinical Psychology, 12,* 36–72.

Bjorck, J. P., & Klewicki, L. L. (in press). The effects of stressor type on projected coping. *Journal of Traumatic Stress.*

Bloom, A. (1987). *The closing of the American mind.* New York: Simon & Schuster.

Bobgan, M., & Bobgan, D. (1987). *Psychoheresy: The psychological seduction of Christianity.* San Francisco: East Gate.

Boehnlein, J. K. (1987). Clinical relevance of grief and mourning among Cambodian refugees. *Social Science and Medicine, 25,* 765–772.

Bohannon, J. R. (1991). Religiosity related to grief levels of bereaved mothers and fathers. *Omega, 23,* 153–159.

Boisen, A. T. (1955). *Religion in crisis and custom: A sociological and psychological study.* Westport, CT: Greenwood Press.

Bolger, N., & Zuckerman, A. (1995). A framework for studying personality in the stress process. *Journal of Personality and Social Psychology, 69,* 890–902.

Bonhoeffer, D. (1971). *Letters and papers from prison.* New York: Collier Books.

Boorstin, D. J. (1983). *The discoverers.* New York: Random House.

Bottoms, B. L., Shaver, P. R., Goodman, F. S., & Qin, J. (1995). In the name of God: A profile of religion-related child abuse. *Journal of Social Issues, 51*, 85–112.

Boudreaux, E., Catz, S., Ryan, L., Amaral-Melendez, M., & Brantley, P. J. (1995). The ways of religious coping scale: Reliability, validity, and scale development. *Assessment, 2*, 233–244.

Bowker, L. H. (1988). Religious victims and their religious leaders: Services delivered to one thousand battered women by the clergy. In A. L. Horton & J. A. Williamson (Eds.), *Abuse and religion: When praying isn't enough* (pp. 229–234). Lexington, KY: Lexington Books.

Bowlby, J. (1969). *Attachment and loss: Vol. I. Attachment.* New York: Basic Books.

Bragan, K. (1977). The psychological gains and losses of religious conversion. *British Journal of Medical Psychology, 50*, 177–180.

Brandstädter, J., & Renner, G. (1990). Tenacious goal pursuit and flexible goal adjustment: Explications and age-related analysis of assimilative and accommodative strategies of coping. *Psychology of Aging, 5*, 58–67.

Bransfield, D. D., Ivy, S. S., Rutledge, D. N., & Wallston, K. (1991). *A religiously-oriented program to promote breast cancer screening.* Paper presented at the meeting of the American Psychological Association, San Francisco, CA.

Brant, C. R., & Pargament, K. I. (1995). *Religious coping with racist and other negative life events among African Americans.* Paper presented at the meeting of the American Psychological Association, New York, NY.

Brehm, J. W. (1966). *A theory of psychological reactance.* New York: Academic Press.

Brenner, E. (1985). *Winning by letting go: Control without compulsion, surrender without defeat.* San Diego: Harcourt Brace Jovanovich.

Brenner, R. R. (1980). *The faith and doubt of holocaust survivors.* New York: Free Press.

Breznitz, S. (1980). The noble challenge of stress. In S. Breznitz (Ed.), *Stress in Israel* (pp. 265–274). New York: Van Nostrand Reinhold.

Brock, T. C., & Balloun, J. L. (1967). Behavioral receptivity to dissonant information. *Journal of Personality and Social Psychology, 6*, 413–428.

Bromley, D. G. (1991). Satanism: The new cult scare. In J. T. Richardson, J. Best, & D. G. Bromley (Eds.), *The satanism scare* (pp. 49–74). New York: Aldine De Gruyter.

Bronfenbrenner, U. (1979). *The ecology of human development: Experiments by nature and design.* Cambridge, MA: Harvard University Press.

Bronowski, J. (1973). *The ascent of man.* Boston: Little, Brown.

Brown, D. R., & Gary, L. E. (1988). Unemployment and psychological distress among black American women. *Sociological Focus, 21*, 209–222.

Brown, G. K., Nicassio, P. M., & Wallston, K. A. (1989). Pain coping strategies and depression in rheumatoid arthritis. *Journal of Consulting and Clinical Psychology, 57*, 652–657.

Brown, L. B. (1966). Egocentric thought in petitionary prayer: A cross-cultural study. *Journal of Social Psychology, 68,* 197–210.

Brown, L. B. (1987). *The psychology of religious belief.* London: Academic Press.

Brutz, J. L., & Allen, C. M. (1986). Religious commitment, peace activism, and marital violence in Quaker families. *Journal of Marriage and the Family, 48,* 491–502.

Buber, M. (1951). *Two types of faith.* New York: Collier Books.

Buber, M. (1970). *I and Thou.* New York: Charles Scribner's Sons.

Bulman, R. J., & Wortman, C. B. (1977). Attributions of blame and coping in the "real world": Severe accident victims react to their lot. *Journal of Personality and Social Psychology, 35,* 351–363.

Burger, J. M. (1989). Negative reactions to increases in perceived personal control. *Journal of Personality and Social Psychology, 56,* 246–256.

Burtt, E. A. (Ed.). (1982). *The teachings of the compassionate Buddha.* New York: Mentor Books.

Butter, E. M. (1997). *Validity of the process evaluation model of religious coping.* Unpublished master's thesis, Bowling Green State University, Bowling Green, OH.

Byrd, R. C. (1988). Positive therapeutic effects of intercessory prayer in a coronary care unit population. *Southern Medical Journal, 81,* 826–829.

Cain, B. S. (1988). Divorce among elderly women: A growing social phenomenon. *Social Casework: The Journal of Contemporary Social Work, 69,* 563–568.

Calhoun, L. G., & Tedeschi, R. G. (1992). *Life crises and religious beliefs: Changed beliefs or assimilated events.* Paper presented at the meeting of the American Psychological Association, Washington, DC.

Calian, C. S. (1981). Christian faith as forgiveness. *Theology Today, 37,* 439–441.

Campbell, E. Q., & Pettigrew, T. F. (1959). Racial and moral crisis: The role of Little Rock ministers. *American Journal of Sociology, 64,* 509–516.

Campbell, J. (1988). *The power of myth.* New York: Doubleday.

Camporessi, R. (1991). *The fear of hell: Images of damnation and salvation in modern Europe.* University Park, PA: Pennsylvania State University Press.

Candler, A. G., Jr. (1951). Self-surrender. In D. W. Soper (Ed.), *These found the way: Thirteen converts to Protestant Christianity* (pp. 51–62). Philadelphia: Westminster Press.

Cannon, W. B. (1939). *The wisdom of the body.* New York: Norton.

Capps, D. E. (1977). Contemporary psychology of religion: The task of theoretical reconstruction. In H. W. Malony (Ed.), *Current perspectives in the psychology of religion* (pp. 36–52). Grand Rapids, MI: William B. Eerdmans.

Capps, D. E. (1981). *Biblical approaches to pastoral counseling.* Philadelphia: Westminster Press.

Capps, D. E. (1990). *Reframing: A new method in pastoral care.* Minneapolis: Fortress Press.

Capps, D. E. (1992). Religion and child abuse: Perfect together. *Journal for the Scientific Study of Religion, 31,* 1–14.

Carey, R. G. (1974). Emotional adjustment in terminal patients: A quantitative approach. *Journal of Counseling Psychology, 21,* 433–439.

Carey, R. G. (1977). The widowed: A year later. *Journal of Counseling Psychology, 24,* 125–131.

Carlson, B. E., & Cervera, N. J. (1991). Incarceration, coping, and support. *Social Work, 36,* 279–285.

Carlson, C. R., Bacaseta, P. E., & Simanton, D. A. (1988). A controlled evaluation of devotional meditation and progressive relaxation. *Journal of Psychology and Theology, 16,* 362–368.

Carlson, D. E. (1988). *Counseling and self-esteem.* Dallas: Word Publishing.

Carson, R. J. (1976). *Mental health centers and local clergy: A source book of sample projects.* Washington, DC: Community Mental Health Institute.

Carver, C. S., Pozo, C., Harris, S. D., Noriega, V., Scheier, M. F., Robinson, D. S., Ketcham, A. S., Moffat, F. L., & Clark, K. C. (1993). How coping mediates the effect of optimism on distress: A study of women with early stage breast cancer. *Journal of Personality and Social Psychology, 65,* 375–390.

Carver, C. S., & Scheier, M. F. (1991). Self-regulation and the self. In J. Strauss & G. R. Goethals (Eds.), *The self: Interdisciplinary approaches* (pp. 239–254). New York: Springer-Verlag.

Carver, C. S., Scheier, M. F., & Weintraub, J. K. (1989). Assessing coping strategies: A theoretically-based approach. *Journal of Personality and Social Psychology, 56,* 267–283.

Casebolt, J. (1990). *The role of religion in problem-solving and decision-making: Reliance on God.* Paper presented at the meeting of the Society for the Scientific Study of Religion, Virginia Beach, VA.

Caudill, W. (1958). *Effects of social and cultural systems in reactions to stress.* New York: Social Science Research Council.

Chalfant, H. P., Heller, P. L., Roberts, A., Briones, D., Aquirre-Hochbaum, S., & Farr, W. (1990). The clergy as a resource for those encountering psychological distress. *Review of Religious Research, 31,* 306–313.

Chidester, D. (1988). *Salvation and suicide: An interpretation of Jim Jones, the Peoples Temple, and Jonestown.* Bloomington: Indiana University Press.

Chidester, D. (1990). *Patterns of transcendence: Religion, death and dying.* Belmont, CA: Wadsworth.

Childs, R. E. (1985). Maternal psychological conflicts associated with the birth of a retarded child. *Maternal–Child Nursing Journal, 14,* 175–182.

Chilton, D. (1987). *Power in the blood: A Christian response to AIDS.* Brentwood, TN: Wolgemuth & Hyatt.

Christensen, A., & Jacobson, N. S. (1994). Who (or what) can do psychotherapy: The status and challenge of nonprofessional therapies. *Psychological Science, 5,* 8–14.

Clark, W. H. (1958). How do social scientists define religion? *Journal of Social Psychology, 47,* 143–147.

Cleary, P. D., & Houts, P. S. (1984, Spring). The psychological impact of the Three Mile Island incident. *Journal of Human Stress,* 28–33.

Cobble, J. F., Jr. (1985). *Faith and crisis in the stages of life.* Peabody, MA: Hendrickson.

Coe, G. A. (1916). *The psychology of religion.* Chicago: University of Chicago Press.

Cohen, E., Mowbray, C. T., Gillette, V., & Thompson, E. (1992). Preventing homelessness: Religious organizations and housing development. In K. I. Pargament, K. I. Maton, & R. E. Hess (Eds.), *Religion and prevention in mental health: Research, vision, and action* (pp. 317–333). New York: Haworth Press.

Cohen, S., & Wills, T. A. (1985). Stress, social support, and the buffering hypothesis. *Psychological Bulletin, 98,* 310–357.

Coleman, S. B., Kaplan, J. D., & Downing, R. W. (1986). Life cycle and loss—The spiritual vacuum of heroin addiction. *Family Process, 25,* 5–23.

Collins, R. L., Taylor, S. E., & Skokan, L. A. (1990). A better world or a shattered vision? Changes in life perspectives following victimization. *Social Cognition, 8,* 263–285.

Collipp, P. J. (1969). The efficacy of prayer: A triple-blind study. *Medical Times, 97,* 201–204.

Colvin, C. R., & Block, J. (1994). Do positive illusions foster mental health? An examination of the Taylor and Brown formulation. *Psychological Bulletin, 116,* 3–20.

Compas, B. E., Forsythe, C. J., & Wagner, B. M. (1988). Consistency and variability in causal attributions and coping with stress. *Cognitive Therapy and Research, 12,* 305–320.

Conway, F., & Siegelman, J. (1982). *Holy terror.* New York: Delta Books.

Conway, K. (1985–1986). Coping with the stress of medical problems among black and white elderly. *International Journal of Aging and Human Development, 21,* 39–48.

Conze, E. (1951). *Buddhism: Its essence and development.* New York: Philosophical Library.

Cook, A. S., & Oltjenbruns, K. A. (1989). *Dying and grieving: Lifespan and family perspectives.* New York: Holt, Rinehart & Winston.

Cook, J. A., & Wimberly, D. W. (1983). If I should die before I wake: Religious commitment and adjustment to the death of a child. *Journal for the Scientific Study of Religion, 22,* 222–238.

Copp, L. A., & Copp, J. D. (1993). Illness and the human spirit. *Quality of Life, 2,* 50–55.

Courtenay, B. C., Poon, L. W., Martin, P., Clayton, G. M., & Johnson, M. A. (1992). Religiosity and adaptation in the oldest-old. *International Journal of Aging and Human Development, 34,* 47–56.

Covalt, N. K. (1960). The meaning of religion to older people. *Geriatrics, 15,* 658–664.

Cox, T. (1980). *Stress.* Baltimore: University Park Press.

Cronbach, L. J. (1975). Beyond the two disciplines of scientific psychology. *American Psychologist, 30,* 116–127.

Croog, S. H., & Levine, S. (1972). Religious identity and response to serious illness: A report on heart patients. *Social Science and Medicine, 6,* 17–32.

Crumm, D. (1991, October 16). Believers rebuild lives, change cities, inspire hope. *Detroit Free Press,* pp. 1a, 8a, 9a.

Cushman, P. (1990). Why the self is empty: Toward a historically situated psychology. *American Psychologist, 45,* 599–611.

Dabrowski, K. (1964). *Positive disintegration.* Boston: Little, Brown.

Daie, N., Witztum, E., Mark, M., & Rabinowitz, S. (1992). The belief in the transmigration of souls: Psychotherapy of a Druze patient with severe anxiety reaction. *British Journal of Medical Psychology, 65,* 119–130.

Dalal, A. K., & Pande, N. (1988). Psychological recovery of accident victims with temporary and permanent disability. *International Journal of Psychology, 23,* 25–40.

Damphouse, K. R., & Crouch, B. M. (1992). Did the devil make them do it? An examination of the etiology of Satanism among juvenile delinquents. *Youth and Society, 24,* 204–227.

D'Antonio, W. V., Newman, W. M., & Wright, S. A. (1982). Religion and family life: How social scientists view the relationships. *Journal for the Scientific Study of Religion, 21,* 218–225.

Darby, B. W., & Schlenker, B. R. (1982). Children's reactions to apologies. *Journal of Personality and Social Psychology, 43,* 742–753.

David, J. P., Ladd, K., & Spilka, B. (1992). *The multidimensionality of prayer and its role as a source of secondary control.* Paper presented at the meeting of the American Psychological Association, Washington, DC.

DeLongis, A., Coyne, J. C., Dakof, G., Folkman, S., & Lazarus, R. S. (1982). Relationship of daily hassles, uplifts, and major life events to health status. *Health Psychology, 1,* 119–136.

Religious scams total $450 million. (1989, August 8). *Detroit Free Press,* 1A, 11A.

Deutsch, A. (1975). Observations on a sidewalk Ashram. *Archives of General Psychiatry, 32,* 166–175.

DeVellis, B. E., DeVellis, R. F., & Spilsbury, J. C. (1988). Parental actions when children are sick: The role of belief in divine influence. *Basic and Applied Social Psychology, 9,* 185–196.

Diamond, E. L. (1982). The role of anger in essential hypertension and coronary heart disease. *Psychological Bulletin, 92,* 410–433.

DiBlasio, F. A., & Benda, B. B. (1991). Practitioners, religion and the use of forgiveness in the clinical setting. *Journal of Psychology and Christianity, 10,* 166–172.

Dienstbier, R. A. (1989). Arousal and physiological toughness: Implications for mental and physical health. *Psychological Bulletin, 96,* 84–100.

Dittes, J. E. (1969). Psychology and religion. In G. Lindzey & E. Aronson (Eds.), *The handbook of social psychology* (2nd ed., Vol. 5, pp. 602–659). Reading, MA: Addison-Wesley.

Domino, G. (1990). Clergy's knowledge of psychopathology. *Journal of Psychology and Theology, 18,* 32–39.

Donahue, M. J. (1985). Intrinsic and extrinsic religiousness: Review and meta-analysis. *Journal of Personality and Social Psychology, 48,* 400–419.

Dooley, D., & Catalano, R. (1980). Economic change as a cause of behavioral disorder. *Psychological Bulletin, 87,* 450–468.

Dor-Shav, N. K., Friedman, B., & Tcherbonogura, R. (1978). Identification, prejudice, and aggression. *Journal of Social Psychology, 104,* 217–222.

Dubow, E. F., & Tisak, J. (1989). The relation between stressful life events and adjustment in elementary school children: The role of social support and social problem-solving skills. *Child Development, 60,* 1412–1423.

Dufton, B. D., & Perlman, D. (1986). Loneliness and religiosity: In the world but not of it. *Journal of Psychology and Theology, 14,* 135–145.

Dunkel-Schetter, C., Feinstein, L. G., Taylor, S. E., & Falker, R. L. (1992). Patterns of coping with cancer. *Health Psychology, 11,* 79–87.

Durkheim, E. (1915). *The elementary forms of the religious life.* New York: Free Press.

Durkheim, E. (1951). *Suicide: A study in sociology* (J. A. Spaulding & G. Simpson, Trans.). New York: Free Press.

Ebaugh, H. R. F. (1988). Leaving Catholic convents: Toward a theory of disengagement. In D. G. Bromley (Ed.), *Falling from the faith: Causes and consequences of religious apostasy* (pp. 100–121). Sage: Newbury Park.

Ebaugh, H. R. F., Richman, K., & Chafetz, J. S. (1984). Life crises among the religiously committed: Do sectarian differences matter? *Journal for the Scientific Study of Religion, 23,* 19–31.

Echemendia, R. J., & Pargament, K. I. (1982). *The psychosocial functions of religion: An elaboration of the I–E dichotomy.* Paper presented at the meeting of the American Psychological Association, Washington, DC.

Eisenbruch, M. (1991). From post-traumatic stress disorder to cultural bereavement: Diagnosis of southeast Asian refugees. *Social Science and Medicine, 33,* 673–680.

Elder, G. H., Jr., & Clipp, E. C. (1989). Combat experience and emotional health: Impairment and resilience in later life. *Journal of Personality, 57,* 312–341.

Elkins, D., Anchor, K. N., & Sandler, H. M. (1979). Relaxation training and prayer behavior as tension reduction techniques. *Behavioral Engineering, 5,* 81–87.

Elkins, D. N. (1995). Psychotherapy and spirituality: Toward a theory of the soul. *Journal of Humanistic Psychology, 35,* 78–98.

Ellis, A. (1986). *The case against religion: A psychotherapist's view and the case against religiosity.* Austin: American Atheist Press.

Ellison, C. G. (1991). Religious involvement and subjective well-being. *Journal of Health and Social Behavior, 32,* 80–89.

Ellison, C. G. (1993). Religious involvement and self-perception among Black Americans. *Social Forces, 71,* 1027–1055.

Ellison, C. G., Bartkowski, J., & Segal, M. (1996). Conservative Protestantism and the parental use of corporal punishment. *Social Forces, 74,* 1003–1028.

Ellison, C. G., & Gay, D. A. (1990). Region, religious commitment, and life satisfaction among black Americans. *Sociological Quarterly, 31,* 123–147.

Ellison, C. G., Gay, D. A., & Glass, T. A. (1989). Does religious commitment contribute to individual life satisfaction? *Social Forces, 68,* 100–123.

Ellison, C. G., & George, L. E. (1994). Religious involvement, social ties, and social support in a Southeastern community. *Journal for the Scientific Study of Religion, 33,* 46–61.

Ellison, C. G., & Sherkat, D. E. (1993). Conservative protestantism and support for corporal punishment. *American Sociological Review, 58,* 138–144.

Ellison, C. G., & Taylor, R. J. (1996). Turning to prayer: Social and situational antecedents of religious coping among African Americans. *Review of Religious Research, 38,* 111–131.

Emblen, J. D. (1992). Religion and spirituality defined according to current use in nursing literature. *Journal of Professional Nursing, 8,* 41–47.

Emrick, C. D. (1987). Alcoholics Anonymous: Affiliation processes and effectiveness as treatment. *Alcoholism: Clinical and Experimental Research, 11,* 416–423.

Eng, E., & Hatch, J. W. (1992). Networking between agencies and black churches: The lay health advisor model. In K. I. Pargament, K. I. Maton, & R. G. Hess (Eds.), *Religion and prevention in mental health: Research, vision, and action* (pp. 293–316). New York: Haworth Press.

Engel, G. L. (1971). Sudden and rapid death during psychological stress: Folklore or folk wisdom? *Annals of Internal Medicine, 74,* 771–782.

Enright, R. D., Eastin, D. L, Golden, S., Serinopoulus, J., & Freedman, S. (1992). Interpersonal forgiveness within the helping professions: An attempt to resolve differences of opinions. *Counseling and Values, 36,* 84–103.

Ensing, D. S. (1991). *The role of religion as a stress buffer: Cross-sectional and longitudinal studies.* Unpublished doctoral dissertation, Bowling Green State University, Bowling Green, OH.

Erikson, E. H. (1980). *Identity and the life cycle.* New York: Norton.

Erin, J. N., Rudin, D., & Njoroge, M. (1991). Religious beliefs of parents of children with visual impairments. *Journal of Visual Impairment and Blindness, 85,* 157–162.

Evans, D. A., & Tyler, F. B. (1976). Is work competence enhancing for the poor? *American Journal of Community Psychology, 4,* 25–33.

Father views starving death of his son a biblical sacrifice. (1989, August 29). *Bowling Green Sentinel-Tribune,* p. 1.

Faust, C. H., & Johnson, T. H. (1935). *Jonathan Edwards: Representative selections, with introduction, bibliography, and notes.* New York: American Book Company.

Fawzy, F. L., Fawzy, N. W., Hyun, C., Elashoff, R., Guthrie, D., Fahey, J. L., & Morton, D. L. (1993). Malignant melanoma: Effects of an earlier structured psychiatric intervention, coping, and affective state on recurrence and survival six years later. *Archives of General Psychiatry, 50,* 681–689.

Fazel, M. K. (1987). *Martyrdom as a means of identity; Iran–Iraq conflict: Roots of a holy war.* Paper presented at the meeting of the Society for the Scientific Study of Religion, Louisville, KY.

Felker, K. (1990). *Gift or gaffe: Perceptions of mothers of children with handicaps to quasi-theological explanations.* Paper presented at the meeting of the American Psychological Association, Washington, DC.

Ferraro, K. F., & Koch, J. R. (1994). Religion and health among black and white adults: Examining social support and consolation. *Journal for the Scientific Study of Religion, 33,* 362–375.

Festinger, L., Riecken, H. W., & Schachter, S. (1956). *When prophecy fails.* New York: Harper & Row.

Fichter, J. H. (1981). *Religion and pain: The spiritual dimensions of health care.* New York: Crossroad.

Fishbein, M., & Ajzen, J. (1975). *Belief, attitude, intention and behavior: An introduction to theory and research.* Reading, MA: Addison-Wesley.

Fitchett, G. (1993a). *Assessing spiritual needs.* Minneapolis: Augsburg Press.

Fitchett, G. (1993b). *Spiritual assessment in pastoral care: A guide to selected resources* (JPCP Monograph, 4). Decatur, GA: Journal of Pastoral Care Publications.

Folkman, S. (1992). Making the case for coping. In B. N. Carpenter (Ed.), *Personal coping: Theory, research, and application* (pp. 31–46). Westport, CT: Praeger.

Folkman, S., Chesney, M. A., Cooke, M., Boccellari, A., & Collette, L. (1994). Caregiver burden in HIV-positive and HIV-negative partners of men with AIDS. *Journal of Consulting and Clinical Psychology, 62,* 746–756.

Folkman, S., Chesney, M. A., Pollack, L., & Coates, T. (1993). Stress, control, coping, and depressive mood in human immunodeficiency virus-positive and -negative gay men in San Francisco. *Journal of Nervous and Mental Disease, 181,* 409–416.

Folkman, S., Chesney, M. A., Pollack, L., & Phillips, C. (1992). Stress, coping, and high-risk sexual behavior. *Health Psychology, 11,* 218–222.

Folkman, S., Lazarus, R. S., Dunkel-Schetter, C., DeLongis, A., & Gruen, R. J. (1986). Dynamics of a stressful encounter: Cognitive appraisals, coping, and encounter outcomes. *Journal of Personality and Social Psychology, 50,* 992–1003.

Fortune, M. M. (1987). *Keeping the faith: Questions and answers for the abused woman.* San Francisco: Harper & Row.

Foster, R. A., & Keating, J. P. (1992). Measuring androcentrism in the Western God concept. *Journal for the Scientific Study of Religion, 31,* 366–375.

Fowers, B. J. (1992). The Cardiac Denial of Impact Scale: A brief self-report research measure. *Journal of Psychosomatic Research, 36,* 469–475.

Fowler, J. W. (1987). *Faith development and pastoral care.* Philadelphia: Fortress Press.

Frankl, V. E. (1984). *Man's search for meaning.* New York: Washington Square Press.

Frankl, V. E. (1986). *The doctor and the soul: From psychotherapy to logotherapy.* New York: Vintage Books.

Frankl, V. E. (1988). *The will to meaning: Foundations and applications of logotherapy.* New York: New American Library.

Franks, K., Templer, D. I., Cappelletty, G. G., & Kauffman, J. (1990–1991). Exploration of death anxiety as a function of religious variables in gay men with and without AIDS. *Omega, 22,* 43–50.

Frazier, P. A., Krasnoff, A. M., & Port, C. L. (1995). *The role of religion in coping with chronic medical conditions.* Paper presented at the meeting of the American Psychological Association, New York, NY.

Freedman, S. R., & Enright, R. D. (1996). Forgiveness as an intervention goal with incest survivors. *Journal of Consulting and Clinical Psychology, 64,* 983–992.

Freedy, J. R., Shaw, D. L., Jarrell, M. P., & Masters, C. R. (1992). Towards an understanding of the psychological impact of natural disasters: An application of the conservation resources stress model. *Journal of Traumatic Stress, 5,* 441–454.

Freud, A. (1966). *The ego and the mechanisms of defense* (Rev. ed.). New York: International Universities Press.

Freud, S. (1923/1961). The ego and the id. In J. Strachey (Ed. and Trans.), *The standard edition of the complete psychological works of Sigmund Freud* (Vol. 19, pp. 12–66). London: Hogarth Press.

Freud, S. (1927/1961). *The future of an illusion.* New York: Norton.

Freud, S. (1928/1961). A religious experience. In J. Strachey (Ed. and Trans.), *The standard edition of the complete psychological works of Sigmund Freud* (Vol. 21, pp. 169–172). London: Hogarth Press.

Freud, S. (1930/1961). *Civilization and its discontents.* New York: Norton.

Friedel, L. A., & Pargament, K. I. (1995). *Coping with controllable and uncontrollable negative events in the work environment.* Paper presented at the meeting of the American Psychological Association, New York, NY.

Friedlander, A. H. (1986). Judaism and the concept of forgiving. *Christian Jewish Relations, 19,* 6–13.

Friedman, E. H. (1985). *Generation to generation: Family process in church and synagogue.* New York: Guilford Press.

Friedman, S. B., Chodoff, P., Mason, J. W., & Hamburg, D. A. (1963). Behavioral observations on parents anticipating the death of a child. *Pediatrics, 32,* 610–625.

Friedrich, W. N., Cohen, D. S., & Wilturner, L. T. (1988). Specific beliefs as moderator variables in maternal coping with mental retardation. *Children's Health Care, 17,* 40–44.

Frijda, N. H. (1988). The laws of emotion. *American Psychologist, 43,* 349–358.

Fromm, E. (1950). *Psychoanalysis and religion.* New Haven: Yale University Press.

Fry, P. S. (1990). A factor analytic investigation of home bound elderly individuals' concerns about death and dying, and their coping responses. *Journal of Clinical Psychology, 46,* 737–748.

Fussell, P. (1994, May 23). How the leaders led. *Newsweek*, pp. 36–38.

Gaer, J. (1958). *The wisdom of the living religions.* London: Skeffington.

Galanter, M. (1980). Psychological induction into the larger group: Findings from a modern religious sect. *American Journal of Psychiatry, 137,* 1574–1579.

Galanter, M. (1982). Charismatic religious sects and psychiatry: An overview. *American Journal of Psychiatry, 139,* 1539–1548.

Galanter, M. (1989). *Cults: Faith healing and coercion.* New York: Oxford University Press.

Galanter, M., Rabkin, R., Rabkin, J., & Deutsch, A. (1979). The "Moonies": A psychological study of conversion and membership in a contemporary religious sect. *American Journal of Psychiatry, 136,* 165–170.

Galileo, G. (1988). Letter to Grand Duchess Christina, 1614. In J. Rohr (Ed.), *Science and religion: Opposing viewpoints* (pp. 17–22). St. Paul: Greenhaven Press.

Gallup, G., Jr., & Castelli, J. (1989). *The people's religion: American faith in the 90's.* New York: Macmillan.

Gard, R. A. (Ed.). (1962). *Buddhism.* New York: Braziller.

Garmezy, N. (1975). The experimental study of children vulnerable to psychopathology. In A. Davis (Ed.), *Child personality and psychopathology: Current topics, Vol. 2* (pp. 171–217). New York: Wiley-Interscience.

Gartrell, C. D., & Shannon, Z. K. (1985). Contacts, cognitions and conversion: A rational choice approach. *Review of Religious Research, 27,* 32–48.

Gass, K. A. (1987). The health of conjugally bereaved older widows: The role of appraisal, coping and resources. *Research in Nursing and Health, 10,* 39–47.

Gates of Prayer: The New Union Prayerbook. (1975). New York: Central Conference of American Rabbis.

Geertz, C. (1966). Religion as a cultural system. In M. Banton (Ed.), *Anthropological approaches to the study of religion* (pp. 1–46). London: Tavistock.

Genia, V. (1990). Interreligious encounter group: A psychospiritual experience for faith development. *Counseling and Values, 35,* 39–51.

Gibbs, H. W., & Achterberg-Lawlis, J. (1978). Spiritual values and death anxiety: Implications for counseling with terminal cancer patients. *Journal of Counseling Psychology, 25,* 563–569.

Gilbert, K. R. (1989). *Religion as a resource for bereaved parents as they cope with the death of their child.* Paper presented at the meeting of the National Council on Family Relations, New Orleans, LA.

Giving and volunteering in the United States. (1988). Washington, DC: Independent Sector.

Glass, D. (1977). Stress, behavior patterns and coronary disease. *American Scientist, 65,* 177–187.

Glick, I. O., Weiss, R. S., & Parkes, C. M. (1974). *The first year of bereavement.* New York: Wiley.

Glock, C. Y., Ringer, B. B., & Babbie, E. R. (1967). *To comfort and to challenge: A dilemma of the contemporary church.* Berkeley: University of California Press.

Glock, C. Y., & Stark, R. (1966). *Christian beliefs and anti-Semitism.* New York: Harper & Row.

Goertzel, V., & Goertzel, M. G. (1962). *Cradles of eminence.* Boston: Little, Brown.

Goldin, J. (Trans.). (1957). *The living Talmud: The wisdom of the fathers and its classical commentaries.* New York: Mentor Books.

Goodman, M., Rubinstein, R. L., Alexander, B. B., & Luborsky, M. (1991). Cultural differences among elderly women in coping with the death of an adult child. *Journal of Gerontology: Social Sciences, 6,* S321–329.

Goodstein, L. (1993, June 10). Put kindness back into public policy, coalitions urge. *Washington Post,* p. A19.

Gordon, D. F. (1974). The Jesus people: An identity synthesis. *Urban Life and Culture, 3,* 159–178.

Gorer, G. (1965). *Death, grief and mourning.* New York: Doubleday.

Gorlow, L., & Schroeder, H. E. (1968). Motives for participating in the religious experience. *Journal for the Scientific Study of Religion, 7,* 241–251.

Gorsuch, R. L. (1968). The conceptualization of God as seen in adjective ratings. *Journal for the Scientific Study of Religion, 7,* 56–64.

Gorsuch, R. L. (1984). Measurement: The boon and bane of investigating religion. *American Psychologist, 39,* 228–236.

Gorsuch, R. L., & Hao, J. Y. (1993). Forgiveness: An exploratory factor analysis and its relationship to religious variables. *Review of Religious Research, 34,* 333–347.

Gorsuch, R. L., & Smith, C. S. (1983). Attributions of responsibility to God: An interaction of religious beliefs and outcomes. *Journal for the Scientific Study of Religion, 22,* 340–352.

Grasmick, H. G., Bursik, R. J., Jr., & Kimpel, M. (1991). Protestant fundamentalism and attitudes toward corporal punishment of children. *Violence and Victims, 6,* 283–298.

Gray, R. E. (1987). Adolescent response to the death of a parent. *Journal of Youth and Adolescence, 16,* 511–525.

Greeley, A. M. (1972). *The denominational society: A sociological approach to religion in America.* Glenview, IL: Scott, Foresman.

Greil, A. L., Porter, K. L., Leitko, T. A., & Riscilli, C. (1989). Why me? Theodicies of infertile women and men. *Sociology of Health and Illness, 11,* 213–229.

Greven, P. (1991). *Spare the child: The religious roots of punishment and the psychological impact of physical abuse.* New York: Knopf.

Grevengoed, N. (1985). *Attributions for death: An examination of the role of religion and the relationship between attributions and mental health.* Unpublished master's thesis, Bowling Green State University, Bowling Green, OH.

Griffin, G. M., & Tobin, D. (1982). *In the midst of life: The Australian response to death.* Carlton, Victoria: Melbourne University Press.

Griffith, E. E. H., Mahy, G. E., & Young, J. L. (1986). Psychological benefits of spiritual Baptist "Mourning,": II. An empirical assessment. *American Journal of Psychiatry, 143,* 226–229.

Griffith, J. L. (1986). Employing the God–family relationship therapy with religious families. *Family Process, 25,* 609–618.

Grinker, R. R., Sr., with the collaboration of Grinker, R. R., Jr., & Timberlake, J. (1962). "Mentally healthy" young males (homoclites). *Archives of General Psychology, 6,* 405–453.

Grinker, R. R., & Spiegel, J. P. (1945). *Men under stress.* Philadelphia: Blakiston.

Grzymala-Moszczynska, H., & Beit-Hallahmi, B. (Eds.). (1996). *Religion, psychopathology, and coping.* Amsterdam, Holland: Rodopi.

Guba, E. G., & Lincoln, Y. S. (1989). *Fourth generation evaluation.* Newbury Park, CA: Sage.

Guidelines for Providers of Psychological Services to Ethnic, Linguistic, and Culturally Diverse Populations. (1993). *American Psychologist, 48,* 45–48.

Gula, R. M. (1984). *To walk together again: The sacrament of reconciliation.* New York: Paulist Press.

Gurin, G., Veroff, J., & Feld, S. (1960). *Americans view their mental health: A nationwide interview survey.* New York: Basic Books.

Haan, N. (1977). *Coping and defending: Processes of self-environment organization.* New York: Academic Press.

Hammann, L. J. (1987). *Exploring the religious labyrinth.* Lanham, MD: University Press of America.

Hannay, D. R. (1980). Religion and health. *Social Science and Medicine, 14A,* 683–685.

Hansen, G. (1992). Religion and marital adjustment. In J. F. Schumaker (Ed.), *Religion and mental health* (pp. 189–198). New York: Oxford University Press.

Harris, N. A., & Spilka, B. (1990). *The sense of control and coping with alcoholism: A multidimensional approach.* Paper presented at the meeting of the Rocky Mountain Psychological Association, Tucson, AZ.

Harris, R. C., Dew, M. A., Lee, A., Amaya, L., Buches, L., Reetz, D., & Coleman, G. (1993). *The role of religion in heart-transplant recipients' health and well-being: Implications for social work professionals.* Unpublished manuscript. University of Pittsburgh, Pittsburgh, PA.

Harris, R. C., Dew, M. A., Lee, A., Amaya, M., Buches, L., Reetz, D., & Coleman, G. (1995). The role of religion in heart-transplant recipients' long-term health and well-being. *Journal of Religion and Health, 34,* 17–32.

Harvey, C. D. H., Barnes, G. E., & Greenwood, L. (1987). Correlates of morale among Canadian widowed persons. *Social Psychiatry, 22,* 65–72.

Hathaway, W. L. (1992). *Religion and the daily coping process: A longitudinal idiographic analysis.* Unpublished doctoral dissertation, Bowling Green State University, Bowling Green, OH.

Hathaway, W. L., & Pargament, K. I. (1990). Intrinsic religiousness, religious coping, and psychosocial competence: A covariance structure analysis. *Journal for the Scientific Study of Religion, 29,* 423–441.

Haugk, K. (1985). *Christian caregiving—a way of life.* Minneapolis: Augsburg Publishing.

Havens, J. (1977). The participant's versus the observer's frame of reference in the psychological study of religion. In H. W. Malony (Ed.), *Current perspectives in the psychology of religion* (pp. 101–115). Grand Rapids, MI: William B. Eerdmans.

Hayden, J., & Przybysz, T. M. (1995). *Adjustment to impending death in incurable metastatic cancer patients.* Paper presented at the meeting of the American Psychological Association, New York, NY.

Hebl, J. H., & Enright, R. D. (1993). Forgiveness as a psychotherapeutic goal with elderly females. *Psychotherapy, 30,* 658–667.

Heiler, F. (1932). *Prayer: A study in the history and psychology of religion.* London: Oxford University Press.

Heirich, M. (1977). Change of heart: A test of some widely held theories about religious conversion. *American Journal of Sociology, 83,* 683–680.

Henderson, C. P., Jr. (1988). Science cannot replace religion. In J. Rohr (Ed.), *Science and religion: Opposing viewpoints* (pp. 72–77). St. Paul, MN: Greenhaven Press.

Here I was sitting at the edge of eternity. (1989). *Life, 12*(10), 28–33, 38, 39.

Heschel, A. J. (1986). *The wisdom of Heschel.* New York: Farrar, Strauss & Giroux.

Hill, P. C. (1994). Toward an attitude process model of religious experience. *Journal for the Scientific Study of Religion, 33,* 303–314.

Hill, P. C., & Butter, E. M. (1995). The role of religion in promoting physical health. *Journal of Psychiatry and Christianity, 14,* 141–155.

Hinkle, L. E. (1974). The concept of "stress" in the biological and social sciences. *International Journal of Psychiatry in Medicine, 5,* 335–357.

Hobart, M. (1985). Is God evil? In D. Parkin (Ed.), *The anthropology of evil* (pp. 165–193). Oxford: Basil Blackwell.

Hobfoll, S. E. (1988). *The ecology of stress.* New York: Hemisphere.

Höffding, H. (1914). *The philosophy of religion.* London: Macmillan.

Hohmann, A. A., & Larson, D. B. (1993). Psychiatric factors predicting use of clergy. In E. L. Worthington Jr. (Ed.), *Psychotherapy and religious values* (pp. 71–84). Grand Rapids, MI: Baker Book House.

Holmes, T. H. (1979). Development and application of a quantitative measure of life change magnitude. In J. E. Barrett, R. M. Rose, & G. L. Klerman (Eds.), *Stress and mental disorder* (pp. 37–54). New York: Raven Press.

Holmes, T. H., & Rahe, R. H. (1967). The social readjustment rating scale. *Journal of Psychosomatic Research, 11,* 213–218.

Hood, R. W., Jr. (1977). Eliciting mystical states of consciousness with semistructured nature experiences. *Journal for the Scientific Study of Religion, 16,* 155–164.

Hood, R. W., Jr. (1978). Anticipatory set and setting: Stress incongruities as elicitors of mystical experience in solitary nature situations. *Journal for the Scientific Study of Religion, 17,* 279–287.

Hood, R. W., Jr., Spilka, B., Hunsberger, B., & Gorsuch, R. (1996). *The psychology of religion: An empirical approach* (2nd ed.). New York: Guilford Press.

Hope, D. (1987). The healing paradox of forgiveness. *Psychotherapy, 24,* 240–244.

Horton, A. L., Wilkins, M. M., & Wright, W. (1988). Women who ended abuse: What religious leaders and religion did for these victims. In A. L. Horton & J. A. Williamson (Eds.), *Abuse and religion: When praying isn't enough* (pp. 235–246). Lexington, MA: Lexington Books.

Hughes, K., with Rita Milios (1990). *God isn't finished with me yet.* Nashville, TN: Winston-Derek.

Hughes, M., McCollum, J., Sheftel, D., & Sanchez, G. (1994). How parents cope with the experience of neonatal intensive care. *Children's Health Care, 23,* 1–14.

Hughes, R. A. (1990). Psychological perspectives on infanticide in a faith healing sect. *Psychotherapy, 27,* 107–115.

Hunsberger, B. (1996). Religious fundamentalism, right-wing authoritarianism, and hostility toward homosexuals in non-Christian religious groups. *International Journal for the Psychology of Religion, 6,* 39–49.

Hunsberger, B., & Brown, L. B. (1984). Religious socialization, apostasy, and the impact of family background. *Journal for the Scientific Study of Religion, 23,* 239–251.

Hunt, R. A., & King, M. (1971). The intrinsic–extrinsic concept: A review and evaluation. *Journal for the Scientific Study of Religion, 10,* 339–356.

Hunter, E. J., McCubbin, H. I., & Metres, P. J., Jr. (1974). Religion and the POW/MIA wife. In H. I. McCubbin, B. B. Dahl, P. J. Metres Jr., E. J. Hunter, & J. A. Plag (Eds.), *Family separation and reunion: Families of prisoners of war and servicemen missing in action* (pp. 85–93). Washington, DC: U.S. Government Printing Office.

Iannaccone, L. R. (1994). Why strict churches are strong. *American Journal of Sociology, 99,* 1180–1211.

Ide, B. A., & Sanli, T. (1992). Health beliefs and behaviors of Saudi women. *Women and Health, 19,* 97–113.

Idler, E. L. (1987). Religious involvement and the health of the elderly: Some hypotheses and an initial test. *Social Forces, 66,* 226–238.

Idler, E. L., & Kasl, S. V. (1992). Religion, disability, depression, and the timing of death. *American Journal of Sociology, 97,* 1052–1079.

Imber-Black, E., & Roberts, J. (1993). *Rituals for our times: Celebrating, healing, and changing our lives, and our relationships.* New York: Harper Perennial.

Jackson, L. E., & Coursey, R. D. (1988). The relationship of God control and internal locus of control to intrinsic religious motivation, coping and purpose in life. *Journal for the Scientific Study of Religion, 27,* 399–410.

Jacobs, P. L. (1984). The older visually impaired person: A vital link in the family and the community. *Journal of Visual Impairment and Blindness, 78,* 154–162.

Jacquet, C. H., Jr. (1986). *Yearbook of American and Canadian churches, 1986.* Nashville: Abingdon Press.

Jacquet C. H., Jr. (Ed.). (1989). *Yearbook of American and Canadian churches, 1989*. Nashville: Abingdon Press.

Jacquet, C. H., Jr., & Jones, A. M. (Eds.). (1991). *Yearbook of American and Canadian churches, 1991*. Nashville, TN: Abingdon Press.

Jaffe, H., Rudin, J., & Rudin, M. (1986). *Why me? Why anyone?* New York: St. Martin's Press.

Jahoda, M. (1958). *Current concepts of positive mental health*. New York: Basic Books.

Jalowiec, A., & Powers, M. J. (1981). Stress and coping in hypertensive and emergency room patients. *Nursing Research, 30,* 10–15.

Jamal, M., & Badawi, J. (1993). Job stress among Muslim immigrants in North America: Moderating effects of religiosity. *Stress Medicine, 9,* 145–151.

James, W. (1902). *The varieties of religious experience: A study in human nature*. New York: Modern Library.

James, W. (1907/1975). *Pragmatism*. Cambridge: Harvard University Press.

Janoff-Bulman, R. (1989). Assumptive worlds and the stress of traumatic events: Applications of the schema construct. *Social Cognition, 7,* 113–136.

Jenkins, R. A. (1992). Toward a psychosocial conceptualization of religion as a resource in cancer care and prevention. In K. I. Pargament, K. I. Maton, & R. E. Hess (Eds.), *Religion and prevention in mental health: Research vision, and action* (pp. 179–194). New York: Haworth Press.

Jenkins, R. A. (1995). Religion and HIV: Implications for research and intervention. *Journal of Social Issues, 51,* 131–144.

Jenkins, R. A., & Pargament, K. I. (1988). Cognitive appraisals in cancer patients. *Social Science and Medicine, 26,* 625–633.

Johnson, D. P., & Mullins, L. C. (1989). Religiosity and loneliness among the elderly. *Journal of Applied Gerontology, 8,* 110–131.

Johnson, P. E. (1959). *Psychology of religion*. Nashville: Abingdon Press.

Johnson, S. C., & Spilka, B. (1991). Coping with breast cancer: The roles of clergy and faith. *Journal of Religion and Health, 30,* 21–33.

Johnson, S. D. (1984). Religion as a defense in a mock jury trial. *Journal of Social Psychology, 125,* 213–220.

Johnson, W. B., DeVries, R., Ridley, C. R., Pettorini, D., & Peterson, D. R. (1994). The comparative efficacy of Christian and secular rational-emotive therapy with Christian clients. *Journal of Psychology and Theology, 22,* 130–140.

Johnson, W. B., & Ridley, C. R. (1992). Brief Christian and non-Christian rational-emotive therapy with depressed Christian clients: An exploratory study. *Counseling and Values, 36,* 220–229.

Jones, J. (1991, September 1). Why are black women scaring off their men? *Washington Post*, Sunday, p. C4.

Jones, S. L., Watson, E. J., & Wolfram, T. J. (1992). Results of the Rech Conference Survey on religious faith and professional psychology. *Journal of Psychology and Theology, 20,* 147–158.

Jones, S. L., & Wilcox, D. A. (1993). Religious values in secular theories of psychotherapy. In E. L. Worthington, Jr. (Ed.), *Psychotherapy and religious values* (pp. 37–61). Grand Rapids, MI: Baker Book House.

Joyce, C. R. B., & Welldon, R. M. C. (1965). The objective efficacy of prayer: A double-blind clinical trial. *Journal of Chronic Disease, 18,* 367–377.

Kahn, R. L., & Antonucci, T. C. (1980). Convoys over the life course: Attachment, roles, and social support. In P. B. Baltes & O. G. Brim (Eds.), *Life span development and behavior* (pp. 253–286). New York: Academic Press.

Kahoe, R. D. (1974). Personality and achievement correlates of intrinsic and extrinsic religious orientations. *Journal of Personality and Social Psychology, 29,* 812–818.

Kaiser, D. (1991). Religious problem-solving styles and guilt. *Journal for the Scientific Study of Religion, 30,* 94–98.

Kaplan, A. (1964). *The conduct of inquiry.* San Francisco: Chandler.

Kaseman, C. M., & Anderson, R. G. (1977). Clergy consultation as a community mental health program. *Community Mental Health Journal, 13,* 84–91.

Kass, J. D., Friedman, R., Leserman, J., Zuttermeister, P. C., & Benson, H. (1991). Health outcomes and a new index of spiritual experience. *Journal for the Scientific Study of Religion, 30,* 203–211.

Keating, A. M., & Fretz, B. R. (1990). Christian anticipations about counselors in response to counselor descriptions. *Journal of Counseling Psychology, 36,* 292–296.

Kelly, E. W., Jr. (1994). The role of religion and spirituality in counselor education: A national survey. *Counselor Education and Supervision, 33,* 227–237.

Kelly, T. A. (1990). The role of values in psychotherapy: A critical review of process and outcome effects. *Clinical Psychology Review, 10,* 171–186.

Kennell, J. E. (1988). *The community church: A study of an inner city church community.* Paper presented at the meeting of the American Psychological Association, Atlanta, GA.

Kesselring, A., Dodd, M. J., Lindsey, A. M., & Strauss, A. L. (1986). Attitudes of patients living in Switzerland about cancer and its treatment. *Cancer Nursing, 9,* 77–85.

Kiecolt-Glaser, J. K., & Glaser, R. (1994). Caregivers, mental health, and immune function. In E. Light, G. Niederehe, & B. D. Lebowitz (Eds.), *Stress effects on family caregivers of Alzheimer's patients: Research and intervention* (pp. 64–75). New York: Springer.

Kinens, J. J. (1989). What is lost shall be found. In J. T. Clemons (Ed.), *Sermons on suicide* (pp. 71–78). Louisville, KY: Westminster/John Knox Press.

King, M. B., & Hunt, R. A. (1969). Measuring the religious variable: Amended findings. *Journal for the Scientific Study of Religion, 8,* 321–323.

Kirkpatrick, L. A. (1989). A psychometric analysis of the Allport–Ross and Feagin measures of intrinsic–extrinsic religious orientation. In M. Lynn & D. Moberg (Eds.), *Research in the social scientific study of religion* (Vol. 1, pp. 1–30). Greenwich, CT: JAI Press.

Kirkpatrick, L. A. (1992). An attachment-theoretical approach to the psychology of religion. *International Journal for the Psychology of Religion, 2,* 3–28.

Kirkpatrick, L. A. (1993a). Fundamentalism, Christian orthodoxy, and intrinsic religious orientation as predictors of discriminatory attitudes. *Journal for the Scientific Study of Religion, 32,* 256–268.

Kirkpatrick, L. A. (1993b). *Loneliness and perceptions of support from God.* Paper presented at the meeting of the American Psychological Association, Toronto, Ontario.

Kirkpatrick, L. A., & Hood, R. W., Jr. (1990). Intrinsic–extrinsic religious orientation: Boon or bane. *Journal for the Scientific Study of Religion, 29,* 442–462.

Kirkpatrick, L. A., Hood, R. W., Jr., & Hartz, G. (1991). Fundamentalist religion conceptualized in terms of Rokeach's theory of the open and closed mind: New perspectives on some old ideas. *Research in the Social Scientific Study of Religion, 3,* 157–179.

Kirkpatrick, L. A., & Shaver, P. R. (1990). Attachment theory and religion: Childhood attachments, religious beliefs and conversions. *Journal for the Scientific Study of Religion, 29,* 315–334.

Kirkpatrick, L. A., & Shaver, P. R. (1992). An attachment-theoretical approach to romantic love and religious belief. *Personality and Social Psychology Bulletin, 18,* 266–275.

Klass, D. (1988). *Parental grief: Solace and resolution.* New York: Springer.

Klinger, E. (1977). *Meaning and void: Inner experience and the incentives in people's lives.* Minneapolis: University of Minnesota Press.

Kloos, B., Horneffer, K., & Moore, T. (1995). Before the beginning: Religious leaders' perceptions of the possibility for mutual beneficial collaboration with psychologists. *Journal of Community Psychology, 23,* 275–291.

Knox, D. H. (1985). *Spirituality: A tool in the assessment and treatment of black alcoholics and their families.* New York: Haworth Press.

Koenig, H. G. (1988). Religious behaviors and death anxiety in later life. *Hospice Journal, 4,* 3–24.

Koenig, H. G. (1994). *Aging and God: Spiritual pathways to mental health in midlife and later years.* New York: Haworth Press.

Koenig, H. G. (1995). Religion and older men in prison. *International Journal of Geriatric Psychiatry, 10,* 219–230.

Koenig, H. G., Cohen, J. J., Blazer, D. G., Kudler, H. S., Krishnan, K. R. R., & Sibert, T. E. (1995). Religious coping and cognitive symptoms of depression in elderly medical patients. *Psychosomatics, 36,* 369–375.

Koenig, H. G., Cohen, H. J., Blazer, F. H., Pieper, C., Meador, K. G., Shelp, F., Goli, V., & DiPasquale, B. (1992). Religious coping and depression among elderly, hospitalized medically ill men. *American Journal of Psychiatry, 149,* 1693–1700.

Koenig, H. G., George, L. K., & Siegler, I. C. (1988). The use of religion and other emotion-regulating coping strategies among older adults. *Gerontologist, 28,* 303–310.

Koenig, H. G., Kvale, J. N., & Ferrel, C. (1988). Religion and well-being in later life. *Gerontologist, 28,* 18–28.

Koenig, H. G., Siegler, I. C., & George, L. K. (1989). Religious and non-religious coping: Impact on adaptation in later life. *Journal of Religion and Aging, 5,* 73–94.

Koenig, H. G., Siegler, I. C., Meador, K., & George, L. K. (1990). Religious coping and personality in later life. *International Journal of Geriatric Psychiatry, 5,* 123–131.

Kohn, M. L. (1972). Class, family, and schizophrenia. *Social Forces, 50,* 295–302.

Koltko, M. E. (1990). How religious beliefs affect psychotherapy: The example of Mormonism. *Psychotherapy, 27,* 132–141.

Kooistra, W. (1990). *An empirical examination of religious doubt among Christian adolescents.* Unpublished doctoral dissertation, Bowling Green State University, Bowling Green, OH.

Koss, J. D. (1987). Expectations and outcomes for patients given mental health care or spiritist healing in Puerto Rico. *American Journal of Psychiatry, 144,* 56–61.

Kotarba, J. A. (1983). Perceptions of death, belief systems and the process of coping with chronic pain. *Social Science and Medicine, 17,* 681–689.

Kowalewski, D., & Leonard, R. (1985). Established banks and established churches: Study of stockholder resolutions. *Review of Religious Research, 27,* 63–76.

Kox, W., Meeus, W., & Hart, H. (1991). Religious conversion of adolescents: Testing the Lofland and Stark model of religious conversion. *Sociological Analysis, 52,* 227–240.

Krause, N. (1991). Stress, religiosity, and abstinence from alcohol. *Psychology and Aging, 6,* 134–144.

Krause, N., & Van Tran, T. (1989). Stress and religious involvement among older blacks. *Journal of Gerontology: Social Sciences, 44,* S4–S13.

Krauss, P., & Goldfischer, M. (1988). *Why me? Coping with grief, loss and change.* Toronto: Bantam Books.

Kremer, J. F., & Stephens, L. (1983). Attributions and arousal as mediators of mitigation's effect on retaliation. *Journal of Personality and Social Psychology, 45,* 335–343.

Kubacka-Jasiecka, D., Dorczak, R., & Opozzynska, M. (1990). *The role of religious values in functioning and mental health of people.* Paper presented at the International Conference on Religion and Mental Health, Jagiellonían University, Cracow, Warsaw.

Kunst, J. L., Tan, S., & Bjorck, J. P. (1994). *Whodunit? Causal attributions for traumatic outcomes.* Unpublished manuscript, Fuller Theological Seminary, Pasadena, CA.

Kushner, H. S. (1981). *When bad things happen to good people.* New York: Schocken Books.

Kushner, H. S. (1989). *Who needs God.* New York: Summit Books.

Lacey, J. J. (1967). Somatic response patterning and stress: Some revisions of activation theory. In M. H. Appley & R. Trumbull (Eds.), *Psychological stress* (pp. 14–42). New York: Appleton-Century Crofts.

LaGrand, L. E. (1985). College student loss and response. In E. S. Zinner (Ed.), *Coping with death on campus: New directions for student services* (Vol. 1, pp. 15–28). San Francisco: Jossey-Bass.

Larson, D. B., Pattison, E. M., Blazer, D. G., Omran, A. R., & Kaplan, B. H. (1986). Systematic analysis of research on religious variables in four major psychiatric journals, 1978–1982. *American Journal of Psychiatry, 143,* 329–334.

Lasker, J. N., Lohmann, J., & Toedter, L. (1989). *The role of religion in bereavement: The case of pregnancy loss.* Paper presented at the meeting of the Society for the Scientific Study of Religion, Salt Lake City, UT.

Latkin, C. A., Hagan, R. A., Littman, R. A., & Sundberg, N. D. (1987). Who lives in Utopia? A brief report on the Rajneeshpuram research project. *Sociological Analysis, 48,* 73–81.

Lazarus, R. S. (1968). Emotions and adaptation: Conceptual and empirical relations. In W. J. Arnold (Ed.), *Nebraska Symposium on Motivation* (pp. 175–266). Lincoln: University of Nebraska Press.

Lazarus, R. S. (1991). *Emotion and adaptation.* New York: Oxford University Press.

Lazarus, R. S., & Folkman, S. (1984). *Stress, appraisal, and coping.* New York: Springer.

Lefcourt, H. M. (1976). *Locus of control: Current trends in theory and research.* Hillsdale, NJ: Erlbaum.

Legere, T. (1984). A spirituality for today. *Studies in Formative Spirituality, 5,* 375–383.

Lehman, D. R., Wortman, C. B., & Williams, A. F. (1987). Long-term effects of losing a spouse or child in a motor vehicle crash. *Journal of Personality and Social Psychology, 52,* 218–231.

Leliaert, R. M. (1989). Spiritual side of "good grief": What happened to holy Saturday. *Death Studies, 13,* 103–117.

Lerner, M. (1994). *Jewish renewal: A path to healing and transformation.* New York: Grosset/Putnam.

Leuba, J. H. (1912). *A psychological study of religion: Its origin, function, and future.* New York: Macmillan.

Levin, J. S. (1984). The role of the black church in community medicine. *Journal of the National Medical Association, 76,* 477–483.

Levin, J. S. (1994). Religion and health: Is there an association, is it valid, and is it causal? *Social Science and Medicine, 38,* 1475–1482.

Levin, J. S., & Vanderpool, H. Y. (1989). Is religion therapeutically significant for hypertension? *Social Science and Medicine, 29,* 69–78.

Levin, T. M., & Zegans, L. S. (1974). Adolescent identity crisis and religious conversion: Implications for psychotherapy. *British Journal of Medical Psychology, 47,* 73–81.

Levine, S. V., & Salter, N. E. (1976). Youth and contemporary religious movements: Psychosocial findings. *Canadian Psychiatric Association Journal, 21*, 411–420.

Lewis, C. S. (1961). *A grief observed*. London: Faber & Faber.

Lewis, K. L., & Epperson, D. L. (1993). Values, pretherapy information and informed consent in Christian counseling. In E. L. Worthington Jr. (Ed.), *Psychotherapy and religious values* (pp. 85–103). Grand Rapids, MI: Baker Book House.

Leyser, Y. (1994). Stress and adaptation in orthodox Jewish families with a disabled child. *American Journal of Orthopsychiatry, 31*, 376–385.

Lilliston, L., Brown, B. M., & Schliebe, H. P. (1982). Perceptions of religious solutions to personal problems of women. *Journal of Clinical Psychology, 38*, 546–549.

Lilliston, L., & Klein, D. G. (1989). *A self-discrepancy reduction model of religious coping*. Paper presented at the meeting of the Society for the Scientific Study of Religion, Salt Lake City, UT.

Lilliston, L., & Klein, D. G. (1990). *A self-discrepancy reduction model of religious coping*. Paper presented at the meeting of the American Psychological Association, Boston, MA.

Lindemann, E. (1944). Symptomatology and management of acute grief. *American Journal of Psychiatry, 101*, 141–148.

Lindenthal, J. J., Myers, J. K., Pepper, M. P., & Stern, M. S. (1970). Mental status and religious behavior. *Journal for the Scientific Study of Religion, 9*, 143–149.

Linebaugh, D. E., & Devivo, P. (1981). The growing emphasis on training pastor-counselors in Protestant seminaries. *Journal of Psychology and Theology, 9*, 266–268.

Linville, P. W. (1987). Self-complexity as a cognitive buffer against stress-related illness and depression. *Journal of Personality and Social Psychology, 52*, 663–676.

Little, D., & Twiss, S. B. (1973). Basic terms in the study of religious ethics. In G. Outka & J. P. Reeder Jr. (Eds.), *Religion and morality: A collection of essays* (pp. 35–77). New York: Anchor Books.

Loewenthal, K. N., & Cornwall, N. (1993). Religiosity and perceived control of life events. *International Journal for the Psychology of Religion, 3*, 39–45.

London, P. (1970). The rescuers: Motivational hypotheses about Christians who saved Jews from the Nazis. In J. Macaulay & L. Berkowitz (Eds.), *Altruism and helping behavior: Social psychological studies of some antecedents and consequences* (pp. 241–250). New York: Academic Press.

Long, D. D., & Miller, B. J. (1991). Suicidal tendency and multiple sclerosis. *Health and Social Work, 16*, 104–109.

Long, J. B. (1975). The death that ends death in Hinduism and Buddhism. In E. Kübler-Ross (Ed.), *Death: The final stage of growth* (pp. 52–72). Englewood Cliffs, NJ: Prentice-Hall.

Lorch, B. R. (1987). Church youth alcohol and education programs. *Journal of Religion and Health, 26*, 106–114.

Loveland, G. G. (1968). The effects of bereavement on certain religious attitudes and behaviors. *Sociological Symposium, 1,* 17–27.

Lovinger, R. J. (1984). *Working with religious issues in psychotherapy.* New York: Aronson.

Maddi, S. R. (1989). *Personality theories: A comparative analysis.* Chicago: Dorsey Press.

Mahedy, W. P. (1986). *Out of the night: The spiritual journey of Vietnam vets.* New York: Ballantine Books.

Malinowski, B. (1944). *A scientific theory of culture and other essays.* Chapel Hill: University of North Carolina Press.

Malony, H. N. (1993). The relevance of "religious diagnosis" for counseling. In E. L. Worthington Jr. (Ed.), *Psychotherapy and religious values* (pp. 105–120). Grand Rapids, MI: Baker Book House.

Manfredi, C., & Pickett, M. (1987). Perceived stressful situations and coping strategies utilized by the elderly. *Journal of Community Health Nursing, 4,* 99–100.

Marmar, C. R., & Horowitz, M. J. (1988). Diagnoses and phase-oriented treatment of post-traumatic stress disorder. In J. P. Wilson, Z. Harel, & B. Kahana (Eds.), *Human adaptation to extreme stress: From the Holocaust to Vietnam* (pp. 81–104). New York: Plenum.

Martin, L. L., & Tesser, A. (1989). Toward a motivational and structural theory of ruminative thought. In J. S. Uleman & J. A. Bargh (Eds.), *The direction of thought: The limits of awareness, intention, and control* (pp. 226–306). New York: Guilford Press.

Martin-Baró, I. (1990). Religion as an instrument of psychological warfare. *Journal of Social Issues, 46,* 93–107.

Maslow, A. (1970). *Motivation and personality* (2nd ed.). New York: Harper & Row.

Matheny, K. B., Aycock, D. W., Pugh, J. L., Curlette, W. L., & Cannella, K. A. S. (1986). Stress coping: A qualitative and quantitative synthesis with implications for treatment. *Counseling Psychologist, 14,* 499–549.

Maton, K. I. (1987). Patterns and psychological correlates of material support within a religious setting: The bidirectional support hypothesis. *American Journal of Community Psychology, 15,* 185–208.

Maton, K. I. (1989a). Community settings as buffers of life stress? Highly supportive churches, mutual help groups, and senior centers. *American Journal of Community Psychology, 17,* 203–232.

Maton, K. I. (1989b). The stress-buffering role of spiritual support: Cross-sectional and prospective investigations. *Journal for the Scientific Study of Religion, 28,* 310–323.

Maton, K. I., & Pargament, K. I. (1987). The roles of religion in prevention and promotion. *Prevention in Human Services, 5,* 161–205.

Maton, K. I., & Rappaport, J. (1984). Empowerment in a religious setting: A multivariate investigation. *Prevention in Human Services, 3,* 37–72.

Maton, K. I., & Seibert, M. (1991). *Third year evaluation of Project RAISE.* (Unpublished evaluation report). Baltimore: University of Maryland.

Maton, K. I., & Wells, E. A. (1995). Religion as a community resource for well-being: Prevention, healing, and empowerment pathways. *Journal of Social Issues, 51,* 177–193.

Matthews, D. A., Larson, D. B., & Barry, C. P. (1993). *The faith factor: An annotated bibliography of clinical research on spiritual subjects.* Bethesda, MD: National Institute for Healthcare Research.

Mattlin, J. A., Wethington, E., & Kessler, R. C. (1990). Situational determinants of coping and coping effectiveness. *Journal of Health and Social Behavior, 31,* 103–122.

May, R. (1970). Psychotherapy and the daimonic. In J. Campbell (Ed.), *Myths, dreams, and religion* (pp. 196–210). New York: Dutton.

McBride, D. C., McCoy, C. B., Chitwood, D. D., Hernandez, E. L., & Mutch, P. M. (1994). Religious institutions as sources of AIDS information for street injection drug users. *Review of Religious Research, 35,* 324–334.

McCrae, R. R. (1984). Situational determinants of coping response: Loss, threat, and challenge. *Journal of Personality and Social Psychology, 46,* 919–928.

McCrae, R. R., & Costa, P. T., Jr. (1986). Personality, coping, and coping effectiveness in an adult sample. *Journal of Personality, 54,* 385–405.

McCullough, M. E. (1995). *Forgiveness as altruism: A social-psychological theory of interpersonal forgiveness and tests of its validity.* Unpublished doctoral dissertation, Virginia Commonwealth University.

McCullough, M. E., & Worthington, E. L., Jr. (1994a). Encouraging clients to forgive people who have hurt them: Review, critique, and research prospectus. *Journal of Psychology and Theology, 22,* 3–20.

McCullough, M. E., & Worthington, E. L., Jr. (1994b). Models of interpersonal forgiveness and their applications to counseling: Review and critique. *Counseling and Values, 39,* 2–14.

McCullough, M. E., & Worthington, E. L., Jr. (1995). Promoting forgiveness: A comparison of two brief psychoeducational group interventions with a waiting list control. *Counseling and Values, 40,* 55–68.

McFadden, S. H. (in press). Religion, spirituality, and aging. In J. E. Birren & K. W. Schaie (Eds.), *Handbook of the psychology of aging* (4th ed.). San Diego: Academic Press.

McFadden, S. H., & Levin, J. S. (1996). Religion, emotions, and health. In C. Magai & S. H. McFadden (Eds.), *Handbook of emotions, adult development, and aging* (pp. 349–365). San Diego: Academic Press.

McGloshen, T. H., & O'Bryant, S. L. (1988). The psychological well-being of older, recent widows. *Psychology of Women Quarterly, 12,* 99–116.

McGrath, J. E. (1970). *Social and psychological factors in stress.* New York: Holt, Rinehart & Winston.

McGuire, M. B. (1988). *Ritual healing in suburban America.* New Brunswick, NJ: Rutgers University Press.

McIntosh, D. N. (1995). Religion as schema, with implications for the relation between religion and coping. *International Journal for the Psychology of Religion, 5,* 1–16.

McIntosh, D. N., Inglehart, M. R., & Pacini, R. (1990). *Flexible and central religious belief systems and adjustment to college.* Paper presented at the meeting of the Midwestern Psychological Association, Chicago, IL.

McIntosh, D. N., Silver, R. C., & Wortman, C. B. (1989). *Parental religious change in response to their child's death.* Paper presented at the meeting of the Society for the Scientific Study of Religion, Salt Lake City, UT.

McIntosh, D. N., Silver, R. C., & Wortman, C. B. (1993). Religion's role in adjustment to a negative life event: Coping with the loss of a child. *Journal of Personality and Social Psychology, 65,* 812–821.

McIntosh, D. N., & Spilka, B. (1990). Religion and physical health: The role of personal faith and control. In M. L. Lynn & D. O. Moberg (Eds.), *Research in the social scientific study of religion* (Vol. 2, pp. 167–194). Greenwich, CT: JAI Press.

McLatchie, L. R., & Draguns, J. G. (1984). Mental health concepts of evangelical Protestants. *Journal of Psychology, 118,* 147–159.

McLoughlin, W. G. (1978). *Revivals, awakenings, and reform: An essay on religion and social change in America, 1607–1977.* Chicago: University of Chicago Press.

McReady, W. C., & Greeley, A. M. (1976). *The ultimate values of the American population* (Vol. 23). Beverly Hills: Sage.

McSherry, E. (1983). The scientific basis of whole person medicine. *Journal of the American Scientific Affiliation, 35,* 217–224.

Mead, M. (1968). The implications of culture change for personality development. In M. Fried (Ed.), *Readings in anthropology: Vol. II. Cultural anthropology* (p. 836). New York: Thomas Y. Crowell.

Meadow, M. J., & Kahoe, R. D. (1984). *Psychology of religion: Religion in individual lives.* New York: Harper & Row.

Meaning of the glorious Koran, The. (1953). (M. M. Pickthall, Trans.). New York: Mentor Books.

Meigs, J. T. (1969). Pastoral care of parents of children with cancer. In W. E. Oates & A. D. Lester (Eds.), *Pastoral care in crucial human situations* (pp. 62–89). Valley Forge, PA: Judson Press.

Melton, J. G. (1986). *Encyclopedic handbook of cults in America.* New York: Garland.

Memorandum on a mass murder. (1990, April 9). *Newsweek,* p. 25.

Menaghan, E. G. (1983). Individual coping efforts: Moderator of the relationship between life stress and mental health outcomes. In H. B. Kaplan (Eds.), *Psychosocial stress: Trends in theory and research* (pp. 157–191). New York: Academic Press.

Menninger, K. (1963). *The vital balance: The life process in mental health and illness.* New York: Viking Press.

Mercer, D., Lorden, R., & Falkenberg, S. (1995). *Mediating effects of religiousness on recovery from victimization.* Paper presented at the meeting of the American Psychological Association, New York, NY.

Meylink, W. D., & Gorsuch, R. L. (1986). New perspectives for clergy–psychologist referrals. *Journal of Psychology and Christianity, 5,* 62–70.

Mickley, J., & Soeken, K. (1993). Religiousness and hope in Hispanic- and Anglo-American women with breast cancer. *Oncology Nursing Forum, 20,* 1171–1177.

Miller, W. R. (1988). Including clients' spiritual perspectives in cognitive-behavioral therapy. In W. R. Miller & J. E. Martin (Eds.), *Behavior therapy and religion: Integrating spiritual and behavioral approaches to change* (pp. 43–55). Newbury Park: Sage.

Millison, M., & Dudley, J. R. (1992). Providing spiritual support: A job for all hospice professionals. *The Hospice Journal, 8,* 49–66.

Minkin, J. S. (1987). *The teachings of Maimonides.* Northvale, NJ: Aronson.

Mitchell, R. E., Cronkite, R. C., & Moos, R. H. (1983). Stress, coping, and depression among married couples. *Journal of Abnormal Psychology, 92,* 433–448.

Moberg, D. (1987). Holy masquerade: Hypocrisy in religion. *Review of Religious Research, 29,* 3–24.

Mondell, S., & Tyler, F. B. (1981). Parental competence and styles of problem solving/play behavior with children. *Developmental Psychology, 17,* 73–79.

Moore, T. (1992). The African American church: A source of empowerment, mutual help, and social change. In K. I. Pargament, K. I. Maton, & R. E. Hess (Eds.), *Religion and prevention in mental health: Research, vision, and action* (pp. 237–258). New York: Haworth Press.

Moos, R. H., Brennan, P. L., Fondacaro, M. R., & Moos, B. S. (1990). Approach and avoidance coping responses among older problem and non-problem drinkers. *Psychology and Aging, 5,* 31–40.

Moos, R. H., Cronkite, R., Billings, A., & Finney, J. (1984). *Health and daily living form manual.* Palo Alto, CA: Social Ecology Laboratory.

Morris, P. A. (1982). The effect of pilgrimage on anxiety, depression and religious attitude. *Psychological Medicine, 12,* 291–294.

Mulhern, S. (1991). Satanism and psychotherapy: A rumor in search of an inquisition. In J. T. Richardson, J. Best, & D. G. Bromley (Eds.), *The satanism scare* (pp. 145–174). New York: Aldine de Gruyter.

Mullen, B., & Suls, J. (1982). The effectiveness of attention and rejection as coping styles: A meta-analysis of temporal differences. *Journal of Psychosomatic Research, 26,* 43–49.

Murphy, L. B. (1974). Coping, vulnerability, and resilience. In D. Hamburg & G. Coelho (Eds.), *Coping and adaptation* (pp. 69–100). New York: Basic Books.

Murphy, L. B., & Moriarty, A. E. (1976). *Vulnerability, coping, and growth: From infancy to adolescence.* New Haven: Yale University Press.

Murray, H. A. (1938). *Explorations in personality: A clinical and experimental study of fifty men of college age.* New York: Oxford University Press.

Narayanan, H. S., Mohan, K. S., & Radhakrishnan, V. K. (1986). The Karma theory of mental illness. *Nimhans Journal, 4,* 61–63.

Neighbors, H. W., Jackson, J. S., Bowman, P. J., & Gurin, G. (1983). Stress, coping, and black mental health: Preliminary findings from a national study. In R. Hess & J. Hermalin (Eds.), *Innovation in prevention* (pp. 5–29). New York: Haworth Press.

Neimeyer, R. A. (1995). An appraisal of constructivist psychotherapies: Contexts and challenges. In M. J. Mahoney (Ed.), *Cognitive and constructive psychotherapies: Theory, research and practice* (pp. 195–208). New York: Springer.

Nelson, A. A., & Wilson, W. P. (1984). The ethics of sharing faith in psychotherapy. *Journal of Psychology and Theology, 12,* 15–23.

Nelson, M. O., & Jones, E. M. (1957). An application of the Q-technique to the study of religious concepts. *Psychological Reports, 3,* 293–297.

Newman, L. E. (1987). The quality of mercy: On the duty to forgive in the Judaic tradition. *Journal of Religious Ethics, 15,* 155–172.

Newman, J. S., & Pargament, K. I. (1990). The role of religion in the problem-solving process. *Review of Religious Research, 31,* 390–404.

Newport, F. (1979, August). The religious switcher in the United States. *American Sociological Review, 44,* 528–552.

Nicholi, A. M. (1974). A new dimension of the youth culture. *American Journal of Psychiatry, 131,* 396–401.

Nielsen, M. E., & Fultz, J. (1991). *Self-complexity and religious orientation, conflict, and belief.* Paper presented at the meeting of the Society for the Scientific Study of Religion, Pittsburgh, PA.

Nino, A. G. (1990). Restoration of the self: A therapeutic paradigm from Augustine's *Confessions. Psychotherapy, 1,* 8–18.

Norris, F. H., & Murrell, S. A. (1988). Prior experience as a moderator of disaster impact on anxiety symptoms in older adults. *American Journal of Community Psychology, 16,* 665–683.

Norton, H., & Slosser, B. (1976). *The miracle of Jimmy Carter.* Plainfield, NJ: Logos International.

Oates, W. E. (1953). *The Bible in pastoral care.* Philadelphia: Westminster Press.

O'Brien, M. E. (1982). Religious faith and adjustment to long-term hemodialysis. *Journal of Religion and Health, 21,* 68–80.

O'Connor, B. P., & Vallerand, R. J. (1990). Religious motivation in the elderly: A French-Canadian replication and an extension. *Journal of Social Psychology, 130,* 51–59.

Oden, T. C. (1983). *Pastoral theology: Essentials of ministry.* San Francisco: Harper & Row.

Osofsky, J. D., & Osofsky, H. J. (1972). The psychological reaction of parents to legalized abortion. *American Journal of Orthopsychiatry, 42,* 48–60.

Otto, R. (1928). *The idea of the holy: An inquiry into the non-rational factor in the idea of the divine and its relation to the rational.* London: Oxford University Press.

Oxman, T. E., Freeman, D. H., Jr., & Manheimer, E. D. (1995). Lack of social participation or religious strength and comfort as risk factors for death after cardiac surgery in the elderly. *Psychosomatic Medicine, 57,* 5–15.

Paden, W. E. (1988). *Religious worlds: The comparative study of religion.* Boston: Beacon Press.

Page One: Major Events 1920–1986 as presented in The New York Times. (1986). New York: New York Times.

Palinkas, L. A. (1982). Ethnicity, identity, and mental health: The use of rhetoric in an immigrant Chinese church. *Journal of Psychoanalytic Anthropology, 5*, 235–258.

Paloutzian, R. F. (1981). Purpose in life and value changes following conversion. *Journal of Personality and Social Psychology, 41*, 1153–1160.

Paloutzian, R. F. (1996). *Invitation to the psychology of religion* (2nd ed.). Boston: Allyn & Bacon.

Pargament, K. I. (1982). The interface among religion, religious support systems and mental health. In D. Biegel & A. Naperstak (Eds.), *Community support systems and mental health* (pp. 161–174). New York: Springer.

Pargament, K. I. (1992). Of means and ends: Religion and the search for significance. *International Journal for the Scientific Study of Religion, 2*, 201–229.

Pargament, K. I., Brannick, M. T., Adamakos, H., Ensing, D. S., Kelemen, M. L., Warren, R. K., Falgout, K., Cook, P., & Myers, J. (1987). Indiscriminate proreligiousness: Conceptualization and measurement. *Journal for the Scientific Study of Religion, 26*, 182–200.

Pargament, K. I., & DeRosa, D. V. (1985). What was that sermon about? Predicting memory for religious messages from cognitive psychology theory. *Journal for the Scientific Study of Religion, 24*, 180–193.

Pargament, K. I., Echemendia, R. J., Johnson, S., Cook, P., McGath, C., Myers, J. G., & Brannick, M. (1987). The conservative church: Psychosocial advantages and disadvantages. *American Journal of Community Psychology, 15*, 269–286.

Pargament, K. I., Ensing, D. S., Falgout, K., Olsen, H., Reilly, B., Van Haitsma, K., & Warren, R. (1990). God help me: I. Religious coping efforts as predictors of the outcomes to significant negative life events. *American Journal of Community Psychology, 18*, 793–824.

Pargament, K. I., Falgout, K., Ensing, D. S., Reilly, B., Silverman, M., Van Haitsma, K. E., Olsen, H., & Warren, R. (1991). The congregation development program: Data-based consultation with churches and synagogues. *Professional Psychology: Research and Practice, 22*, 393–404.

Pargament, K. I., & Hahn, J. (1986). God and the just world: Causal and coping attributions to God in health situations. *Journal for the Scientific Study of Religion, 25*, 193–207.

Pargament, K. I., Ishler, K., Dubow, E., Stanik, P., Rouiller, R., Crowe, P., Cullman, E., Albert, M., & Royster, B. J. (1994). Methods of religious coping with the Gulf War: Cross-sectional and longitudinal analyses. *Journal for the Scientific Study of Religion, 33*, 347–361.

Pargament, K. I., Johnson, S. M., Echemendia, R. J., & Silverman, W. H. (1985). The limits of fit: Examining the implications of person–environment congruence within different religious settings. *Journal of Community Psychology, 13*, 20–30.

Pargament, K. I., Kennell, J., Hathaway, W., Grevengoed, N., Newman, J., & Jones, W. (1988). Religion and the problem-solving process: Three styles of coping. *Journal for the Scientific Study of Religion, 27*, 90–104.

Pargament, K. I., Maton, K. I., & Hess, R. E. (Eds.). (1992). *Religion and prevention in mental health: Research, vision, and action.* New York: Haworth Press.

Pargament, K. I., & Myers, J. (1982). *The individual–systems spiral: A foundation of value for action in community psychology.* Paper presented at the meeting of the American Psychological Association, Washington, D. C.

Pargament, K. I., Olsen, H., Reilly, B., Falgout, K., Ensing, D., & Van Haitsma, K. (1992a). *Studies of the ecology of religious coping.* Unpublished manuscript, Bowling Green State University, Bowling Green, OH.

Pargament, K. I., Olsen, H., Reilly, B., Falgout, K., Ensing, D., & Van Haitsma, K. (1992b). God help me (II): The relationship of religious orientations to religious coping with negative life events. *Journal for the Scientific Study of Religion, 31,* 504–513.

Pargament, K. I., & Park, C. L. (1995). Merely a defense? The variety of religious means and ends. *Journal of Social Issues, 51,* 13–32.

Pargament, K. I., Royster, B. J. T., Albert, M., Crowe, P., Cullman, E. P., Holley, R., Schaefer, D., Sytniak, M., & Wood, M. (1990). *A qualitative approach to the study of religion and coping: Four tentative conclusions.* Paper presented at the meeting of the American Psychological Association, Boston, MA.

Pargament, K. I., & Silverman, W. H. (1982). Exploring some correlates of sermon impact on Catholic parishioners. *Review of Religious Research, 24,* 33–39.

Pargament, K. I., Silverman, W., Johnson, S., Echemendia, R., & Snyder, S. (1983). The psychosocial climate of religious congregations. *American Journal of Community Psychology, 11,* 351–381.

Pargament, K. I., Smith, B., & Brant, C. (1995). *Religious and nonreligious coping methods with the 1993 Midwest flood.* Paper presented at the meeting of the Society for the Scientific Study of Religion, St. Louis, MO.

Pargament, K. I., Smith, B., & Koenig, H. G. (1996). *Religious coping with the Oklahoma City bombing: The brief RCOPE.* Paper presented at the meeting of the American Psychological Association, Toronto.

Pargament, K. I., Steele, R., & Tyler, F. B. (1979). Religious participation, religious motivation, and individual psychosocial competence. *Journal for the Scientific Study of Religion, 18,* 412–419.

Pargament, K. I., & Sullivan, M. S. (1981). *Examining attributions of control across diverse personal situations: A psychosocial perspective.* Paper presented at the meeting of the American Psychological Association, Los Angeles, CA.

Pargament, K. I., Sullivan, M. S., Balzer, W. E., Van Haitsma, K. S., & Raymark, P. H. (1995). The many meanings of religiousness: A policy capturing approach. *Journal of Personality, 63,* 953–983.

Pargament, K. I., Sullivan, M. S., Tyler, F. B., & Steele, R. E. (1982). Patterns of attribution of control and individual psychosocial competence. *Psychological Reports, 51,* 1243–1252.

Pargament, K. I., Tyler, F., & Steele, R. (1979a). The church/synagogue and the psychosocial competence of the member: An initial inquiry into a neglected dimension. *American Journal of Community Psychology, 7,* 649–664.

Pargament, K. I., Tyler, F. B., & Steele, R. E. (1979b). Is fit it? The relationship between church/synagogue member fit and the psychosocial competence of the member. *Journal of Community Psychology, 7,* 243–252.

Pargament, K. I., Zinnbauer, B. J., Scott, A., Butter, E. M., Zerowin, J., & Stanik, P. (in press). Red flags and religious coping: Identifying some religious warning signs among people in crisis. *Journal of Clinical Psychology.*

Park, C. L., & Cohen, L. H. (1993). Religious and nonreligious coping with the death of a friend. *Cognitive Therapy and Research, 17,* 561–577.

Park, C. L., Cohen, L. H., & Herb, L. (1990). Intrinsic religiousness and religious coping as life stress moderators for Catholics vs. Protestants. *Journal of Personality and Social Psychology, 59,* 562–574.

Park, C. L., Cohen, L. H., & Murch, R. L. (1996). Assessment and prediction of stress-related growth. *Journal of Personality, 64,* 71–105.

Park, C. L., & Folkman, S. (in press). Meaning in the context of stress and coping. *Review of General Psychology.*

Patton, J. (1985). *Is human forgiveness possible? A pastoral care perspective.* Nashville: Abingdon Press.

Payne, D. (1982). *Life after divorce.* New York: Pilgrim Press.

Payne, R., Bergin, A. E., Bielema, K. A., & Jenkins, P. H. (1992). Review of religion and mental health: Prevention and the enhancement of psychosocial functioning. In K. I. Pargament, K. I. Maton, & R. E. Hess (Eds.), *Religion and prevention: Research, vision, and action* (pp. 57–82). New York: Haworth Press.

Payne, E. C., Kravitz, A. R., Notman, M. T., & Anderson, J. V. (1976). Outcome following therapeutic abortion. *Archives of General Psychology, 33,* 725–733.

Pearlin, L. I. (1982). The social contexts of stress. In L. Goldberger & S. Breznitz (Eds.), *Handbook of stress: Theoretical and clinical aspects* (pp. 367–379). New York: Free Press.

Pearlin, L. I., & Schooler, C. (1978). The structure of coping. *Journal of Health and Social Behavior, 19,* 2–21.

Pecheur, D. R., & Edwards, K. J. (1984). A comparison of secular and religious versions of cognitive therapy with depressed Christian college students. *Journal of Psychology and Theology, 12,* 45–54.

Peck, D. L. (1988). Religious conviction, coping, and hope: The relation between a functional corrector and a future prospect among life-without-parole inmates. *Case Analyses, 2,* 201–219.

Pennebaker, J. W., & Beall, S. (1986). Confronting a traumatic event: Toward an understanding of inhibition and disease. *Journal of Abnormal Psychology, 95,* 274–281.

Pennebaker, J. W., Hughes, C. F., & O'Heeron, R. C. (1987). The psychophysiology of compassion: Linking inhibitory and psychosomatic processes. *Journal of Personality and Social Psychology, 52,* 781–793.

Peterson, C., Seligman, M. E. P., & Vaillant, G. E. (1988). Pessimistic explanatory style is a risk factor for physical illness: A thirty-five year longitudinal study. *Journal of Personality and Social Psychology, 55,* 23–27.

Phillips, A. (1986). Forgiveness reconsidered. *Christian Jewish Relations, 19*, 14–21.

Piaget, J. (1954). *The construction of reality in the child.* New York: Basic Books.

Pingleton, J. P. (1989). The role and function of forgiveness in the psychotherapeutic process. *Journal of Psychology and Theology, 17*, 27–35.

Plante, T. G., & Manuel, G. M. (1992). The Persian Gulf War: Civilian war related stress and the influence of age, religious faith, and war attitudes. *Journal of Clinical Psychology, 48*, 178–182.

Poggie, J. J., Jr., Pollnac, R., & Gersuny, C. (1976). Risk as a basis for taboos among fishermen in southern New England. *Journal for the Scientific Study of Religion, 15*, 252–267.

Pollner, M. (1989). Divine relations, social relations, and well-being. *Journal of Health and Social Behavior, 30*, 92–104.

Poloma, M. M., & Gallup, G. H., Jr. (1991). *Varieties of prayer: A survey report.* Philadelphia: Trinity Press International.

Pratt, J. B. (1946). *The religious consciousness: A psychological study.* New York: Macmillan.

Pressman, P., Lyons, J. S., Larson, D. B., & Gartner, J. (1992). Religion, anxiety, and the fear of death. In J. F. Schumaker (Ed.), *Religion and mental health* (pp. 98–109). New York: Oxford University Press.

Pressman, P., Lyons, J. S., Larson, D. B., & Strain, J. J. (1990). Religious belief, depression, and ambulation status in elderly women with broken hips. *American Journal of Psychiatry, 147*, 758–760.

Prest, L. A., & Keller, J. F. (1993). Spirituality and family therapy: Spiritual beliefs, myths, and metaphors. *Journal of Marital and Family Therapy, 19*, 137–148.

Price, R. H., Cowen, E. L., Lorion, R. P., & Ramos-McKay, J. (1988). *14 ounces of prevention.* Washington, DC: American Psychological Association.

Propst, L. R. (1980). The comparative efficacy of religious and nonreligious imagery for the treatment of mild depression in religious individuals. *Cognitive Therapy and Research, 4*, 167–178.

Propst, L. R. (1988). *Psychotherapy in a religious framework: Spirituality in the emotional healing process.* New York: Human Services Press.

Propst, L. R. (1991). *The crucified God: Chosen suffering as a path to healing.* John G. Finch Symposium Lecture at Fuller Theological Seminary, Pasadena, CA.

Propst, L. R., Ostrom, R., Watkins, P., Dean, T., & Mashburn, D. (1992). Comparative efficacy of religious and nonreligious cognitive-behavioral therapy for the treatment of clinical depression in religious individuals. *Journal of Consulting and Clinical Psychology, 60*, 94–103.

Proudfoot, W., & Shaver, P. (1975). Attribution theory and the psychology of religion. *Journal for the Scientific Study of Religion, 14*, 317–330.

Pruyser, P. W. (1968). *A dynamic psychology of religion.* New York: Harper & Row.

Pruyser, P. W. (1976). *The minister as diagnostician: Personal problems in pastoral perspective.* Philadelphia: Westminster Press.

Pruyser, P. W. (1977). The seamy side of current religious beliefs. *Bulletin of the Menninger Clinic, 41,* 329–348.

Purisman, R., & Maoz, B. (1977). Adjustment and war bereavement—Some considerations. *British Journal of Medical Psychology, 50,* 1–9.

Rabins, P. V., Fitting, M. D., Eastham, J., & Zabora, J. (1990). Emotional adaptation over time in care-givers for chronically ill elderly people. *Age and Ageing, 19,* 185–190.

Rabkin, J. G., & Streuning, E. L. (1976). Life events, stress, and illness. *Science, 194,* 1013–1020.

Ragan, C., Malony, H. N., & Beit-Hallahmi, B. (1980). Psychologists and religion: Professional factors associated with personal belief. *Review of Religious Research, 21,* 208–217.

Raleigh, E. D. H. (1992). Sources of hope in chronic illness. *Oncology Nursing Forum, 19,* 443–448.

Rappaport, J. (1977). *Community psychology: Values, research, and action.* New York: Holt, Rinehart & Winston.

Rappaport, J. (1981). In praise of paradox: A social policy of empowerment over prevention. *American Journal of Community Psychology, 9,* 1–26.

Ratliff, J. B. (1989). *When you are facing change.* Louisville: Westminster/John Knox Press.

Regier, D. A., Boyd, J. H., Burke, J. D., Rae, D. S., Myers, J. K., Kramer, M., Robins, C. N., George, L. K., Karno, M., & Locke, B. Z. (1988). One month prevalence of mental disorders in the U. S. *Archives of General Psychiatry, 45,* 977–986.

Religious scams total $450 million. (1989, August 8). *Detroit Free Press,* 1A, 11A.

Rettino, E., & Rettino, D. (1985). *Kid's praise 5: Psalty's camping adventure* [Record]. Costa Mesa, CA: Maranthal Music.

Reynolds, D. K., & Nelson, F. L. (1981). Personality, life situation, and life expectancy. *Suicide and Life-Threatening Behavior, 11,* 99–110.

Richards, P. S., Owen, L., & Stein, S. (1993). A religiously oriented group counseling intervention for self-defeating perfectionism: A pilot study. *Counseling and Values, 37,* 96–104.

Richardson, J. T. (Ed.). (1978). *Conversion careers: In and out of the new religions* (Vol. 47). Beverly Hills, CA: Sage.

Richardson, J. T. (1985). The active vs. passive convert: Paradigm conflict in conversion/recruitment research. *Journal for the Scientific Study of Religion, 24,* 163–179.

Richardson, J. T. (1993). Religiosity as deviance: Negative religious bias in and misuse of the DSM III. *Deviant Behavior: An Interdisciplinary Journal, 14,* 1–21.

Riegel, K. F. (1975). Adult life crises: A dialectic interpretation of development. In N. Datan & L. H. Ginsberg (Eds.), *Life span developmental psychology: Normative life crises* (pp. 99–128). New York: Academic Press.

Riley, J. W., Jr. (1968). Death and bereavement. In D. Sills (Ed.), *International encyclopedia of the social sciences* (Vol. 4, pp. 19–26). New York: Macmillan.

Ritzema, R. J. (1979). Attribution to supernatural causation: An important component of religious commitment. *Journal of Psychology and Theology, 7*, 286–293.

Ritzema, R. J., & Young, C. (1983). Causal schemata and the attribution of supernatural causality. *Journal of Psychology and Theology, 11*, 36–43.

Robbins, T., & Anthony, D. (1979). The sociology of contemporary religious movements. *Annual Review of Sociology, 5*, 75–89.

Roberts, B., & Thorsheim, H. (1987). A partnership approach to consultation: The process and results of a major primary prevention field experiment. In J. Kelly & R. Hess (Eds.), *The ecology of prevention: Illustrating mental health consultation* (pp. 151–186). New York: Haworth Press.

Roberts, J. (1988). Setting the frame: Definition, functions, and typology of rituals. In E. Imber-Black, J. Roberts, & R. A. Whiting (Eds.), *Rituals in family and family therapy* (pp. 3–46). New York: Norton.

Robertson, N. (1988). *Getting better: Inside alcoholic anonymous.* New York: Fawcett Crest.

Rofe, Y., & Lewin, I. (1980). Daydreaming in a war environment. *Journal of Mental Imagery, 4*, 59–75.

Rokeach, M. (1968). *Beliefs, attitudes, and values: A theory of organization and change.* San Francisco: Jossey-Bass.

Rokeach, M. (1973). *The nature of human values.* New York: Free Press.

Rosenak, C. M., & Hamden, O. M. (1992). Forgiveness in the psychotherapeutic process: Clinical applications. *Journal of Psychology and Christianity, 11*, 188–197.

Rosenberg, M. (1962). The dissonant religious context and emotional disturbance. *American Journal of Sociology, 68*, 1–10.

Rosenblatt, P. C., Walsh, H. P., & Jackson, D. A. (1976). *Grief and mourning in cross-cultural perspective.* New Haven, CT: HRAF Press.

Rosenstiel, A. K., & Keefe, F. J. (1983). The use of coping strategies in chronic low back pain patients: Relationship to patient characteristics and current adjustment. *Pain, 17*, 33–44.

Rosik, C. H. (1989). The impact of religious orientation in conjugal bereavement among older adults. *International Journal of Aging and Human Development, 28*, 251–260.

Ross, C. E. (1990). Religion and psychological distress. *Journal for the Scientific Study of Religion, 29*, 236–245.

Rosten, L. (1972). *Leo Rosten's treasury of Jewish quotations.* New York: McGraw-Hill.

Roth, S., & Cohen, L. J. (1986). Approach, avoidance, and coping with stress. *American Psychologist, 41*, 813–819.

Rothbaum, B. O., & Jackson, J. (1990). Religious influence on menstrual attitudes and symptoms. *Women and Health, 16*, 63–78.

Rowe, J. O., Halling, S., Davies, E., Leifer, M., Powers, D., & Van Bronkhorst, J. (1989). The psychology of forgiving another: A dialogical research approach. In R. S. Valle & S. Halling (Eds.), *Existential-phenomenological perspectives in psychology: Exploring the breadth of human experience* (pp. 233–244). New York: Plenum Press.

Rubin, Z., & Peplau, L. A. (1975). Who believes in a just world? *Journal of Social Issues, 31,* 65–89.

Rupp, J. (1988). *Praying our goodbyes.* Notre Dame, IN: Ave Maria Press.

Rupp, J. (1990). *Walking with God through grief and loss.* St. Meinrad, IN: Abbey Press.

Rutledge, J., & Spilka, B. (1993). *Coping with intimacy: A problem for the single adult Mormon.* Paper presented at the meeting of the American Psychological Association, Toronto.

Ryan, R. M., Rigby, S., & King, K. (1993). Two types of religious internalization and their relations to religious orientations and mental health. *Journal of Personality and Social Psychology, 65,* 586–596.

Rychlak, J. E. (1981). *Introduction to personality and psychotherapy.* Boston: Houghton-Mifflin.

Rye, M. S. (1996). *Forgiveness and mental health: An integration of philosophy, religion, and psychology.* Unpublished manuscript, Bowling Green State University, Bowling Green, OH.

Sacks, O. (1988). The divine curse. *Life Magazine, 11,* 94–103.

Sales, S. M. (1972). Economic threat as a determinant of conversion rates in authoritarian and nonauthoritarian churches. *Journal of Personality and Social Psychology, 23,* 420–428.

Salzman, L. (1953). The psychology of religious and ideological conversion. *Psychiatry, 16,* 177–187.

Sanders, C. M. (1979–1980). A comparison of adult bereavement in the death of a spouse, child, and parent. *Omega, 10,* 303–322.

Sappington, A. A. (1990). Recent psychological approaches to the free will versus determinism issue. *Psychological Bulletin, 108,* 19–29.

Sargant, W. (1957). *Battle for the mind.* Garden City, NY: Doubleday.

Sattler, D. N., Hamby, B. A., Winkler, J. M., & Kaiser, C. (1994). *Hurricane Iniki: Psychological functioning following disaster.* Paper presented at the meeting of the American Psychological Association, Los Angeles, CA.

Saucer, P. R. (1991). Evangelical renewal therapy: A proposal for integration of religious values into psychotherapy. *Psychological Reports, 69,* 1099–1106.

Saudia, T. L., Kinney, M. R., Brown, K. C., & Young-Ward, L. (1991). Health locus of control and helpfulness of prayer. *Heart and Lung, 20,* 60–65.

Schaefer, C. A., & Gorsuch, R. L. (1991). Psychological adjustment and religiousness: The multivariate belief-motivation theory of religiousness. *Journal for the Scientific Study of Religion, 30,* 448–461.

Schafer, R. L. (1984). Pastoral accompaniment of the cancer patient. *Journal of Religion and Health, 23,* 138–148.

Scheie, D. M., Markham, J., Mayer, S. E., Slettom, J., & Williams, T. (1991). *Religious institutions as partners in community based program development: Findings from year one of the Lilly Endowment Program.* Minneapolis, MN: Rainbow Research.

Schimmel, S. (1980). Education of the emotions in Jewish devotional literature: Anger and its control. *Journal of Religious Ethics, 8,* 259–276.

Schneirla, T. C. (1959). An evolutionary and developmental theory of biphasic processes underlying approach and withdrawal. *Nebraska Symposium on Motivation* (pp. 1–42). Lincoln: University of Nebraska Press.

Schoenrade, P., & Leavitt, C. (1989). *Coping with mortality: Religious beliefs and personal priorities as responses.* Paper presented at the meeting of the Society for the Scientific Study of Religion, Salt Lake City, UT.

Schulz, R., & Williamson, G. M. (1994). Health effects of caregiving: Prevalence of mental and physical illness in Alzheimer's caregivers. In E. Light, G. Niederhe, & B. D. Lebowitz (Eds.), *Stress effects on family caregivers of Alzheimer's patients: Research and intervention* (pp. 38–63). New York: Springer.

Schumaker, J. F. (Ed.). (1992). *Religion and mental health.* New York: Oxford University Press.

Schwab, J. J., & Schwab M. E. (1978). *Sociocultural roots of mental illness: An epidemiologic survey.* New York: Plenum Medical Book.

Schwab, R., & Petersen, K. U. (1991). Religiousness: Its relation to loneliness, neuroticism, and subjective well-being. *Journal for the Scientific Study of Religion, 29,* 335–345.

Schwartz, L. L., & Kaslow, F. W. (1979). Religious cults, the individual and the family. *Journal of Marital and Family Therapy, 5,* 15–26.

Sears, S. F., Jr., & Greene, A. F. (1994). Religious coping and the threat of heart transplantation. *Journal of Religion and Health, 33,* 221–229.

Seeman, T. (1991). Personal control and coronary artery disease: How generalized expectancies about control may influence disease risk. *Journal of Psychosomatic Medicine, 35,* 661–669.

Segall, M., & Wykle, M. (1988–1989). The black family's experience with dementia. *Journal of Applied Social Sciences, 13,* 170–191.

Seggar, J., & Kunz, P. (1972). Conversion: Evaluation of a step-like process for problem-solving. *Review of Religious Research, 13,* 178–184.

Seldes, G. (1985). *The great thoughts.* New York: Ballantine Books.

Selye, H. (1976). *The stress of life* (Rev. ed.). New York: McGraw-Hill.

Selye, H. (1982). History and present status of the stress concept. In G. Goldberger & S. Breznitz (Eds.), *Handbook of stress: Theoretical and clinical aspects* (pp. 7–20). New York: Free Press.

Sethi, S., & Seligman, M. E. P. (1993). Optimism and fundamentalism. *Psychological Science, 4,* 256–259.

Shafranske, E. P. (Ed.). (1996). *Religion and the clinical practice of psychology.* Washington, DC: APA Books.

Shafranske, E. P., & Gorsuch, R. L. (1984). Factors associated with perceptions of spirituality in psychotherapy. *Journal of Transpersonal Psychology, 16,* 231–241.

Shafranske, E. P., & Malony, H. N. (1990). Clinical psychologists' religious and spiritual orientations and their practice of psychotherapy. *Psychotherapy, 27,* 72–78.

Shams, M., & Jackson, P. R. (1993). Religiosity as predictor of well-being and moderator of the psychological impact of unemployment. *British Journal of Medical Psychology, 66,* 341–352.

Sharansky, N. (1988). *Fear no evil* (S. Hoffman, Trans.). New York: Vintage Books.

Shaver, P., Lenauer, M., & Sadd, S. (1980). Religiousness, conversion, and subjective well-being: The "healthy-minded" religion of modern American women. *American Journal of Psychiatry, 131,* 1563–1568.

She defies court's order for C-section, gives birth naturally. (1993, December 3), *Toledo Blade* p. 3.

Sherkat, D. E., & Reed, M. D. (1992). The effects of religion and social support on self-esteem and depression among the suddenly bereaved. *Social Indicator Research, 26,* 259–275.

Shontz, F. C. (1975). *The psychological aspects of physical illness and disability.* New York: Macmillan.

Shrimali, S., & Broota, K. A. (1987). Effect of surgical stress on belief in God and superstition: An in situ investigation. *Journal of Personality and Clinical Studies, 3,* 135–138.

Siegel, B. S. (1986). *Love, medicine, and miracles: Lessons learned about self-healing from a surgeon's experience with exceptional patients.* New York: Harper & Row.

Siegel, J. M., & Kuykendall, D. H. (1990). Loss, widowhood and psychological distress among the elderly. *Journal of Consulting and Clinical Psychology, 58,* 519–524.

Sijuwade, P. O. (1994). Sex differences in stress, illness and coping resources among the Nigerian elderly. *Social Behavior and Personality, 22,* 239–260.

Silber, E., Coelho, G. V., Murphy, E. D., Hamburg, D. A., Pearlin, L. I., & Rosenberg, H. (1961). Competent adolescents coping with college decisions. *Archives of General Psychiatry, 5,* 517–537.

Silver, R. L., & Wortman, C. B. (1980). Coping with undesirable life events. In J. Garber & M. E. P. Seligman (Eds.), *Human helplessness: Theory and applications* (pp. 279–375). New York: Academic Press.

Simmonds, R. B. (1977). Conversion or addiction: Consequences of joining a Jesus Movement group. *American Behavioral Scientist, 20,* 909–924.

Simon, S. B., & Simon, S. (1990). *Forgiveness: How to make peace with your past and get on with your life.* New York: Basic Books.

Simons, R. L., & West, G. E. (1984–1985). Life changes, coping resources, and health among the elderly. *International Journal of Aging and Human Development, 20,* 173–189.

Singer, M. T. (1979). Coming out of the cults. *Psychology Today, 12,* 72–82.

Singer, P. B. (1983). *In prison you came to me.* New York: Pilgrim Press.

Smedes, L. B. (1996). *The art of forgiving.* Nashville, TN: Moorings.

Smith, D. K., Nehemkis, A. M., & Charter, R. A. (1983–1984). Fear of death, death attitudes, and religious conviction in the terminally ill. *International Journal of Psychiatry in Medicine, 13,* 221–232.

Smith, H. (1958). *The religions of man.* New York: Harper & Row.

Smith, J. E. (1968). *Experience and God.* New York: Oxford University Press.

Smith, M. B. (1966). Explorations in competence: A study of Peace Corps teachers in Ghana. *American Psychologist, 21,* 556–566.

Smith, T. W., Allred, K. D., Morrison, C. A., & Carlson, S. D. (1989). Cardiovascular reactivity and interpersonal influence: Active coping in a social context. *Journal of Personality and Social Psychology, 56,* 209–218.

Snow, D. A., & Machalek, R. (1984). The sociology of conversion. *Annual Review of Sociology, 10,* 167–190.

Sodestron, K. E., & Martinson, I. M. (1987). Patients' spiritual coping strategies: A study of nurse and patient perspectives. *Oncology Nursing Forum, 14,* 41–46.

Sonnenblick, M., Friedlander, Y., & Steinberg, A. (1993). Disassociation between the wishes of terminally ill parents and decisions by their offspring. *Journal of the American Geriatric Society, 41,* 599–604.

Soper, D. W. (1951). At the end of self, God. In D. W. Soper (Ed.), *These found the way: Thirteen converts to Protestant Christianity* (pp. 173–175). Philadelphia: Westminster Press.

Sorrentino, R. M., & Hardy, J. (1974). Religiousness and derogation of an innocent victim. *Journal of Personality, 42,* 372–382.

Speisman, J. C., Lazarus, R. S., Mordkoff, A. M., & Davison, L. A. (1964). The experimental reduction of stress based on ego-defense theory. *Journal of Abnormal and Social Psychology, 68,* 367–380.

Spellman, C. M., Baskett, G, D., & Byrne, D. (1971). Manifest anxiety as a contributing factor in religious conversion. *Journal of Consulting and Clinical Psychology, 36,* 245–247.

Spencer, S. J., & McIntosh, D. N. (1990, August). *Extremity and importance in attitude structure: Attitudes as self-schemata.* Paper presented at the meeting of the American Psychological Association, Boston, MA.

Spero, M. H. (1985). The reality and the image of God in psychotherapy. *American Journal of Psychotherapy, 39,* 75–85.

Spilka, B. (1993, August). *Spirituality: Problems and directions in operationalizing a fuzzy concept.* Paper presented at the meeting of the American Psychological Association, Toronto, Canada.

Spilka, B., Armatas, P., & Nussbaum, J. (1964). The concept of God: A factor-analytic approach. *Review of Religious Research, 6,* 28–36.

Spilka, B., & Bridges, R. A. (1992). Religious perspectives on prevention: The role of theology. In K. I. Pargament, K. I. Maton, & R. E. Hess (Eds.), *Religion and prevention in mental health: Research, vision, and action* (pp. 19–36). New York: Haworth Press.

Spilka, B., Hood, R. W., Jr., & Gorsuch, R. L. (1985). *The psychology of religion: An empirical approach.* Englewood Cliffs, NJ: Prentice-Hall.

Spilka, B., & Schmidt, G. (1983). General attribution theory for the psychology of religion: The influence of event-character on attributions to God. *Journal for the Scientific Study of Religion, 22,* 326–339.

Spilka, B., Shaver, P., & Kirkpatrick, L. (1985). A general attribution theory for the psychology of religion. *Journal for the Scientific Study of Religion, 24,* 1–20.

Spinoza, B. (1957). *The ethics of Spinoza: The road to inner freedom* (Dagobert R. Runes, Ed.). Secaucus, NJ: Citadel Press.

Spiro, M. (1966). Religion: Problems of definition and explanation. In M. Banton (Ed.), *Anthropological approaches to the study of religion* (pp. 85–126). London: Tavistock.

Spiro, M. (1978). *Burmese supernaturalism*. Philadelphia: Institute for the Study of Human Issues.

Spitz, R. A. (1945). Hospitalism: An inquiry into the genesis of psychiatric conditions in early childhood. *Psychoanalytic Study of the Child, 1,* 53–74.

Starbuck, E. D. (1899). *The psychology of religion*. New York: Scribner.

Stark, R., & Bainbridge, W. S. (1985). *The future of religion: Secularization, revival, and cult formation*. Berkeley: University of California Press.

Stark, R., & Glock, C. Y. (1970). *American piety: The nature of religious commitment*. Berkeley: University of California Press.

Steinberg, M. (1975). *Basic Judaism*. New York: Harcourt Brace Jovanovich.

Steinitz, L. Y. (1981). The local church as support for the elderly. *Journal of Gerontological Social Work, 4,* 43–53.

Steinsaltz, A. (1976). *The essential Talmud*. New York: Basic Books.

Stephenson, P. H. (1983–1984). "He died too quick!" The process of dying in a Hutterian colony. *Omega, 14,* 127–134.

Stern, M. J., & Pascale, L. (1979). Psychosocial adaptation post-myocardial infarction: The spouse's dilemma. *Journal of Psychosomatic Research, 23,* 83–87.

Stern, M. J., Pascale, L., & Ackerman, A. (1977). Life adjustment post myocardial infarction: Determining predictive variables. *Archives of Internal Medicine, 137,* 1680–1685.

Stinnett, N. (1979). Strengthening families. *Family Perspective, 13,* 3–9.

Stone, A. A., & Neale, J. M. (1984). New measures of daily coping: Development and preliminary results. *Journal of Personality and Social Psychology, 46,* 892–906.

Stouffer, S. A., Comsdaine, A. A., Comsdaine, M. H., Williams, R. W., Jr., Smith, M. B., Janis, J. L., Star, S. A., & Cottrell, L. S., Jr. (1965). *The American soldier: Combat and its aftermath* (Vol. 2). New York: Wiley.

Straus, R. A. (1979). Religious conversion as a personal and collective accomplishment. *Sociological Analysis, 40,* 158–165.

Strauss, R., & Bacon, S. D. (1953). *Drinking in college*. New Haven: Yale University Press.

Streng, F. J. (1976). *Understanding religious life*. Encino, CA: Dickenson.

Strunk, O., Jr. (1977). Humanistic religious psychology: A new chapter in the psychology of religion. In H. Malony (Ed.), *Current perspectives in the psychology of religion* (pp. 27–35). Grand Rapids, MI: William B. Eerdmans.

Sturgeon, R. S., & Hamley, R. W. (1979). Religion and anxiety. *Journal of Social Psychology, 108,* 137–138.

Swanson, G. E. (1960). *The birth of the gods*. Ann Arbor: University of Michigan Press.

Tamburrino, M. B., Franco, K. N., Campbell, N. B., Pontz, J. E., Evans, C. L., & Jurs, S. G. (1990). Postabortion dysphoria and religion. *Southern Medical Journal, 83,* 736–738.

Tan, S. Y. (1990). *Lay counseling: Equipping Christians for a helping ministry.* Grand Rapids, MI: Zondervan.

Tarjanyi, J. (1990, May 26). When religion becomes holy obsession. *Toledo Blade,* p. 18.

Tate, E. D., & Miller, G. R. (1971). Differences in value systems of persons with varying religious orientations. *Journal for the Scientific Study of Religion, 10,* 357–365.

Taylor, D. (1985). Theological thoughts about evil. In D. Parkin (Ed.), *The anthropology of evil* (pp. 26–41). Oxford: Basil Blackwell.

Taylor, E. J., & Amanta, M. (1994a). Cancer nurses' perceptions on spiritual care: Implications for pastoral care. *Journal of Pastoral Care, 48,* 259–265.

Taylor, E. J., & Amanta, M. (1994b). Midwifery to the soul while the body dies: Spiritual care among hospice nurses. *American Journal of Hospice and Palliative Care, 11,* 28–35.

Taylor, R. J., & Chatters, L. M. (1988). Church members as a source of informal social support. *Review of Religious Research, 30,* 193–203.

Taylor, S. E., & Brown, J. D. (1988). Illusion and well-being: A social psychological perspective on mental health. *Psychological Bulletin, 103,* 193–210.

Taylor, S. E., & Brown, J. D. (1994). Positive illusions and well-living revisited: Separating fact from fiction. *Psychological Bulletin, 116,* 21–27.

Tedeschi, R. G., & Calhoun, L. G. (1995). *Trauma and transformation: Growing in the aftermath of suffering.* Thousand Oaks, CA: Sage.

Ten Boom, C. (1971). *The hiding place.* Toronto: Bantam Books.

Thoits, P. A. (1986). Social support as coping assistance. *Journal of Consulting and Clinical Psychology, 54,* 416–423.

Thompson, M. P., & Vardaman, P. J. (in press). The role of religion in coping with loss of a family member in homicide. *Journal for the Scientific Study of Religion.*

Thompson, S. C., Sobolew-Shubin, A., Galbraith, M. E., Schwankovsky, L., & Cruzen, D. (1993). Maintaining perceptions of control: Finding perceived control in low control circumstances. *Journal of Personality and Social Psychology, 64,* 293–304.

Thompson, W. E. (1981). The Oklahoma Amish: Survival of an ethnic subculture. *Ethnicity, 8,* 476–487.

Thumma, S. (1991). Seeking to be converted: An examination of recent conversion studies and theories. *Pastoral Psychology, 39,* 185–194.

Tillich, P. (1951). *Systematic theology* (Vol. 1). Chicago: University of Chicago Press.

Tjelveit, A. C. (1986). The ethics of value conversion in psychotherapy: Appropriate and inappropriate therapist influence on client values. *Clinical Psychology Review, 6,* 515–537.

Toch, H. H. (1955). Crisis situations and ideological revelations. *Public Opinion Quarterly, 19,* 53–67.

Toh, Y. M., & Tan, S. Y. (in press). The effectiveness of church-based lay counselors: A controlled outcome study. *Journal of Psychology and Christianity.*

Trainer, M. F. (1981). *Forgiveness: Intrinsic, role-expected, expedient, in the context of divorce.* Unpublished doctoral dissertation, Boston University, Boston.

Travisano, R. V. (1970). Alternation and conversion as qualitatively different transformations. In G. P. Stone & H. A. Farberman (Eds.), *Social psychology through symbolic interaction* (pp. 594–606). Waltham, MA: Ginn-Blaisdell.

Truax, C. B. (1966). Reinforcement and nonreinforcement in Rogerian psychotherapy. *Journal of Abnormal Psychology, 71,* 1–9.

Twain, M. (1974). *Letters from the earth.* New York: Perennial Library.

Tyler, F. B. (1970). The shaping of the science. *American Psychologist, 25,* 219–226.

Tyler, F. B. (1978). Individual psychosocial competence: A personality configuration. *Educational and Psychological Measurement, 38,* 309–323.

Tyler, F. B., Moran, J. A., Gatz, M. A., & Gease, E. I. (1982). Individual psychosocial competence and aging. *Academic Psychology Bulletin, 4,* 503–514.

Tyler, F. B., Pargament, K. I., & Gatz, M. (1983). The resource collaborator role: A model for interactions involving psychologists. *American Psychologist, 38,* 388–398.

Tyler, F. B., Brome, D. R., & Williams, J. E. (1991). *Ethnic validity, ecology, and psychotherapy: A psychosocial competence model.* New York: Plenum.

Tylor, E. B. (1968). The science of culture. In M. H. Fried (Ed.), *Readings in anthropology: Cultural anthropology* (Vol. 2, pp. 1–18). New York: Thomas Y. Crowell.

Ullman, C. (1982). Cognitive and emotional antecedents of religious conversion. *Journal of Personality and Social Psychology, 43,* 183–192.

Ullman, C. (1988). Psychological well-being among converts in traditional and nontraditional religious groups. *Psychiatry, 51,* 312–322.

Upanishads: Breath of the eternal, The. (1975). (S. Prabhavananda & F. Manchester, Trans.). New York: Mentor Books.

VandeCreek, L., Pargament, K., Cowell, B., Belavich, T., Brant, C., Friedel, L., & Perez, L. (1995). *The vigil: Religion and the search for control in the hospital waiting room.* Paper presented at the meeting of the American Psychological Association, New York, NY.

van Gennep, A. (1960). *The rites of passage* (M. B. Vizedom & G. L. Caffee, Trans.). Chicago: University of Chicago Press.

Veroff, J., Douvan, E., & Kulka, R. A. (1981). *The inner American: A self-portrait from 1957 to 1976.* New York: Basic Books.

Veroff, J., Kulka, P. A., & Douvan, E. (1981). *Mental health in America: Patterns of help seeking from 1957 to 1976.* New York: Basic Books.

Vetter, G. B., & Green, M. (1932–1933). Personality and group factors in the making of atheists. *Journal of Abnormal and Social Psychology, 27,* 179–194.

Victor, J. S. (1991). The dynamics of rumor-panics about satanic cults. In J. T. Richardson, J. Best, & D. G. Bromley (Eds.), *The satanism scare* (pp. 221–236). New York: Aldine de Gruyter.

Videka-Sherman, L. (1982). Coping with the death of a child: A study over time. *American Journal of Orthopsychiatry, 52*, 688–698.

Vitaliano, P. P., DeWolfe, D. J., Maiuro, R. D., Russo, J., & Katon, W. (1990). Appraised changeability of a stressor as a modifier of the relationship between coping and depression: A test of the hypothesis of fit. *Journal of Personality and Social Psychology, 59*, 582–592.

Vitz, P. C. (1977). *Psychology as religion: The cult of self-worship.* Grand Rapids, MI: William B. Eerdmans.

von Bertalanffy, L. (1968). *General systems theory: Foundation, development, and applications.* New York: Braziller.

Waldfogel, S., & Wolpe, P. R. (1993). Using awareness of religious factors to enhance interventions in consultation-liaison psychiatry. *Hospital and Community Psychiatry, 44*, 473–477.

Wall, K. (1994). Prescription: Prayer. *Physician, 6*, 17.

Walters, R. P. (1983). *Forgive and be free: Healing the wounds of past and present.* Grand Rapids, MI: Zondervan.

Watson, P. J., Hood, R. W., Jr., Foster, S. G., & Morris, R. J. (1988). Sin, depression and narcissism. *Review of Religious Research, 29*, 295–305.

Watson, P. J., Hood, R. W., Jr., Morris, R. J., & Hall, J. R. (1984). Empathy, religious orientation and social desirability. *Journal of Psychology, 117*, 211–216.

Watson, P. J., Hood, R. W., Jr., Morris, R. J., & Hall, J. R. (1985). Religiosity, sin, and self-esteem. *Journal of Psychology and Theology, 13*, 116–128.

Watson, P. J., Morris, R. J., & Hood, R. W., Jr. (1988). Sin and self-functioning: Part 3. The psychology and ideology of irrational beliefs. *Journal of Psychology and Theology, 16*, 348–361.

Watson, P. J., Morris, R. J., & Hood, R. W., Jr. (1989). Interactional factor correlations with means and end religiousness. *Journal for the Scientific Study of Religion, 28*, 337–347.

Watzlawick, P. (1988). *Ultra-solutions or how to fail most successfully.* New York: Norton.

Weaver, A. J., Koenig, H. G., & Larson, D. B. (1997). Marriage and family therapists and the clergy: A need for clinical collaboration, training, and research. *Journal of Marital and Family Therapy, 23*, 13–25.

Weidman, S. (1989). *Intermarriage: The challenge of living with differences between Christians and Jews.* New York: Free Press.

Weinborn, M. (1995). *A means and ends approach to religious orientation.* Unpublished master's thesis, Bowling Green State University, Bowling Green, OH.

Weiner, B., Graham, S., Peters, O., & Zmuidinas, M. (1991). Public confession and forgiveness. *Journal of Personality, 59*, 281–312.

Weisner, T. S., Belzer, L., & Stolze, L. (1991). Religion and families of children with developmental delays. *American Journal of Mental Retardation, 95*, 647–662.

Welch, M. R., & Barrish, J. (1982). Bringing religious motivation back in: A multivariate analysis of motivational predictors of student religiosity. *Review of Religious Research, 23,* 357–369.

Welford, A. T. (1947). Is religious behavior dependent upon affect or frustration? *Journal of Abnormal and Social Psychology, 42,* 310–319.

Wells, E. A., & Maton, K. I. (1992). *Social justice religious motivation.* Paper presented at the meeting of the American Psychological Association, Washington, DC.

Wheaton, B. (1983). Stress, personal coping resources, and psychiatric symptoms: An investigation of interactive models. *Journal of Health and Social Behavior, 24,* 208–229.

Wheaton, B. (1985). Models for the stress-buffering functions of coping resources. *Journal of Health and Social Behavior, 26,* 352–364.

Whipple, V. (1987). Counseling battered women from fundamentalist churches. *Journal of Marital and Family Therapy, 13,* 251–258.

White, R. W. (1963). Ego and reality in psychoanalytic theory. *Psychological Issues, 3,* 1–210.

White, R. W. (1974). Strategies of adaptation: An attempt at systematic description. In G. V. Coelho, P. A. Hamburg, & J. E. Adams (Eds.), *Coping and adaptation* (pp. 47–68). New York: Basic Books.

Whitehead, E. E., & Whitehead, J. D. (1979). *Christian life patterns: The psychological challenges and religious invitation of adult life.* Garden City, NY: Doubleday.

Wicks, J. W. (1990). *1990 Greater Toledo Area Survey.* Bowling Green, Ohio: Population and Society Research Center.

Wiesel, E. (1992, April 19). When passion is dangerous. *Parade Magazine,* pp. 20–21.

Wiesenthal, S. (1976). *The sunflower.* New York: Schocken Books.

Wikan, U. (1988). Bereavement and loss in two Muslim communities: Egypt and Bali compared. *Social Science and Medicine, 27,* 451–460.

Wilber, K. (1995). *Sex, ecology, spirituality: The spirit of evolution.* Boston: Shambhala.

Williams, D. R., Larson, D., Buckler, R. E., Heckmann, R. C., & Pyle, C. M. (1991). Religion and psychological distress in a community sample. *Social Science and Medicine, 32,* 1257–1262.

Willits, F. K., & Crider, D. M. (1988). Religion and well-being: Men and women in the middle years. *Review of Religious Research, 29,* 281–294.

Wilson, M. R., & Filsinger, E. E. (1986). Religiosity and marital adjustment: Multidimensional relationships. *Journal of Marriage and the Family, 48,* 147–151.

Wilson, W. P. (1972). Mental health benefits of religious salvation. *Diseases of the Nervous System, 33,* 382–386.

Winger, D., & Hunsberger, B. (1988). Clergy counseling practices, Christian orthodoxy and problem solving styles. *Journal of Psychology and Theology, 16,* 41–48.

Witter, B. A., Stock, W. A., Okun, M. A., & Haring, M. J. (1985). Religion and subjective well-being in adulthood: A quantitative synthesis. *Review of Religious Research, 26,* 332–342.

Witztum, E., Greenberg, D., & Dasberg, H. (1990). Mental illness and religious change. *British Journal of Medical Psychology, 63,* 33–41.

Wood, J. B., & Parham, I. A. (1990). Coping with perceived burden: Ethnic and cultural issues in Alzheimer's family caregiving. *Journal of Applied Gerontology, 9,* 325–329.

Wooton, R. J., & Allen, D. F. (1983). Dramatic religious conversion and schizophrenic decompensation. *Journal of Religion and Health, 22,* 212–220.

Worthington, E. L., Jr. (1989). Religious faith across the lifespan: Implications for counseling and research. *Counseling Psychologist, 17,* 555–612.

Worthington, E. L., Jr. (1990). *Counseling before marriage.* Dallas: Word.

Worthington, E. L., Jr., Dupont, P. D., Berry, J. T., & Duncan, L. A. (1988). Christian therapists' and clients' perceptions of religious psychotherapy in private and agency settings. *Journal of Psychology and Theology, 16,* 282–293.

Worthington, E. L., Jr., Kurusu, T. A., McCullough, M. E., & Sandage, S. J. (1996). Empirical research on religion and psychotherapeutic processes and outcomes: A 10-year review and research prospectus. *Psychological Bulletin, 119,* 448–487.

Worthington, E. L., Jr., & Scott, G. G. (1983) Goal selection for counseling with potentially religious clients by professional and student counselors in explicitly Christian or secular settings. *Journal of Psychology and Theology, 11,* 318–329.

Wright, S., Pratt, C., & Schmall, V. (1985). Spiritual support for caregivers of dementia patients. *Journal of Religion and Health, 24,* 31–38.

Wulff, D. M. (1997). *Psychology of religion: Classic and contemporary* (2nd ed.). New York: Wiley.

Wuthnow, R. (1976). *The consciousness reformation.* Berkeley: University of California.

Wyrtzen, J. C. (1996). *Pastoral counseling: A national mental health resource.* Fairfax, VA: American Association of Pastoral Counselors.

Yalom, I. D. (1980). *Existential psychotherapy.* New York: Basic Books.

Yancey, P. (1977). *Where is God when it hurts?* Grand Rapids, MI: Zondervan.

Yates, J. W., Chalmer, B. J., St. James, P., Follansbee, M., & McKegney, F. B. (1981). Religion in patients with advanced cancer. *Medical and Pediatric Oncology, 9,* 121–128.

Yelsma, P., & Montambo, L. (1990). Patients' and spouses' religious problem-solving styles and their physiological health. *Psychological Reports, 66,* 857–858.

Yinger, J. M. (1970). *The scientific study of religion.* London: Macmillan.

York, G. Y. (1987). Religious-based denial in the NICU: Implications for social work. *Social Work in Health Care, 12,* 31–45.

Young, K. (1926). The psychology of hymns. *Journal of Abnormal and Social Psychology, 20,* 391–406.

Zeidner, M., & Hammer, A. L. (1992). Coping with missile attack: Resources, strategies, and outcomes. *Journal of Personality, 60,* 709–746.

Zerowin, J. (1996). *Religious coping with death among Jews.* Unpublished master's thesis, Bowling Green State University, Bowling Green, OH.

Zerubavel, E. (1991). *The fine line: Making distinctions in everyday life.* New York: Free Press.

Zinnbauer, B. J., & Pargament, K. I. (1995). *Spiritual conversion: A study of religious change among college students.* Paper presented at the meeting of the Society for the Scientific Study of Religion, St. Louis, MO.

Zinnbauer, B. J., & Pargament, K. I. (1996). *When worlds collide: On the integration of religion, spirituality, and psychotherapy.* Unpublished manuscript, Bowling Green State University, Bowling Green, OH.

Zinnbauer, B. I., Pargament, K. I., Cowell, B., Rye, M., & Scott, A. B. (1996). *Religion and spirituality: Unfuzzying the fuzzy.* Paper presented at the meeting of the American Psychological Association, Toronto, Canada.

Zuckerman, D. M., Kasl, S. V., & Ostfeld, A. M. (1984). Psychosocial predictors of mortality among the elderly poor. *American Journal of Epidemiology, 119,* 410–423.

Author Index

Subject Index